WHIPLASH:
evidence base for clinical practice

WHIPLASH:
evidence base for clinical practice

Michele Sterling and Justin Kenardy

CHURCHILL LIVINGSTONE
ELSEVIER

Sydney Edinburgh London New York Philadelphia St Louis Toronto

2011

ELSEVIER

Churchill Livingstone
is an imprint of Elsevier

Elsevier Australia. ACN 001 002 357
(a division of Reed International Books Australia Pty Ltd)
Tower 1, 475 Victoria Avenue, Chatswood, NSW 2067

National Library of Australia Cataloguing-in-Publication Data

---

Sterling, Michele.

Whiplash: evidence base for clinical practice / Michele Sterling; Justin Kenardy

9780729539463 (pbk.)

Whiplash injuries
Cervical vertebrae – wounds and injuries
Neck – wounds and injuries

Kenardy, Justin.

614.5973

Publisher: Melinda McEvoy
Developmental Editor: Rebecca Cornell
Publishing Services Manager: Helena Klijn
Project Coordinator: Karen Griffiths
Edited by Carolyn Pike
Proofread by Tim Learner
Line art by Rod Maclean
Design by Lisa Petroff
Index by Bob Sanny
Typeset by TNQ Books and Journals Pvt. Ltd.
Printed by 1010 Printing International Ltd.

Contents

Foreword

The field of pain management is currently undergoing unprecedented positive change and, in this environment, this book makes a valuable contribution to currently evolving initiatives. Only recently has the magnitude of the problem of chronic pain been documented. In all industrialised countries, one in five persons suffers chronic pain at an annual cost to the economy of the order of A$1.85m per 1 million population and at huge personal cost to individuals, families and communities. On the basis of rigorous epidemiological studies in Australia, chronic pain has been reported to be the third most costly health problem—and yet this chronic condition is best described as the largest 'unrecognised' health problem worldwide. Chronic pain is not even included in healthcare plans to focus on chronic disease management in most countries. Indeed, it is not understood that new evidence points strongly to chronic pain as a disease entity, comprising physical, psychological and environmental elements.

In 2010, an Australian National Pain Summit was held in response to the foregoing evidence of a compelling need to improve the management of all forms of pain (acute, chronic and cancer). The Summit was the culmination of the extensive cooperative work of 150 healthcare, consumer and community organisations leading to the unanimous support of a comprehensive National Pain Strategy (www.painsummit.org.au). Several regional governments in Australia, notably Queensland (the home state of the editors of this text), have moved quickly to provide financial support for implementation of the recommendations of the National Pain Strategy, which focuses on six key goals:

1. people in pain as a national health priority
2. knowledgeable, empowered and supported consumers
3. access to skilled professionals and best-practice evidence-based care
4. access to multidisciplinary care at all levels
5. quality improvement and evaluation
6. research.

Many other countries are taking similar initiatives.

At an international level, the International Association for the Study of Pain (IASP) hosted an International Pain Summit (IPS) in conjunction with the IASP World Congress on Pain in Montreal, Canada, September, 2010. The outcome of the Summit was the development of two documents: 'Desirable characteristics of national pain strategies' and 'The Declaration of Montreal: access to pain management is a fundamental human right'.

In this rapidly evolving national and international milieu, this text on whiplash-associated disorders, by Michele Sterling and Justin Kenardy, is very timely and apt. As the editors point out in the introduction, the term 'whiplash' has been much debated and is controversial, with quite fierce disagreement—to the detriment of patients, their carers, families, insurers and the economy. I suspect that current worldwide initiatives described above will help this situation, because 'whiplash' is a complex pain condition and such conditions are now beginning to receive the attention that they deserve.

As outlined in the Australian National Pain Strategy goals, one of the keys to further progress is goal three—access to best-practice evidence-based care. This text comprehensively presents the available evidence base for understanding and treating whiplash. Primarily aimed at health practitioners, I have no doubt that consumers will take an interest in the book's contents. I particularly draw the potential reader's attention to the editors' focus on 'whiplash' as comprising a variable number of problems in the major domains of *physical*, *psychological* and *environmental*. Not surprisingly, the authors are a distinguished multidisciplinary group of clinicians and researchers—each having provided key knowledge of this condition and its treatment.

Although there is as yet no definitive understanding of the causes of whiplash, much more knowledge has accumulated over the past 10–15 years—some derived from new insights into other chronic pain conditions. It may seem surprising that treatments for this condition are often ineffective but, again, steady progress is being made.

The great value of a text of this quality and comprehensiveness is that it allows us to see clearly where we are at present and to rationally plan the research, education, quality improvement and evaluation that needs to be done, while utilising current evidence as a basis for best practice. The editors are to be congratulated on an excellent resource for clinicians, patients, carers and the healthcare industry, as well as health insurers and workers compensation insurers.

Professor **Michael J Cousins AM**
MD DSc FANZCA FRCA FFPMANZCA FAChPM (RACP)
Professor & Head,
Pain Management Research Institute
University of Sydney
Royal North Shore Hospital

Prev Chair, National Pain Summit, Australia
Prev Chair, International Pain Summit, IASP

Contributors

Jan Buitenhuis PhD, MD
Medical Advisor, Univé Insurance
Lecturer and Research Associate, Department of Social Medicine, University Medical Centre Groningen, University of Groningen, Groningen, The Netherlands

Luke Connelly BA (Econ), MEconSt, PhD
Professor of Health Economics, School of Medicine, Faculty of Health Sciences and School of Economics, Faculty of Business, Economics and Law; Associate Director, Centre for National Research on Disability and Rehabilitation Medicine (CONROD); Director, Australian Centre for Economic Research on Health, University of Queensland, Brisbane, Queensland, Australia

Michele Curatolo PhD, MD
Professor and Head of the Division of Pain Therapy, Department of Anesthesiology and Pain Therapy, University of Bern, Bern, Switzerland

Peter de Jong PhD
Department of Clinical Psychology, University of Groningen, The Netherlands

James Elliot PhD
Assistant Professor, Department of Physical Therapy and Human Movement Sciences, Feinberg School of Medicine, Northwestern University, Chicago, USA

Deborah Falla PhD
Associate Professor, Centre for Sensory–Motor Interaction, Department of Health Science and Technology, Aalborg University, Aalborg, Denmark

Ian Freckelton SC
Professor, Faculty of Law, Department of Forensic Medicine, School of Psychology, Psychiatry and Psychological Medicine, Monash University, Melbourne, Victoria, Australia
Adjunct Professor, National Institute of Public Health and Mental Health Research, Auckland University of Technology, Auckland, New Zealand

Lena Holm BSc, PhD Post Doc
Unit of Epidemiology, Institute of Environmental Medicine, Karolinska Institutet, Stockholm, Sweden

Jan Jaspers PhD
Department of Medical Psychology, University Medical Centre Groningen, University of Groningen, Groningen, The Netherlands

Gwendolen Jull MPhty, FACP, PhD, GradDipManipTher, DipPhty
Director, Centre of Clinical Research Excellence in Spinal Pain, Injury and Health; Head of Cervical Spine Research Unit, Division of Physiotherapy, University of Queensland, Brisbane, Queensland, Australia

Justin Kenardy BSc (Hons), PhD, FAPS
Professor, Schools of Psychology and Medicine; Deputy Director, Centre of National Research on Disability and Rehabilitation Medicine, University of Queensland; Chief Investigator, Centre of Clinical Research Excellence in Spinal Pain, Injury and Health, Brisbane, Queensland, Australia

Samuel MacLean MD, MPH
Assistant Professor, Department of Anaesthesiology; Director, TRYUMPH Research Program, Centre for Neurosensory Disorders, University of North Carolina School of Medicine, Chapel Hill, North Carolina, USA

Dennis J. Maiman PhD, MD
Professor and Chair, Department of Neurosurgery, Medical College of Wisconsin, Milwaukee, Wisconsin, USA

Brian McGuire BA, MClinPsych, DipCrim, DipHealthSc, PhD, AFPsSI, Reg Psychol (PsSI), AFBPsS (Psychol)
Senior Lecturer, School of Psychology; Joint Director, Centre of Pain Research, National University of Ireland, Galway, Ireland

Frank A. Pintar PhD
Professor, Department of Neurosurgery, Medical College of Wisconsin; Adjunct Professor of Biomedical Engineering, Marquette University; Director, Neuroscience Research Laboratories, VA Medical Centre, Milwaukee, Wisconsin, USA

Trudy Rebbeck BAppSc (Phty), MAppSc (ManipPhty), PhD, FACP
Discipline of Physiotherapy, University of Sydney, Sydney, New South Wales, Australia

Natalie Spearing BSN, MBA, RN
Centre of National Research on Disability and Rehabilitation Medicine, University of Queensland, Brisbane, Queensland, Australia

Brian Stemper PhD
Associate Professor, Department of Neurosurgery, Medical College of Wisconsin; Adjunct Professor of Biomedical Engineering, Marquette University, Milwaukee, Wisconsin, USA

Michele Sterling BPhty, MPhty, PhD, GradDipManipPhysio, FACP
Associate Professor, Schools of Medicine and Health and Rehabilitation Science; Chief Investigator, Centre of Clinical Research Excellence in Spinal Pain, Injury and Health; Associate Director, Centre of National Research on Disability and Rehabilitation Medicine, University of Queensland, Brisbane, Queensland, Australia

Julia Treleaven BPhty, PhD
Lecturer, Division of Physiotherapy, School of Health and Rehabilitation Sciences; Senior Researcher, Centre of Clinical Research Excellence in Spinal Pain, Injury and Health, University of Queensland, Brisbane, Queensland, Australia

Gerbrig Versteegen PhD
Pain Expertise Centre, University Medical Centre Groningen, University of Groningen, Groningen, The Netherlands

Narayan Yoganandan PhD
Professor and Chairman of Biomedical Engineering, Department of Neurosurgery, Medical College of Wisconsin; Adjunct Professor of Biomedical Engineering, Marquette University, Milwaukee, Wisconsin, USA

Reviewers

Marianne Bennison BSc (Hons) Ost Med
Practice Education Lead Osteopathy and Senior Lecturer, Oxford Brookes University, Oxford, UK

Carol Fawkes PGCert (EBM), MSc, DO, Lic Ac, MBAcC
Research Development Officer – Osteopathy, School of Health Professions, University of Brighton, Brighton, UK

Navine G Haworth DC, DICCP, GCTTL
Lecturer, Health Sciences, RMIT University, Melbourne, Victoria, Australia

Mr Stephen Makinde BSc (Hons) Ost. Med., MSc Clinical Neuro.

Susan Slade PhD
Department of Physiotherapy, Monash University, Melbourne, Victoria, Australia

Dr Gordon Waddington PhD, MAppSc (SportsPhysio), MExSpSc
Professor of Physiotherapy, Associate Dean Research, Faculty of Health, University of Canberra, Canberra, ACT, Australia

Acknowledgments

As editors, we would foremostly like to thank the contributors to this book. We are indebted to them for sharing their research and clinical expertise in order to achieve our goal of a broad and thorough view of whiplash associated disorders.

We would also like to thank the people who donated their valuable time to be participants in the many research studies described in this book. Without their efforts the understanding of this condition would not have moved forward.

Research cannot progress without financial support and we thank the following bodies for research support: National Health and Medical Research Council of Australia (NHMRC); Australian Research Council (ARC); Centre of National Research on Disability and Rehabilitation Medicine (CONROD), The University of Queensland; Physiotherapy Research Foundation of Australia; Motor Accident Insurance Commission Queensland (MAIC); Suncorp Metway General Insurance, Queensland.

Finally we would like to thank our families for the understanding and patience during the preparation of this book.

Michele Sterling and Justin Kenardy

Introduction

Michele Sterling and Justin Kenardy

Whiplash associated disorders (WAD) are a common, disabling and costly condition that occur usually as a consequence of a motor vehicle crash (MVC). While the figures vary depending on the cohort studied, current understanding is that up to 50% of people who experience a whiplash injury will never fully recover,[1] and up to 30% will remain moderately to severely disabled by their condition.[2, 3] The associated costs secondary to whiplash injury, including medical care, disability, lost work productivity, as well as personal costs, are substantial. Claims for personal injury after whiplash cost more than £3 billion per year in the United Kingdom,[4] while data from the United States are even more staggering, with costs reaching US$230 billion per annum.[5] In Australia, whiplash injury accounts for the vast majority of submitted claims, as well as the greatest incurred costs in the Queensland compulsory third party scheme.[6] In Queensland, the economic costs related to whiplash injury are substantial and exceeded $500 million from 1994 to 2001;[7] in New South Wales in the period 1989–1998, 50,000 whiplash claims were made, costing approximately $1.5 billion.[8]

Whiplash is one of the most debated and controversial painful musculoskeletal conditions. This is, in part, due to the often compensable nature of the injury and the fact that a precise pathoanatomical diagnosis is not usually achievable, at least with current imaging techniques. Whiplash has had a tumultuous history since Harold Crowe first coined the term in 1928, a term he later regretted.[9] Many have argued about the legitimacy of the condition, with some even maintaining that it is a condition of deception, folly and greed,[10] and others that it is merely symptom 'amplification'.[11] Others (in relation to pain in general) have criticised this perspective. They maintain that when the presentation does not fit the clinician's prototypical construct of the condition in question, the patient's entire presentation is deemed to be inappropriate, thus throwing the metaphorical baby out with the bath water. Instead of a more empirical approach, this prescriptive reasoning process allows clinicians to make moral or ethical claims about the patient's behaviour.[12] In recent times, perhaps coincidentally but in parallel with the growth in empirical literature about whiplash, critics have become less vocal.

In 1995, the Quebec Task Force called for more research into the whiplash condition[13] and the scientific community have responded. Although we are little closer to being able to identify an injured peripheral structure, it is generally accepted that there is an initial peripheral injury of some kind to the neck following whiplash.[14] However, even if identification were easy and obvious, there is doubt it would improve management directions and outcomes. This is because of the lack of correspondence between imaging results and pain and disability in whiplash.[15, 16] Instead the focus of current research has been to identify manifestations of the condition that may be amenable to treatment interventions. There is now much data available indicating that whiplash is a legitimate condition characterised by a wide range of physiological and psychological manifestations.

In general, whiplash, whether in the acute or chronic stage of the condition, is resistant to treatment interventions. To date, no conservative treatment approach has shown substantial benefits for those who develop chronic moderate-to-severe symptoms following whiplash injury. Two recent randomised controlled trials (RCT) of physical rehabilitation approaches demonstrated only very marginal effects. Stewart et al.[17] showed only a 2 point decrease (on a 10 point scale) in pain levels immediately after a six-week functional exercise management intervention but with no significant effects at more long-term follow-ups. Similarly, a recent RCT showed only modest effects (pain and disability scores decreased by just clinically relevant amounts) with a more neck specific exercise approach.[18] Importantly in this study, those participants with moderate-to-severe symptoms and features indicative of augmented central nociceptive processing showed no statistically significant improvement with the intervention. Other forms of treatment fare little better, with approaches such as cognitive behavioural therapy[19] and phasic coordination type exercises[20] providing only modest benefits to pain and disability. With respect to acute whiplash, while the maintenance of activity and some form of exercise seem superior to rest and immobilisation with a collar, a significant proportion of injured people still develop chronic pain and disability.[21–23]

One reason for these modest effects may be due to the heterogenous nature of the whiplash condition. Most treatment trials have investigated relatively non-specific approaches to treatment without taking the varied nature of the condition into account. It would appear that WAD is a more complex condition than previously assumed. Recent investigations have begun to provide insight into the characteristics of the whiplash condition, both physiological and psychological, which allows speculation of potential underlying processes that may contribute to the pain and disability of whiplash and its propensity to chronicity. It is hoped that researchers will take this heterogeneity into account in their design of future clinical trials.

Additionally, most people with whiplash injuries and clinicians involved in their management have to work with a compensable system of some kind. This places additional pressures on, not only injured individuals and treatment providers, but also those involved in administering claims systems, policy makers and those in the medicolegal field. It would seem likely that system or environmental factors will complicate the whiplash presentation and the outcomes following injury, and this has been an area of vigorous debate.[24]

This book aims to bring together current knowledge of the whiplash condition that will allow all stakeholders involved in the management of patients with whiplash, from clinicians to policy makers, to gain greater understanding of this condition. The book includes perspectives from a wide range of disciplines that we hope will ultimately lead to improved outcomes for injured people.

STRUCTURE OF THE BOOK

In this book, the spectrum of the current evidence base for whiplash is covered. The book begins with a discussion of the epidemiology and magnitude of the problem of whiplash and the clinical presentation of the condition, including knowledge of the clinical pathway following injury. Our understanding of the mechanism of injury to the neck sustained in an MVC has progressed a long way since the rather simplistic flexion/hyperextension mechanism previously described, and Chapter 3 synthesises the knowledge in this area and outlines the implications for potential pathological lesions. Chapter 4 explores the evidence supporting the presence of peripheral lesions.

Probably, most progress of recent times has been the advances made in understanding the physiological and psychological factors underlying the whiplash condition. Chapters 5–8 bring together current evidence of these processes. It is now clear that some injured people will display features indicative of augmented central nociceptive processing mechanisms or central hyperexcitability and that these factors seem to play a role in the transition to chronicity. Chapter 5 outlines these changes. There is also a growing literature demonstrating that changes in muscle and motor function occur following whiplash injury and these dysfunctions have implications for the nature of exercise prescription. Additionally, postural control changes, including proprioceptive deficits, disturbed eye movement control and balance loss are common, particularly in those individuals who also report dizziness in association with their neck pain. The identification of these changes has led to the development of specific exercise programs designed to ameliorate them. In 1995, when the Quebec Task Force conducted their review, few studies were available that investigated the psychological responses to whiplash injury. The situation is now quite different and pain-related behaviours and psychological responses are present in cases of both acute and chronic WAD. Further to this, psychological distress associated with the MVC or post-traumatic stress symptoms have been shown to be present in people with whiplash to much the same extent as with other more severe types of trauma where the injured person is hospitalised. Such factors are often overlooked in the management of whiplash, but should be considered as they appear to be important in the maintenance of pain and disability.

A further unexplored area is that of the physiological stress response to the injury (and pain) and its potential role in outcomes following whiplash. Research in this area is relatively new for whiplash and Chapter 9 outlines the current evidence and future exciting developments in this area.

The identification of early prognostic indicators, which is dealt with in Chapter 10, is important in order to identify injured people at risk of poor recovery and to develop and institute appropriate early management that may be directed at modifiable risk factors. Chapters 11–13 outline the evidence and implications of current knowledge on the management of WAD. It is not the aim of these chapters to be systematic reviews of specific interventions, but rather to synthesise the knowledge outlined in the earlier chapters and the implications for current and future management approaches. As most whiplash-injured people will initially seek care in the primary care environment, Chapter 11 on acute WAD provides suggestions for assessment and management for practitioners who may not necessarily see many patients with whiplash. Chapters 12 and 13 discuss physical and psychological treatment options for patients with chronic WAD. We acknowledge that these aspects of management should not be dichotomised and, in Chapter 17, case descriptions bring together the physical and psychological management approaches. It is hoped that this will facilitate clinical translation of the knowledge discussed in the earlier chapters of the book.

The whiplash-injured person is often negotiating a compensation system of some description, although the exact nature of which will depend upon the specific jurisdiction. It is generally considered that compensation and litigation factors have a detrimental influence on outcomes following injury.[25] For these reasons, Chapters 14 and 16 are dedicated to the evidence and thoughtful discussion of compensation and litigation related issues in whiplash. Chapter 16 deals with the controversial issue of malingering.

Finally, Chapter 18 draws together the main themes of the book. Although knowledge of whiplash has increased markedly in the last 15 years, it is still incomplete as outcomes for injured people are far from optimal. Future directions for research are discussed, with the aim in mind to improve health outcomes and decrease personal and economic costs associated with this intriguing and challenging condition.

References

1. Carroll L, Holm L, Hogg-Johnson S, et al. Course and prognostic factors for neck pain in whiplash-associated disorders (WAD). Results of the Bone and Joint Decade 2000–2010 Task Force on Neck Pain and its Associated Disorders. *Spine* 2008;33(42):583–92.
2. Rebbeck T, Sindhusake D, Cameron I, et al. A prospective cohort study of health outcomes following whiplash associated disorders in an Australian population. *Inj Prev* 2006;12:93–8.
3. Sterling M, Jull G, Kenardy J. Physical and psychological predictors of outcome following whiplash injury maintain predictive capacity at long term follow-up. *Pain* 2006;122:102–8.
4. Joslin C, Khan S, Bannister G. Long-term disability after neck injury. A comparative study. *J Bone Joint Surg (Br)* 2004;86(7):1032–4.
5. Blincoe L, Seay A, Zaloshnja E, et al. Economic impact of motor vehicle crashes 2000. Washington, DC: US Department of Transportation, National Highway Traffic Safety Administration, 2002.
6. Motor Accident Insurance Commission. Annual report. Brisbane: MAIC, 2009.
7. Motor Accident Insurance Commission. Whiplash: review of CTP Queensland data to 31 Dec 2001. Brisbane: MAIC, 2002.
8. Motor Accident Authority. Whiplash and the NSW Motor Accidents Scheme. Statistical information paper no. 7. Sydney: MAA, 1999.
9. Crowe H. A new diagnostic sign in neck injuries. *Calif Med* 1964;100:12–13.
10. Malleson A. Whiplash and other useful illnesses. Quebec: McGill-Queen's University Press, 2002.
11. Ferrari R. Whiplash and symptom amplification. *Pain* 2001;89:293–4.
12. Cronje R, Williamson O. Is pain ever normal? *Clin J Pain* 2006;22(8):692–9.
13. Spitzer WO, Skovron ML, Salmi LR, et al. Scientific monograph of Quebec Task Force on Whiplash Associated Disorders: redefining "Whiplash" and its management. *Spine* 1995;20(8 Suppl):1S–73S.
14. Siegmund G, Winkelstein BA, Ivancic PC, et al. The anatomy and biomechanics of acute and chronic whiplash injury. *Traffic Inj Prev* 2009;10(2):101–12.
15. Elliott J, Sterling M, Noteboom T, et al. The clinical presentation of chronic whiplash and the relationship to findings of MRI fatty infiltrates in the cervical extensor musculature: a preliminary investigation. *Eur Spine J* 2009;18(9):1371–8.
16. Ichihara D, Okado E, Chiba K, et al. Longitudinal magnetic resonance imaging study on whiplash injury patients: minimum 10-year follow-up. *J Orthop Sc* 2009;14(5):602–10.
17. Stewart M, Maher C, Refshauge K, et al. Randomised controlled trial of exercise for chronic whiplash associated disorders. *Pain* 2007;128(1–2):59–68.
18. Jull G, Sterling M, Kenardy J, Beller E. Does the presence of sensory hypersensitivity influence outcomes of physical rehabilitation for chronic whiplash? A preliminary RCT. *Pain* 2007;129(2): 28–34.
19. Soderlund A, Lindberg P. Cognitive behavioural components in physiotherapy management of chronic whiplash associated disorders (WAD): a randomised group study. *G Ital Med Lav Ergon* 2007;29(1 Suppl A):A5–11.
20. Fitz-Ritson D. Phasic exercises for cervical rehabilitation after "whiplash" trauma. *J Man Phys Ther* 1995;18(1):21–4.
21. Provinciali L, Baroni M, Illuminati L, Ceravolo MG. Multimodal treatment to prevent the late whiplash syndrome. *Scand J Rehab Med* 1996;28(2):105–11.

22. Rosenfeld M, Seferiadis A, Carllson J, Gunnarsson R. Active intervention in patients with whiplash associated disorders improves long-term prognosis: a randomised controlled clinical trial. *Spine* 2003;28(22):2491–8.
23. Rosenfeld M, Seferiadis A, Gunnarsson R. Active involvement and intervention in patients exposed to whiplash trauma in automobile crashes reduces costs. *Spine* 2006;31(16):1799–804.
24. Merskey H, Teasell R, Nussbaum D. Science, whiplash, insurance and minimising pain. *J Whiplash Rel Dis* 2003;2(2):5–12.
25. Cameron P, Gabbe B. Editorial: the effect of compensation claims on outcomes after injury. *Injury* 2009;40:905–6.

CHAPTER 1
Epidemiology of whiplash associated disorders

Lena Holm

DEFINITIONS

The term *whiplash injury* has been used since the late 1920s, when H. E. Crowe coined the term at a medical meeting in San Francisco.[1] It was originally described as an injury mechanism to the neck, but was later also used to define the actual symptoms after such an event. The first known case report was published in the *Journal of the American Medical Association* in 1953, when Gay and Abbot described 50 patients who had been exposed to whiplash mechanism in car collisions.[2] It was reported that the majority had been exposed to rear-end collisions and that the majority were also examined between one and 24 months after the collision, thus representing a mix of patients with acute or persistent symptoms. Cervical pain with radiation into the occipital region of the skull, shoulder girdle or upper extremities were reported as common symptoms, but irritability, poor concentration and subjective vertigo were also described.

People who are exposed to energy transfer to the neck, in sports, falls or other mishaps, may also experience cervical pain.[3–5] After such events, however, it is less common that the injury is labelled 'whiplash', but instead other terms, such as neck strain, neck sprain or simply neck injury, are used. The term *whiplash associated disorder* (WAD) was introduced in 1995 by the Quebec Task Force (QTF), who published the first systematic review on whiplash injuries.[6] The term was intended to reflect that whiplash is an injury mechanism, and the consequences of the mechanism were the spectrum of symptoms (disorders). The QTF formulated the following conceptual definition:

> Whiplash is an acceleration-deceleration mechanism of energy transfer to the neck. It may result from rear-end or side-impact motor vehicle collisions, but can also occur during diving or other mishaps. The impact may result in bony or soft-tissue injuries (whiplash injury) which in turn may lead to a variety of clinical manifestations (whiplash-associated disorders).[6]

The reason for excluding frontal collisions from the definition is not discussed in the report and is likely to be an error, since it is known that 25–30% of whiplash injury occurs in such impact direction.[7–9]

The QTF also suggested a classification of WAD into five categories based on clinical signs and symptoms (see Chapter 2). This classification is mostly used to classify WAD in the acute phase.

Since the publication of the QTF findings, the term WAD has been increasingly used in the medical literature, and it is also a frequently used term in insurance medicine.

CUMULATIVE INCIDENCE OF AND RISK FACTORS FOR WAD

Cumulative incidence

The *cumulative incidence* is the number of new cases of an event or outcome occurring in a population over a certain time period. Some evidence from the literature indicates that the incidence of WAD differs between countries. There is also some evidence that the incidence of WAD has increased from the beginning of the 1990s to after the year 2000, with the annual incidence for the latter period being about 300 per 100,000 inhabitants in studies where emergency setting visits are used. In some instances, the increase is between three and tenfold.[10–12] It is not known if this increase is partly due to a change in care-seeking behaviour.

There are also some indications from administrative insurance claims databases in different European countries (e.g. Norway, the Netherlands and Sweden) of a reduction in the number of WAD claims, whereas such decreases have not been seen in Denmark or the United Kingdom. Sweden, for instance, has seen a 33% decrease in personal motor vehicle crash (MVC) injury claims between 2002 and 2008. The relative decrease is similar between the incidence of WAD and other types of injuries, with WAD constituting about 50% of all MVC injury claims. This decrease is not due to a reduction in the number of MVCs, and nor has the insurance system in Sweden changed. Instead, this decrease is likely to be due to a combination of reasons. For example, some car manufacturers have developed whiplash-protection devices for new car models, which presumably will result in fewer cases of WAD as a result of rear-end collisions. Secondly, during the second half of the 1990s, police personnel in Sweden showed an increased awareness that there is no need to advise car occupants to seek healthcare if no symptoms are present. Thirdly, the mass media focus in Sweden on whiplash has decreased substantially from over 800 articles in the beginning of the 2000s to only about 200 articles in 2008.

Incidence calculation through insurance claims may be prone to other forms of bias. For instance, insurance systems where there are no benefits for the person responsible for a collision may underestimate the frequency of injuries, since fewer claims would be reported. This would also happen with insurance systems where insurance claim access is limited, or where payments for compensation result in a significant increase in the insurance premium. On the other hand, healthcare data may also be prone to bias, since such data only captures those who seek the type of healthcare utilisation in question (e.g. emergency care).

Risk factors for onset of WAD

A *risk factor* for an outcome (i.e. disease/injury) is a factor that is independently associated with the outcome or condition in question. Knowledge of the aetiology (cause) of WAD is limited. One reason for this is the difficulty in obtaining accurate and appropriate denominators to calculate risks. Rather than using persons exposed to collisions as the denominator, researchers have used proxies, such as registered licensed drivers,[6] population censuses,[13, 14] or persons involved in collisions where at least one person was injured.[9] Some studies have adjusted for possible confounding factors, while others have not. A *confounding factor* is an independent risk factor for the outcome and is also associated with the exposure/risk factor of interest. Examples of possible confounding factors include gender, age, pre-collision physical and mental health, and severity and direction of crash impact.

Risk factors for WAD reported in published studies include presence of neck pain prior to the collision,[15, 16] being the driver or the front-seat passenger (compared to rear-seat passenger), and being exposed to a rear-end collision or frontal collision rather than a side collision.[9] Female gender has been suggested to be associated with a slightly higher incidence of WAD in some studies,[9, 6, 13] but other studies have found no gender differences.[11, 14] All these studies have weaknesses, primarily, the lack of 'true' denominators and/or the limited possibility to control for potential confounding factors.

One possible risk factor for WAD is the severity of the crash (impact). The biomechanical research on WAD is mainly based on experimental studies using cadavers, volunteers and simulation experiments. So far, the injury mechanism has not been established as a known risk factor. Reasons for this may be that there are different injury mechanisms occurring with different crash types. Car occupant acceleration, velocity and rebound are all factors that should be considered.[17] In much of the research, a major focus is on rear-end injury mechanisms despite consistent findings that rear-end collisions are only responsible for 40–55% of all cases of WAD in MVCs.[8, 18] However, there are some promising results from actual rear-end collisions in that the redesign of headrests and seats so that head/neck extension is limited in rear-end collisions has reduced the incidence of WAD.[19, 20] Before firm conclusions about the magnitude of such preventive interventions can be drawn, larger studies with well-defined outcome measures and controls for potential confounding factors are needed.

COURSE AND PROGNOSIS OF WAD AFTER A MOTOR VEHICLE CRASH

Course of recovery

Understanding the course and prognosis in WAD is critical. Will people recover from this common injury? If so, when? If the injury is transient and self-limiting, there would be no need for major prevention and intervention strategies. The natural course and prognosis of WAD has been a controversial matter. Some claim that the prognosis is solely determined by the physical injury and its severity, and that pre- and post-psychosocial factors are not relevant in recovery.[21–23] Others claim that persistent WAD is mainly a 'psycho-cultural' illness, and refer to studies from Lithuania and Greece where there is no or little awareness or reporting of WAD resulting from a whiplash mechanism.[24–26] Studies from these countries report that 2% or less of study participants report long-lasting symptoms after car collisions.[15, 27] However, drawing firm conclusions based on the findings of these studies is inappropriate, since 'psycho-cultural' factors were not studied per se. Nevertheless, when persons who do not experience neck pain following a car collision have been asked to report on which symptoms they would expect after neck injury or minor head injury, those from Lithuania and

Greece do not expect to have as many symptoms or do not have as long-lasting symptoms compared to persons in Canada.[28–30]

In the majority of studies, the recovery rate is substantially lower than recovery rates reported in Greece and Lithuania. Some report a 66–68% recovery rate at one year after the injury,[31, 32] whereas others report a less than 40% recovery rate at a similar time point.[33, 34] Differences in recovery rates are at least partially due to selection bias. For instance, in the study by Miettinen et al., only 58% of the invited study population was followed up 12 months post injury, so it was unknown what the recovery rate was for the 42% of participants who could not be contacted at follow-up.[33]

Prognostic factors

A *prognostic factor* is a factor that is independently associated with the prognosis, and which can contribute to or work against recovery from a condition. Some factors known to contribute to a poor prognosis in WAD are similar to those for other forms of persistent neck pain. These factors include, among others, passive coping strategies, poor mental health, high level of stress, high pain intensity and more 'associated' symptoms, such as arm pain, headache and nausea.[35–40] Similar to the literature on neck pain in the general population, gender does not seem to be a clear prognostic factor in WAD, after adjustments have been made for psychosocial factors.[41] This suggests that the observed poor prognosis in females in some studies might be explained in terms of the psychosocial factors rather than the biological factors of gender. Furthermore, societal factors, such as insurance systems with possibilities to claim for pain and suffering,[37] and extensive healthcare utilisation in the early stage of the injury,[42] have been suggested to be associated with delayed recovery in WAD.

Surprisingly, the bulk of evidence suggests that crash-related factors (e.g. impact direction, awareness of collision, head position) are not associated with the prognosis.[41]

There is evidence that people's lowered expectations of recovery and return to work, assessed early in the process of recovery, are an important predictor for long-lasting WAD, even after controlling for other factors, such as prior health, pain intensity, pain areas and acute post-traumatic stress symptoms.[43–45] An *expectation* is defined as a degree of belief that some event will occur,[46] and is also explained by some as being tied to an outcome, such as a recovery state or return to work, rather than the individual behaviours required to achieve that outcome (self-efficacy expectations).[47] It is believed to be influenced by personal and psychological features, such as anxiety, self-efficacy, coping abilities and fear, and recent studies have demonstrated that in those with WAD, initial pain, depressive symptomatology, and some crash and demographic factors were associated with recovery and return-to-work expectation.[48]

Health expectations are postulated to be primarily learned from the cultural environment, and based on 'prior knowledge'. The mechanism by which expectations influence emotional and physical reactions may also actually affect the autonomic nervous system, involving biochemical processes, which may explain some of the power observed in studies of the placebo and nocebo effect.[49, 50] These mechanisms help to explain why persons who strongly anticipate they will recover really do, and why strong expectations about bad health actually lead to bad health. A concept that is closely related to expectations is a person's belief—the lens through which a person views the world—which is shaped by the environment. In a study where injured persons were asked about their belief of the origin of their neck pain (causal belief), those who believed that something serious had happened to their neck had greater perceived disability during follow-up compared to those who did not have such beliefs.[51]

WAD and widespread pain

One important aspect about the course of recovery from WAD is whether the neck injury is a trigger for subsequent widespread body pain. This has been suggested from cross-sectional studies, but knowing whether widespread pain came before the neck injury remains unclear from this type of study design.[52, 53] A potential aetiological explanation is a neurophysiological disturbance in the peripheral and central nervous system, which, in some instances, leads to an increased sensitivity to pain in other 'uninjured' areas.[54, 55] Another possible explanation for widespread pain is that new tissue damage may result from an altered pattern of movement in the body due to the neck pain. The exact aetiology of widespread pain is probably complex and multifactorial, but there are no indications that it would be specific to WAD. It can also occur after surgical intervention or any tissue damage.[54] In addition, large prospective studies on pain of other aetiology have demonstrated that psychosocial factors at work, repetitive strains or other physical strains at work, awareness of symptoms and illness behaviour may increase the risk of development of widespread pain.[56–58] Thus, it seems that biological as well as psychological and social factors contribute to the development of widespread pain.

Prospective studies on WAD and its association with widespread pain are sparse and the evidence is not clear. The results from one study suggest a relationship between the onset of neck pain or other associated symptoms as well as self-perceived injury severity, after an MVC, and subsequent widespread pain.[59] However, age, gender, health behaviour and somatic symptoms prior to collision were at least as important. Another study investigated the incidence of onset of more extensive pain during 12 months follow-up of WAD claimants, and associated factors with such an outcome.[60] In that study, a less conservative definition of widespread pain was used and would probably have resulted in a higher incidence. The main conclusions were that widespread pain was common over a 12-month period (21%), but most improved over the follow-up period. Female gender, poor prior health, greater initial symptomatology (including pain intensity) and more depressive symptoms were associated with the development of extensive pain. The authors also found that local neck/spinal pain was rare after a traffic collision—only 11% of eligible WAD claimants had local neck/back pain, raising the question of the potential cause of widespread pain in other studies.

Work absenteeism and work disability

Many persons with acute WAD also have some absence from work, and no clear difference occurs between 'blue' and 'white' collar workers. In one population-based study, 46% of persons had been off work due to the injury.[8] A similar figure (49%) was seen in a Dutch study.[61] The majority of people returned to work within a few days and only 4–9% were reported to be off work at six months post injury.[32, 62] In a study from the Netherlands, factors associated with not returning to work were older age and concentration problems.[63] There was no association between degree of manual labour ('blue' or 'white' collar work) or education level and not returning to work.

AN EPIDEMIOLOGICAL APPROACH TO AETIOLOGY

In epidemiology, one of the aims is to assess the independent association between a potential risk or prognostic factor. It is, however, extremely important to keep in mind that in most diseases and injuries, a multifactorial causal model is needed to understand the onset and prognosis.

This can effectively be discussed using the 'pie' model, or the component cause model, introduced to epidemiologists by Rothman.[64] In Figure 1.1, some prognostic factors that may be involved in recovery from WAD are introduced in two different 'pie' models.

According to the 'pie' model, all *contributing causes* in one of the *sufficient causes*, or 'pie', *are* needed, in order to recover from WAD. Each *sufficient cause* represents one of presumably several alternative routes leading to recovery. The interactions between *contributing causes* are illustrated as separate 'pie slices' included in the same 'pie'. Slices in one 'pie' are said to interact, because it is their joint action that leads to recovery. The six outlined examples given in Figure 1.1 represent both 'biological', 'psychological' and 'social' factors. The other B's, P's and S in the figure represent other factors that are important for the prognosis. In real life, of course, different distributions of biological, psychological and social factors occur among different people.

In the literature, there is no recognised single *contributing cause* that is considered *necessary* for recovery from WAD. Neither has any *sufficient cause* been identified. Instead, several *contributing causes* (i.e. factors that affect the causes for recovery) have been found. When linking this 'pie' model to the evidence of prognostic factors in WAD, numerous sets of possible 'individual pies' become obvious. In summary, several different *sufficient causes* for recovery from WAD exist; in other words, several alternative routes lead to recovery.

In research, the effect of individual *contributing causes*, or risk factors, are usually investigated for the condition in question. Complete *sufficient causes* usually do not lend themselves to studies because few of these scenarios actually exist (exceptions include bacterial infection). Still, it is important to keep the 'pie' model in mind when interpreting and discussing empirical results on risk and prognosis. A single contributing cause may otherwise be confused for a *sufficient cause*. The whole picture of specific sets of *sufficient causes* is seldom discussed in the research of WAD or in other contexts.

The causal process is more complicated than explained by the 'pie' model, since effects are likely to depend on other factors that happen simultaneously. For instance, some persons in pain may call for support from family members or workmates, which in turn may change the person's future pain perception and behaviour (positively or negatively). In other instances, pain intensity may cause depressed mood, or depressed mood may cause more pain (bidirectional). Nevertheless, this component cause model is

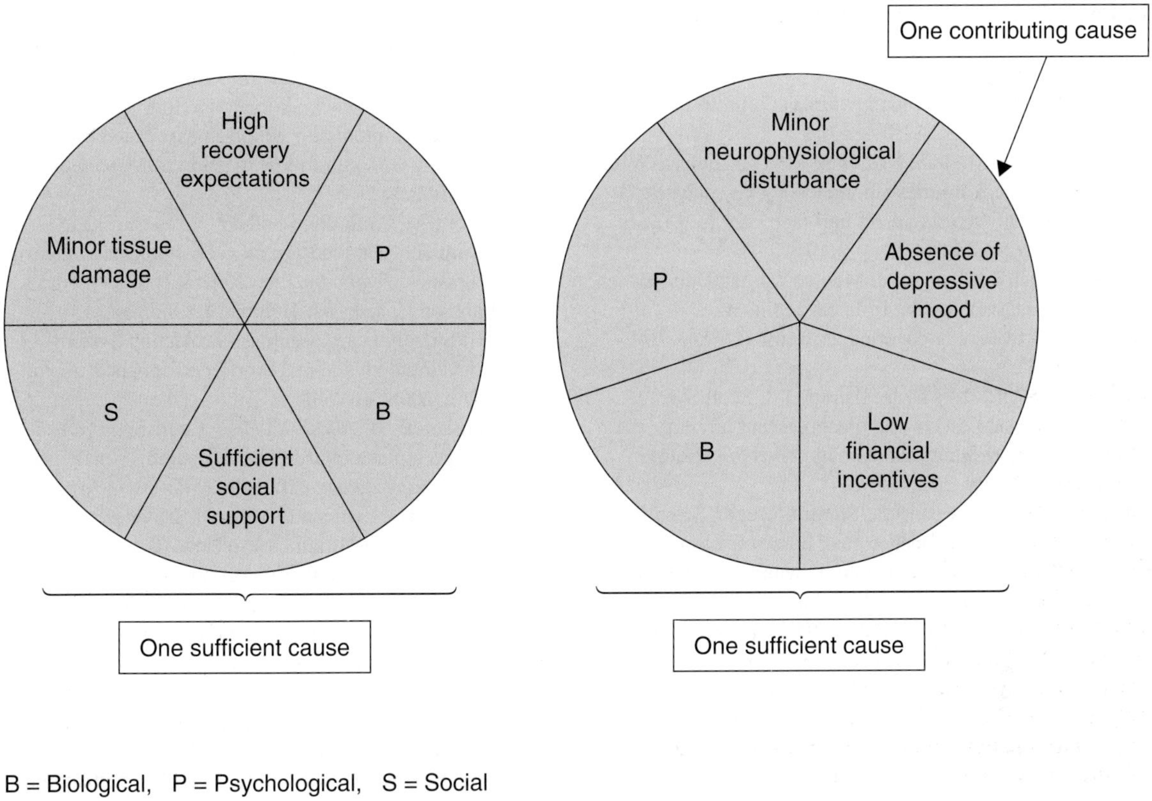

Figure 1.1 The 'pie' model—examples of factors related to recovery from WAD.

a fruitful way to conceptualise WAD as it visualises the multifactorial nature of WAD and how biological, psychological and social factors may interact.

THE ECONOMIC BURDEN OF WAD

Little is known about the individual and societal economic burden of WAD. For instance, little is known about the prevalence of long-lasting work disability due to WAD, which is probably the most costly part. This burden is probably largely dependent on the legislation in different countries. In 2002, an independent and temporary Commission on Whiplash-Related Injuries was formed in Sweden, initiated by the four largest motor vehicle insurers. The mandate of the 3-year Commission was an examination of the problems of WAD from road safety, medical care, insurance and societal aspects.[65] One of the conclusions of the final report was that the yearly cost for society and for the insurance industry was approximately SEK 1.5 billion (US$201 million), while projected costs (i.e. what new cases of WAD arising in a particular year will cost society and insurers by the time the person reaches retirement age) amounted to SEK 4.6 billion (US$648 million). These calculations were based on an annual incidence of 30,000 WAD cases (324 per 100,000 inhabitants) in the year 2002. Since the report's publication, the number of WAD cases have decreased dramatically to about 16,000 claims in 2008 (173 per 100,000 inhabitants), which, of course, has an impact on the overall costs.

Comparable data has not been found, but there is some evidence from a study that addressed the incidence of WAD in 10 European countries.[66] The administrative data suggest that the total claims cost in Switzerland was 500 million Swiss francs (US$467 million). Switzerland's population is 80% that of Sweden. Expenditures in addition to the claims cost was not reported in that study.

SUMMARY

In summary, as in almost all other diseases and injuries, factors that are involved in the risk or prognosis of WAD are multifactorial and constitute a web of biological, psychological and social components.

References

1. Crowe H. A new diagnostic sign in neck injuries. *Calif Med* 1964;100:12–13.
2. Gay J, Abbott K. Common whiplash injuries of the neck. *JAMA* 1953;152:1698–704.
3. Benson BW, Mohtadi NG, Rose MS, Meeuwisse WH. Head and neck injuries among ice hockey players wearing full face shields vs half face shields. *JAMA* 1999;282(24):2328–32.
4. Versteegen GJ, Kingma J, Meijler WJ, ten Duis HJ. Neck sprain not arising from car accidents: a retrospective study covering 25 years. *Eur Spine J* 1998;7(3):201–5.
5. Lorish TR, Rizzo TD, Jr., Ilstrup DM, Scott SG. Injuries in adolescent and preadolescent boys at two large wrestling tournaments. *Am J Sports Med* 1992;20(2):199–202.
6. Spitzer WO, Skovron ML, Salmi LR, et al. Scientific monograph of the Quebec Task Force on whiplash-associated disorders: redefining "whiplash" and its management. *Spine* 1995;20(8 Suppl):1S–73S.
7. Holm LW, Carroll LJ, Cassidy JD, Ahlbom A. Factors influencing neck pain intensity in whiplash-associated disorders in Sweden. *Clin J Pain* 2007;23(7):591–7.
8. Ferrari R, Russell AS, Carroll LJ, Cassidy JD. A re-examination of the whiplash-associated disorders (WAD) as a systemic illness. *Ann Rheum Dis* 2005:1337–42.
9. Berglund A, Alfredsson L, Jensen I, et al. Occupant- and crash-related factors associated with the risk of whiplash injury. *Ann Epidemiol* 2003;13(1):66–72.
10. Bylund P-O, Björnstig U. Sick leave and disability pension among passenger car occupants injured in urban traffic. *Spine* 1998;23(9):1023–8.
11. Versteegen GJ, Kingma J, Meijler WJ, ten Duis HJ. Neck sprain in patients injured in car accidents: a retrospective study covering the period 1970–1994. *Eur Spine J* 1998;7(3):195–200.
12. Björnstig U, Hildingson C, Toolanen G. Soft-tissue injury of the neck in hospital based material. *Spine* 1990;18(4):263–7.
13. Quinlan KP, Annest JL, Myers B, et al. Neck strains and sprains among motor vehicle occupants—United States, 2000. *Accid Anal Prev* 2004;36(1):21–7.
14. Bring G, Bjornstig U, Westman G. Gender patterns in minor head and neck injuries: an analysis of casualty register data. *Accid Anal Prev* 1996;28(3):359–69.
15. Obelieniene D, Schrader H, Bovim G, et al. Pain after whiplash: a prospective controlled inception cohort study. *J Neurol Neurosurg Psychiatry* 1999;66:279–83.
16. Wiles NJ, Jones GT, Silman AJ, Macfarlane GJ. Onset of neck pain after a motor vehicle accident: a case-control study. *J Rheumatol* 2005;32(8):1576–83.
17. Sendur P, Thibodeau R, Burge J, Tencer A. Parametric analysis of vehicle design influence on the four phases of whiplash motion. *Traffic Inj Prev* 2005;6(3):258–66.
18. Crutebo S, Nilsson C, Skillgate E, Holm LW. The course of symptoms for whiplash-associated disorders in Sweden: 6-month followup study. *J Rheumatol* 2010;37(7):1527–33.
19. Farmer CM, Wells JK, Lund AK. Effects of head restraint and seat redesign on neck injury risk in rear-end crashes. *Traffic Inj Prev* 2003;4(2):83–90.
20. Jakobsson L, Isaksson-Hellman I, Lindman M. WHIPS (Volvo cars' Whiplash Protection System)—the development and real-world performance. *Traffic Inj Prev* 2008;9(6):600–5.
21. Johansson B. *Whiplashskador har entydig organisk grund* [Whiplash injuries has an unambiguous organic basis]. *Läkartidningen* 2001;98(25):3061–2.
22. Freeman MD, Centeno C. "Alar, Transverse, and Apical Ligament Strain Due to Head-Turned Rear Impact" by Maak et al. *Spine* 2006;31(17):2030.
23. Freeman M, Croft A, Rossignol A, et al. A review and methodologic critique of the literature refuting whiplash syndrome. *Spine* 1999;24(1):86–98.
24. Ferrari R, Shorter E. From railway spine to whiplash—the recycling of nervous irritation. *Med Sci Monit* 2003;9(11):HY27–37.
25. Ferrari R, Kwan O, Russell AS, et al. The best approach to the problem of whiplash? One ticket to Lithuania please. *Clin Exp Rheumatol* 1999;17:321–6.
26. Ferrari R. Myths of whiplash. *Surgeon* 2003;1(2):99, 101–3.
27. Partheni M, Constantoyannis C, Ferrari R, et al. A prospective cohort study of the outcome of acute whiplash injury in Greece. *Clin Exp Rheumatol* 2000;18:67–70.
28. Ferrari R, Constantoyannis C, Papadakis N. Cross-cultural study of symptom expectation following minor head injury in Canada and Greece. *Clin Neurol Neurosurg* 2001;103(4):254–9.
29. Ferrari R, Obelieniene D, Russell AS, et al. Symptoms expectation after minor head injury. A comparative study between Canada and Lithuania. *Clin Neurol Neurosurg* 2001;103:184–94.
30. Ferrari R, Obelieniene D, Russell A, et al. Laypersons′ expectation of the sequelae of whiplash injury. A cross-cultural comparative study between Canada and Lithuania. *Med Sci Monit* 2002;8(11):728–34.
31. Kivioja J, Jensen I, Lindgren U. Early coping strategies do not influence the prognosis after whiplash injuries. *Injury* 2005;36(8):935–40.
32. Sterner Y, Toolanen G, Gerdle B, Hildingsson C. The incidence of whiplash trauma and the effect of different factors on recovery. *J Spinal Disord Tech* 2003;16(2):195–9.

33. Miettinen T, Airaksinen O, Lindgren KA, Leino E. Whiplash injuries in Finland—the possibility of some sociodemographic and psychosocial factors to predict the outcome after one year. *Disabil Rehabil* 2004;26(23):1367–72.
34. Gargan MF, Bannister GC. The rate of recovery following whiplash injury. *Eur Spine J* 1994;3(3):162–4.
35. Croft PR, Lewis M, Papageorgiou AC, et al. Risk factors for neck pain: a longitudinal study in the general population. *Pain* 2001;93(3):317–25.
36. Bot SD, van der Waal JM, Terwee CB, et al. Predictors of outcome in neck and shoulder symptoms: a cohort study in general practice. *Spine* 2005;30(16):E459–70.
37. Cassidy JD, Carroll L, Côté P, et al. Effect of eliminating compensation for pain and suffering on the outcome of insurance claims for whiplash injury. *N Engl J Med* 2000;342(16):1179–86.
38. Carroll LJ, Cassidy JD, Côté P. The role of pain coping strategies in prognosis after whiplash injury: passive coping predicts slowed recovery. *Pain* 2006;124:18–26.
39. Côté P, Cassidy JD, Carroll L, et al. A systematic review of the prognosis of acute whiplash and a new conceptual framework to synthesize the literature. *Spine* 2001;26(19):E445–58.
40. Carstensen TB, Frostholm L, Oernboel E, et al. Post-trauma ratings of pre-collision pain and psychological distress predict poor outcome following acute whiplash trauma: a 12-month follow-up study. *Pain* 2008;139(2):248–59.
41. Carroll LJ, Holm LW, Hogg-Johnson S, et al. Course and prognostic factors for neck pain in whiplash-associated disorders (WAD): results of the Bone and Joint Decade 2000-2010 Task Force on Neck Pain and Its Associated Disorders. *Eur Spine J* 2008;17 (Suppl 1):S83–92.
42. Côté P, Hogg-Johnson S, Cassidy JD, et al. Initial patterns of clinical care and recovery from whiplash injuries: a population-based cohort study. *Arch Intern Med* 2005;165(19):2257–63.
43. Holm LW, Carroll LJ, Cassidy JD, et al. Expectations for recovery important in the prognosis of whiplash injuries. *PLoS Med* 2008;5(5):e105.
44. Carroll LJ, Holm LW, Ferrari R, et al. Recovery in whiplash-associated disorders: do you get what you expect? *J Rheumatol* 2009;36(5):1063–70.
45. Ozegovic D, Carroll LJ, David Cassidy J. Does expecting mean achieving? The association between expecting to return to work and recovery in whiplash associated disorders: a population-based prospective cohort study. *Eur Spine J* 2009;18(6):893–9.
46. Kirsch I. How expectancies shape experience. Washington, DC: The American Psychology Association, 1999.
47. Janzen JA, Silvius J, Jacobs S, et al. What is a health expectation? Developing a pragmatic conceptual model from psychological theory. *Health Expect* 2006;9(1):37–48.
48. Ozegovic D, Carroll L, Cassidy J. Factors associated with return to work expectations in a population based WAD cohort. *J Rehabil Med* 2010;42;66–73.
49. Pariente J, White P, Frackowiak RS, Lewith G. Expectancy and belief modulate the neuronal substrates of pain treated by acupuncture. *Neuroimage* 2005;25(4):1161–7.
50. Beauregard M. Effect of mind on brain activity: evidence from neuroimaging studies of psychotherapy and placebo effect. *Nord J Psychiatry* 2009;63(1):5–16.
51. Buitenhuis J, de Jong PJ, Jaspers JP, Groothoff JW. Catastrophizing and causal beliefs in whiplash. *Spine* 2008;33(22):2427–33.
52. Buskila D, Neuman L, Vaisberg G, et al. Increased rates of fibromyalgia following cervical spine injury. *Arthritis Rheum* 1997;40(3):446–52.
53. McLean SA, Williams DA, Clauw DJ. Fibromyalgia after motor vehicle collision: evidence and implications. *Traffic Inj Prev* 2005;6(2):97–104.
54. Melzack R, Coderre TJ, Katz J, Vaccarino AL. Central neuroplasticity and pathological pain. *Ann N Y Acad Sci* 2001;933:157–74.
55. Meeus M, Nijs J. Central sensitization: a biopsychosocial explanation for chronic widespread pain in patients with fibromyalgia and chronic fatigue syndrome. *Clin Rheumatol* 2006:465–73.
56. McBeth J, Harkness EF, Silman AJ, Macfarlane GJ. The role of workplace low-level mechanical trauma, posture and environment in the onset of chronic widespread pain. *Rheumatology (Oxford)* 2003;42(12):1486–94.
57. McBeth J, Macfarlane GJ, Benjamin S, Silman AJ. Features of somatization predict the onset of chronic widespread pain. *Arthritis Rheum* 2001;44(4):940–6.
58. Harkness EF, Macfarlane GJ, Nahit E, et al. Mechanical injury and psychosocial factors in the work place predict the onset of widespread body pain: a two-year prospective study among cohorts of newly employed workers. *Arthritis Rheum* 2004;50(5): 1655–64.
59. Wynne-Jones G, Jones GT, Wiles NJ, et al. Predicting new onset of widespread pain following a motor vehicle collision. *J Rheumatol* 2006;33(5):968–74.
60. Holm LW, Carroll LJ, Cassidy JD, et al. Widespread pain following whiplash-associated disorders: incidence, course, and risk factors. *J Rheumatol* 2006;34(1):193–200.
61. Hendriks EJ, Scholten-Peeters GG, van der Windt DA, et al. Prognostic factors for poor recovery in acute whiplash patients. *Pain* 2005;114(3):408–16.

62. Kasch, H, Bach F, Jensen T. Handicap after acute whiplash injury: a 1-year prospective study of risk factors. *Neurology* 2001;56(12):1637–43.
63. Buitenhuis J, de Jong PJ, Jaspers JP, Groothoff JW. Work disability after whiplash: a prospective cohort study. *Spine* 2009;34(3):262–7.
64. Rothman K. Epidemiology: an introduction. New York: Oxford University Press, 2002.
65. The Swedish Commission on Whiplash-Related Injuries. The Whiplash Commission Final Report, 2009. Online. Available at: http://www.whiplashkommissionen.se/english/english.htm, viewed 20 August 2010.
66. Chappuis G, Soltermann B. Number and cost of claims linked to minor cervical trauma in Europe: results from the comparative study by CEA, AREDOC and CEREDOC. *Eur Spine J* 2008;17(10):1350–7.

CHAPTER 2
Clinical presentation of whiplash associated disorders

Michele Sterling

Symptoms following whiplash injury can be diverse in nature. The predominant symptom is neck pain and it is present in almost all patients,[1] with some patients also reporting neck stiffness.[2] In addition, headache has been reported in 50–90% of patients, shoulder and arm pain in 40–70% of patients and back pain (thoracic and/or lumbar regions) in 35% of injured people.[1, 3, 4] Paraesthesia and/or anaesthesia, usually in the upper limbs, presents in up to 20% of patients.[2] Apart from pain, other common symptoms include dizziness, visual and auditory disturbances, temporomandibular joint pain, photophobia and fatigue.[1, 2, 5] Symptoms of dizziness have been shown to be related to postural control disturbances, including proprioceptive deficits, disturbed eye movement control and balance loss,[5–7] and these are discussed in depth in Chapter 7. Cognitive difficulties, such as the loss of concentration and memory, are also common, although the cause of these difficulties remains elusive and there is no evidence to date that they are related to a diffuse brain injury.[8] Possible other causes include pain intensity, psychological factors, such as anxiety, or medication usage.[8]

PATTERNS OF RECOVERY

The onset of symptoms may occur immediately or, in many patients, may be delayed for up to 12–15 hours.[2, 9] Recent systematic review data indicate that up to 50% of injured people will not have fully recovered one year post injury.[10] Prospective studies that have followed whiplash-injured people from soon after injury to either recovery or the development of chronic symptoms indicate that rapid improvement occurs in the first three months with little, if any, change after this period.[11] However, these conclusions were based on the pooling of mean data from just nine cohorts using various measurement tools and assumed a linear pattern of change.

More sophisticated statistical techniques are available to measure longitudinal data. The recent development of more advanced statistical modelling tools that take advantage of data sources with repeated measures allows for empirical estimation of the development of certain processes over time.[12] Group-based trajectory models are designed to identify clusters of individuals following similar progressions of some behaviour or outcome over time.[13] Most statistical approaches assume linear relationships of variables over time but this may not necessarily be the case. Trajectory models also allow exploration of non-linear changes in symptoms that might, for example, be more rapid initially or less rapid at later stages.

Using these types of analyses, a recent study demonstrated a general pattern of decline in pain/disability levels (measured with the Neck Disability Index[14]) over 12 months following whiplash injury. However, three distinct patterns of predicted recovery (trajectories) were identified (Fig 2.1):

1. initial milder pain/disability but full recovery—45% of participants were predicted to follow this trajectory
2. initial moderate pain/disability with recovery to mild levels—39% of participants were predicted to follow this trajectory
3. initial severe levels of pain/disability persisting at chronic moderate-to-severe levels for the 12 month study period—16% of participants were predicted to follow this trajectory.[15]

In this study, the majority of injured people were predicted to have some degree of persistent symptoms (55%) at 12 months.[15] These findings are consistent with recent systematic reviews that indicate a general decrease in symptoms following injury but that a significant proportion (approximately 50%) of people will have ongoing symptoms at one year post motor vehicle crash (MVC).[10]

Psychological distress in various forms, such as anxiety, post-traumatic stress symptoms, depressive symptoms and pain-related distress,[17–19] are also commonly reported by those with acute and chronic whiplash; these are discussed in depth in Chapter 8. However, few studies have documented the psychological recovery pathways following injury. In the study described above, trajectory based modelling

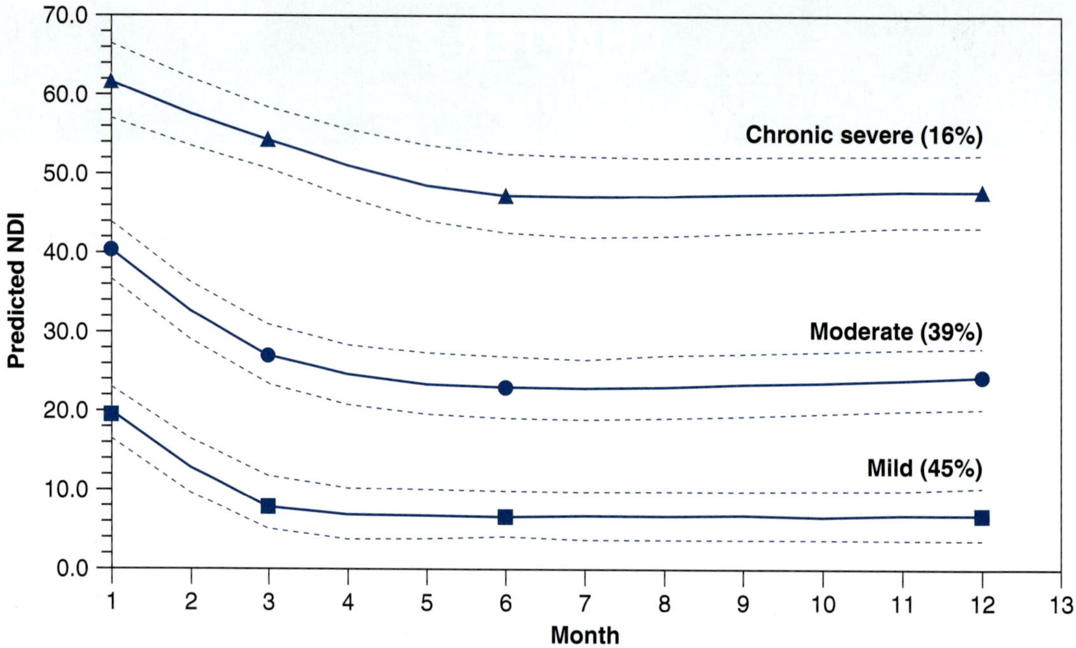

Figure 2.1 Predicted Neck Disability Index (NDI) trajectories with 95% confidence limits and predicted probability of membership (%). Suggested cut-offs for the NDI are: 0–8% (no pain and disability); 10–28% (mild pain and disability); 30–48% (moderate pain and disability); 50–68% (severe pain and disability); and >70% complete disability.[16] With permission.

was also used to identify recovery pathways for symptoms of post-traumatic stress disorder (PTSD) using the symptom severity score of the Posttraumatic Stress Diagnostic Scale (PDS).[20] It was demonstrated that 40% of whiplash-injured individuals were estimated to show psychological resilience to the injury, while 43% were estimated to have initial moderate PTSD symptoms declining to subclinical levels by three months and 17% showed persistent moderate-to-severe symptoms for at least 12 months (Fig 2.2). The symptom severity score of the PDS was used in the analyses, but this tool also yields a PTSD diagnosis if specific criteria are met following a minimum period of one month post injury.[20] In this study, at three months post MVC, 22.3% of participants met the criteria for a probable PTSD diagnosis, with this percentage decreasing to 17.1% by 12 months. These data are interesting in that they are similar to that documented for people with more severe traumatic injury that required hospitalisation or admission to intensive care[21] and are somewhat unexpected for whiplash, which is considered a more 'minor' injury.

Thus, in general, while there seems to be a general decline in both pain and disability and psychological symptoms following injury, clear and distinct recovery or non-recovery pathways can be identified.

Inspection of these trajectories (Figs 2.1 and 2.2) also reveals that most recovery, if it occurs, takes place in the first two to three months following the initial injury, with the condition plateauing after this time. These data are in agreement with those of a recent systematic review[11] and indicate the importance of management in the acute/subacute stage in order to prevent the development of a chronic pain condition. The exception to this is the chronic moderate-to-severe PTSD trajectory where there appeared to be a worsening of symptoms at around six months. It is likely that individuals who may follow this trajectory will require specific psychological intervention to prevent this course. Such management approaches are often not provided to people with whiplash.[23, 24]

PHYSICAL AND PSYCHOLOGICAL CHARACTERISTICS

Most whiplash-injured people who present for treatment will display some physical and psychological signs associated with their neck pain condition. These

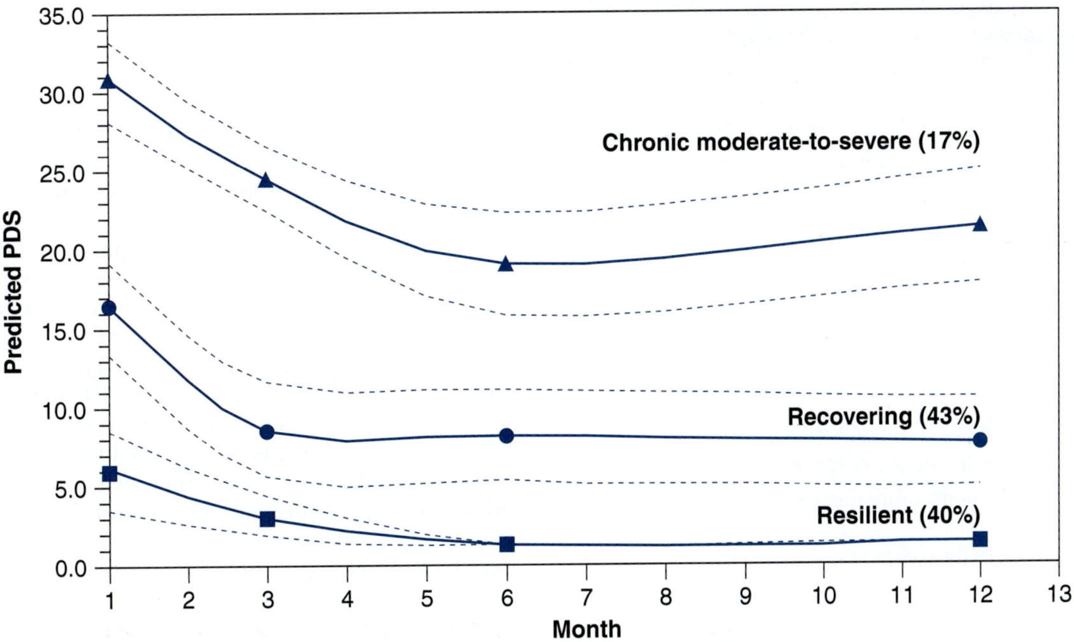

Figure 2.2 Predicted PDS trajectories with 95% confidence limits and predicted probability of membership (%). Suggested cut-offs for the PDS total symptom severity score are: 0 no rating, 1–10 mild; 11–20 moderate; 21–35 moderate-to-severe; and ≥36 severe.[22] With permission.

are commonly in the form of decreased range of neck movement, local hyperalgesia over the cervical spine and possibly some psychological distress.[25] Approximately 20–30% of those injured will display a more complex presentation comprising: sensory disturbances such as allodynia and widespread hyperalgesia in the neck region but also at remote sites such as the lower limbs; spinal cord hyperexcitability via heightened flexor withdrawal responses; more marked loss of neck movement; motor control deficits, including altered patterns of muscle recruitment in the neck and shoulder girdles; and greater levels of psychological distress.[23] Readers are referred to Chapters 5–8 for a detailed discussion of these characteristics and their assessment.

CLASSIFICATION SYSTEMS FOR WAD

The varied nature of symptoms reported following whiplash injury lends itself to suggest that a classification system of the condition would be useful in order to guide both research investigation and treatment decision-making. In 1995, the Quebec Task Force (QTF) developed the Quebec classification of WAD.[26] The authors proposed this classification system (Table 2.1) in order to facilitate the evaluation of research and to provide clinicians with useful guidelines for making decisions about therapeutic management. It classified patients with whiplash according to the type and severity of signs and symptoms observed shortly after the injury.[26]

Since its release, the QTF classification has been criticised. Much of this criticism has pointed out that while the QTF review of WAD rejected many articles that did not meet rigorous scientific criteria, the guidelines themselves suffered from the same faults—they were adopted and promoted without scientific validation.[27] The QTF classification system has demonstrated predictive capacity in that increasing grades of WAD predicted increasingly higher pain intensities and disability two years later.[10, 28] Walton et al.[28] reported that the size of effect was significant when WAD grades II and III were compared against grades I and 0, and that this effect was consistent at various follow-up time points. However, the system is symptom-based with the inclusion of rather nebulous and non-specific items, such as ‘point tenderness’ and ‘movement loss’. Patients classified as WAD II, the most common QTF grade, have been shown to manifest a broad range of physical impairments

Table 2.1 Quebec Task Force classification (grade) of whiplash associated disorders (WAD)[24]

Grade	Clinical presentation
0	No complaint about neck pain No physical signs
I	Neck complaint of pain, stiffness or tenderness only No physical signs
II	Neck complaint Musculoskeletal signs, including: • decreased range of movement • point tenderness
III	Neck complaint Neurological signs, including: • decreased or absent deep tendon reflexes • muscle weakness • sensory deficits
IV	Neck complaint and fracture or dislocation

and psychological distress, and it has been argued that this grade could be refined.[29] Even though the QTF recognised the shortcomings of their classification system, it was probably the best that could be developed at the time due to the fact that knowledge about WAD was virtually limited to patient-reported signs and symptoms.

Other classification systems have been proposed but are yet to be validated. One of these adapted the QTF system to include additional measures of sensory and motor function, as well as measures of psychological distress, in order to take into account recent developments in the knowledge and understanding of these features in acute WAD.[28] This system is illustrated in Table 2.2. In this system, the WAD II grade is divided into three subcategories. Patients with WAD IIA demonstrate what could be termed a 'less complex' presentation with some physical sign but little or no psychological distress; patients with WAD IIB have the additional presence of psychological distress; and patients with WAD IIC show more widespread sensory disturbances indicative of augmented central nociceptive processing changes and greater levels of distress and/or symptoms of post-traumatic stress.[30]

Recently, another system was proposed that includes not only whiplash but also other cervical spine conditions, such as non-traumatic neck pain and radiculopathy.[31] These authors recommend that people seeking care for neck pain should be triaged into one of four groups: grade I neck pain with no signs of major pathology and no or little interference with daily activities; grade II neck pain with no signs of major pathology, but interference with daily activities; grade III neck pain with neurologic signs of nerve compression; grade IV neck pain with signs of major pathology.[32] The authors maintain that this approach will direct interventions.[32] However, this system also seems non-specific and again the grade II classification is extremely broad, with data suggesting varied outcomes in this group from full recovery to chronic pain development.[30] Additionally, there is evidence that non-traumatic neck pain shows different features to both WAD and cervical radiculopathy,[33, 34] particularly in the sensory manifestations of the various conditions. This may also be the case for the psychological features of neck pain conditions where post-traumatic stress symptoms would seem to be unlikely in neck pain of a non-traumatic nature but are common in WAD. These differences may reflect different underlying mechanisms for various neck pain conditions, suggesting that combining all conditions into one classification system may not be advisable. As with other classification models, this system also requires validation before it can be accepted.

CONCLUSIONS

The clinical presentation of whiplash can be diverse. While neck pain and/or stiffness are the cardinal symptoms, numerous other symptoms have been reported. The clinical pathway following whiplash injury has been explored and distinct trajectories for recovery of pain and disability, as well as for psychological distress (post-traumatic stress), have been identified. Consistent data also demonstrate most recovery to occur in the first two to three months following injury, with a plateauing of symptoms after this time, indicating the potential importance for early interventions applied in this interval. Various classification systems for WAD have been proposed but these require validation before acceptance into general clinical practice.

Table 2.2 Proposed new classification system (grade) for acute whiplash associated disorders (WAD)[28]

Grade	Clinical presentation
WAD 0	No complaint about neck pain No physical signs
WAD I	Neck complaint of pain, stiffness or tenderness only No physical signs
WAD IIA	Neck pain Motor impairment • Decreased ROM • Altered muscle recruitment patterns Sensory impairment • Local cervical mechanical hyperalgesia
WAD IIB	Neck pain Motor impairment • Decreased ROM • Altered motor function and postural control Sensory impairment • Local cervical mechanical hyperalgesia Psychological distress
WAD IIC	Neck pain Motor impairment • Decreased ROM • Altered motor function and postural control Sensory impairment • Local cervical mechanical hyperalgesia • Generalised sensory hypersensitivity • Some may show SNS disturbances Psychological distress • Elevated levels of acute post-traumatic stress
WAD III	Neck pain Motor impairment • Decreased ROM • Altered motor function and postural control Sensory impairment • Local cervical mechanical hyperalgesia • Generalised sensory hypersensitivity • Some may show SNS disturbances Psychological distress • Elevated levels of acute post-traumatic stress (IES scale)

(Continued)

Table 2.2 Proposed new classification system (grade) for acute whiplash associated disorders (WAD)[28]—cont'd

Grade	Clinical presentation
	Neurological signs of conduction loss, including: • decreased or absent deep tendon reflexes • muscle weakness • sensory deficits
WAD IV	Fracture or dislocation

IES, Impact of Events; ROM, range of movement; SNS, sympathetic nervous system.

References

1. Stovner L. The nosologic status of the whiplash syndrome: a critical review based on a methodological approach. *Spine* 1996;21(23):2735–46.
2. Sterner Y, Gerdle B. Acute and chronic whiplash disorders: a review. *J Rehabil Med* 2004;36:193–209.
3. Radanov B, Sturzenegger M, Di Stefano G. Long-term outcome after whiplash injury. A 2-year follow-up considering features of injury mechanism and somatic, radiologic, and psychological findings. *Medicine* 1995;74(5):281–97.
4. Sterling M, Treleaven J, Edwards S, Jull G. Pressure pain thresholds in chronic whiplash associated disorder: further evidence of altered central pain processing. *J Musculoskeletal Pain* 2002;10(3):69–81.
5. Treleaven J, Jull G, Sterling M. Dizziness and unsteadiness following whiplash injury: characteristic features and relationship with cervical joint position error. *J Rehabil* 2003;34:1–8.
6. Treleaven J, Jull G, Low Choy N. Standing balance in persistent whiplash: a comparison between subjects with and without dizziness. *J Rehabil Med* 2005;37:224–9.
7. Treleaven J, Jull G, Low Choy N. Smooth pursuit neck torsion test in whiplash associated disorders: relationship to self-reports of neck pain and disability, dizziness and anxiety. *J Rehabil Med* 2005;37:219–23.
8. Sturzenegger M, Radaonov B, Winter P, et al. MRI-based brain volumetry in chronic whiplash patients: no evidence for traumatic brain injury. *Acta Neurol Scand* 2008;117:49–54.
9. Hildingsson C, Toolanen G. Outcome after soft-tissue injury of the cervical spine: a prospective study of 93 car-accident victims. *Acta Orthop Scand* 1990;61(4):357–9.
10. Carroll L, Holm L, Hogg-Johnson S, et al. Course and prognostic factors for neck pain in whiplash-associated disorders (WAD). Results of the Bone and Joint Decade 2000–2010 Task Force on Neck Pain and Its Associated Disorders. *Spine* 2008;33(42):583–92.
11. Kamper S, Rebbeck T, Maher C, et al. Course and prognostic factors of whiplash: a systematic review and meta-analysis. *Pain* 2008;138(3):617–29.
12. Taylor D, Ezell M, Kuchibhatla M, et al. Identifying trajectories of depressive symptoms for women caring for their husbands with dementia. *J Am Geriatric Soc* 2008;56:322–7.
13. Jones B, Nagin D. Advances in group-based trajectory modeling and an SAS procedure. *Sociol Methods Res* 2007;35(4):542–71.
14. Vernon H, Mior S. The Neck Disability Index: A study of reliability and validity. *J Manip Physiol Ther* 1991;14(7):409–15.
15. Sterling M, Hendrikz J, Kenardy J. Developmental trajectories of pain/disability and PTSD symptoms following whiplash injury. *Pain* 2010;150(1): 22–8.
16. MacDermid J, Walton D, Avery S, et al. Measurement properties of the neck disability index: a systematic review. *J Orthop Sports Phys Ther* 2009;39(5): 400–17.
17. Buitenhuis J, DeJong J, Jaspers J, Groothoff J. Relationship between posttraumatic stress disorder symptoms and the course of whiplash complaints. *J Psychosom Res* 2006;61(3):681–9.
18. Phillips L, Carroll L, Cassidy D, Côté P. Whiplash-associated disorders: who gets depressed? Who stays depressed? *Eur Spine J* 2010;19(6):945–56.
19. Sterling M, Kenardy J, Jull G, Vicenzino B. The development of psychological changes following whiplash injury. *Pain* 2003;106(3):481–9.
20. Foa E. Posttraumatic Stress Diagnostic Scale: Manual. Minneapolis: Pearson; 1995.
21. O'Donnell M, Creamer M, Bryant R, et al. Posttraumatic disorders following injury: an empirical and methodological review. *Clin Psychol Rev* 2003;23:587–603.
22. McCarthy S. Posttraumatic stress diagnostic scale (PDS). *Occupational Med* 2008;58:379–180.

23. Côté P, Hogg-Johnson S, Cassidy D, et al. Initial patterns of clinical care and recovery from whiplash injuries. *Arch Int Med* 2005;165:2257–63.
24. Sterling M, Jull G, Vicenzino B, et al. Physical and psychological factors predict outcome following whiplash injury. *Pain* 2005;114:141–8.
25. Sterling M, Kenardy J. Physical and psychological aspects of whiplash: important considerations for primary care assessment. *Man Ther* 2008;13(2): 93–102.
26. Spitzer WO, Skovron ML, Salmi LR, et al. Scientific monograph of Quebec Task Force on Whiplash associated Disorders: redefining "Whiplash" and its management. *Spine* 1995;20(8 Suppl):1S–73S.
27. Freeman M, Croft A, Rossignol A. "Whiplash associated disorders: redefining whiplash and its management" by the Quebec Task Force. A critical evaluation. *Spine* 1998;23(9):1043–9.
28. Walton D, Pretty J, MacDermid J, Teasell R. Risk factors for persistent problems following whiplash injury: results of a systematic review and meta-analysis. *J Orthop Sports Phys Ther* 2009;39(5):334–50.
29. Hartling L, Brison R, Ardern C, Pickett W. Prognostic value of the Quebec classification of whiplash associated disorders. *Spine* 2001;26(1):36–41.
30. Sterling M. A proposed new classification system for whiplash associated disorders: implications for assessment and management. *Man Ther* 2004;9(2): 60–70.
31. Guzman J, Hurwitz E, Carroll L, et al. A new conceptual model of neck pain. *Eur Spine J* 2008;17(Suppl 1):S14–S23.
32. Guzman J, Haldeman S, Carroll L, et al. Clinical practice implications of the Bone and Joint Decade 2000–2010 Task Force on Neck Pain and Its Associated Disorders. *Spine* 2008;33(4S):S199–S213.
33. Chien A, Eliav E, Sterling M. Whiplash (grade ii) and cervical radiculopathy share a similar sensory presentation: an investigation using quantitative sensory testing. *Clin J Pain* 2008;24(7):595–603.
34. Scott D, Jull G, Sterling M. Sensory hypersensitivity is a feature of chronic whiplash associated disorders but not chronic idiopathic neck pain. *Clin J Pain* 2005;21(2):175–81.

CHAPTER 3
Mechanism of injury

Brian D. Stemper, Narayan Yoganandan, Frank A. Pintar, Dennis J. Maiman

Injuries to the human body from external dynamic exposure occur due to the application of abnormal loads or motions that exceed physiological limits. Specific to motor vehicle rear-impact crashes, abnormal motions of the head–neck complex during the application of posterior–anterior acceleration to the seated occupant have been used to understand the biomechanical mechanism of injury, develop metrics to quantify trauma and, from a clinical point of view, determine structures that sustain the injury to explore improved treatment options. The focus of this chapter is to briefly discuss the kinematics, injury theories, injury metrics, and vehicle- and occupant-related factors involved in rear impact–induced injury.

HEAD–NECK KINEMATICS: GLOBAL AND SEGMENTAL

Low-speed automotive rear-impact collisions induce motions to the human head–neck complex that are unique to other loading vectors. These motions have been used to propose various injury mechanisms and injury criteria in over 50 years of biomechanical research. Mechanisms describe the method by which tissues are injured, whereas criteria define quantifiable thresholds for specific injury types. From an overall vehicle-to-occupant interaction perspective, the impact event begins when the target vehicle is struck from behind and the automotive seat accelerates forward with approximately the same pulse as the vehicle itself because of its attachment to the vehicle frame. The seat back forces the occupant's thorax forward, inducing a posterior–anterior acceleration of the head–neck complex via the inertial loading mechanism. The head initially remains stationary due to its inertia. Anterior displacement of the thorax relative to the head is termed retraction or head lag. With continued anterior movement of the thorax, axial load is transferred up the cervical spine and the head begins to rotate backward into extension. The head eventually strikes the head restraint and rebounds forward into flexion. Therefore, the three phases of the impact event are retraction, extension and rebound.

From a local perspective of the head–neck complex kinematics, as the head translates posteriorly during the retraction phase, the cervical spine compensates for the differential motion between the head and thorax by developing a transient non-physiological S-shaped curve. This kinematic signature is characterised by flexion at the cranial (C0–C2) segments and extension at caudal segments (C4–C7). Rear impact–induced injuries (commonly termed whiplash injuries) occur during this phase. Following the retraction phase, the entire cervical column sustains physiological C-shaped extension curvature that lasts until the head rebounds and the cervical column transitions into flexion curvature. The mechanisms of injury during these three phases of kinematics are described below.

INJURY THEORIES

Hyperextension theory: anterior column injury

Global hyperextension of the head–neck forms the basis of the *hyperextension theory* (Fig 3.1). Development of this theory was based on experiments using human volunteers, post-mortem human subjects (PMHSs), anthropomorphic test devices and primates.[1–4] Clinical studies have reported that hyperextension most commonly results in anterior cervical column injuries in the form of anterior longitudinal ligament and intervertebral disc ruptures.[5–11] These injuries were reproduced during rear-impact experiments. For example, hyperextension-type injuries occurred in anaesthetised primates in simulated automotive rear-impact collisions.[1] The primates were placed supine on a steel platform without head restraint, and the platform was accelerated by a guided drop tower. The initial platform height varied from 0.6 m to 12 m. Another study documented cervical spinal injuries consistent with the hyperextension mechanism by subjecting PMHSs to single-application rear impacts at a change in velocity of 15 or 25 km/h.[12] Sled tests were conducted with PMHSs

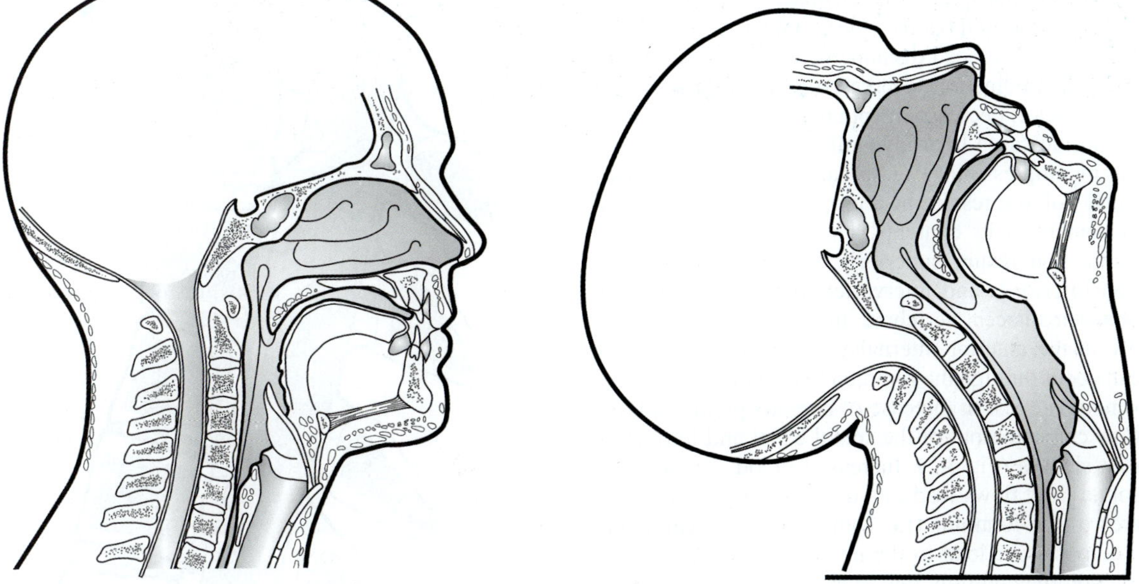

Figure 3.1 Globalised hyperextension of the head–neck complex results in tension of anterior vertebral column tissues, such as the anterior longitudinal ligament and intervertebral disc.

seated upright in a rigid seat without head restraint. Two out of the three PMHSs subjected to high-velocity tests sustained anterior longitudinal ligament and disc ruptures. Likewise, a study subjecting PMHSs to multiple rear impacts using a relatively rigid seat demonstrated similar injury patterns in specimens following tests without head restraints.[13] Anterior disc separation and tears of the annulus and anterior ligaments were identified in two out of the three PMHSs exposed to impacts between 11.0 and 15.5 km/h.

Injuries in the studies cited above occurred without the presence of a head restraint. However, these safety devices were introduced into passenger vehicles in the United States in 1969 with the intent of preventing head–neck hyperextension during rear-impact collisions. Therefore, based on global head–neck kinematics and using the hyperextension mechanism, it is difficult to explain the most commonly reported symptoms of posterior neck pain and headache reported in a majority of contemporary cases of rear-impact collisions. In the absence of global head–neck hyperextension, localised or segmental hyperextension may lead to injuries that result in neck pain. In particular, extension in lower cervical segments (C4–C7) may exceed local tissue thresholds and result in tension injury to anterior soft tissues. Some clinical studies using data derived from vehicles equipped with head restraints seem to support this assertion by continuing to report the presence of anterior cervical column injuries, including anterior longitudinal ligament ruptures, horizontal avulsion of vertebral end plates, and separation of the intervertebral disc from vertebral bodies.[5, 14–16] Experimental and computational literature has provided some additional support. Tests using PMHSs subjected to multiple impacts in a rigid seat with a head restraint have reported similar hyperextension-type injuries.[13] A computational modelling study showed that segmental anterior longitudinal ligament strains can approach catastrophic failure levels during the retraction phase, before head-to-head-restraint contact.[17] This finding is particularly relevant as it demonstrated that global head–neck hyperextension is not required to induce local hyperextension-type injuries.

Hydrodynamic theory: nerve root injury

Increased hydrodynamic pressure in the spinal canal during cervical spine bending forms the basis of the *hydrodynamic theory*.[18, 19] This theory centres around the fact that length and cross-sectional area of the spinal canal increase during flexion and decrease during extension.[20] During extension motion, as experienced during automotive rear-impact collisions, decreased cross-sectional area can be attributed to protrusion of the ligamentum flava into the canal space due to laxity from the reduced distance between adjacent laminae. In combination, decreased length and area lead to an overall decrease in spinal canal volume, resulting in increased hydrodynamic pressure. Because of the incompressibility of spinal fluids, the decreased canal volume results in a proportional outward displacement of its contents. The canal outlets are the foramen magnum superiorly, cervicothoracic junction inferiorly, and intervertebral foramina laterally between adjacent vertebrae. In the case of blood supply in the anterior internal venous plexus, the flow can occur through the foramen to the anterior external venous plexus. In the case of cerebrospinal fluid, the flow can occur out of the spinal canal and into nerve root sleeves (Fig 3.2). Increased blood and cerebrospinal fluid flows lead to a decreased cross-sectional area of the foramina (i.e. stenosis), which can apply a compressive load to the nerve root. Depending on the volume and flow rate, the compressive load may exceed tolerance, resulting in transient or chronic dysfunction of the affected root(s).

Nerve root pain from compressive radiculopathy is commonly reported by occupants involved in automotive rear-impact collisions. In particular, sharp pain and paraesthesia in the neck, shoulders and upper back are associated with compression of the nerve roots.[21] Clinical rear impact studies have reported consistent findings. For example, neck, shoulder and back pain were reported by 92%, 49% and 39% of referred patients, respectively, following whiplash injury.[22] However, pain directly attributed to the nerve roots (radicular pain) was present in only 15% of patients. Another study reported that neck pain was present in 100% of consecutive patients involved in an automotive rear-impact collision.[23] Forty-eight per cent of those patients reported concomitant paraesthesia symptoms. Other clinical and epidemiological studies have reported similar findings, although this list is not comprehensive.[24–27] While cervical nerve roots may be injured during automotive rear-impact collisions, nerve root injury can only explain some of the symptoms involved in whiplash associated disorders (WAD).

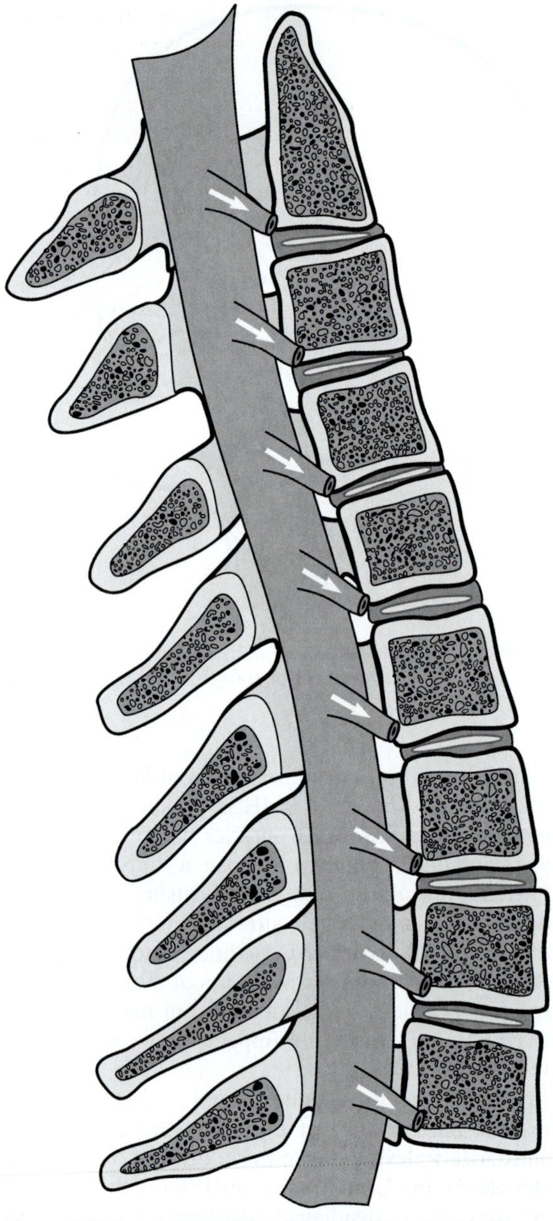

Figure 3.2 Retraction of the head relative to the thorax leads to decreased spinal canal volume, which forces cerebrospinal fluid out of the canal through the nerve root sleeves. This can lead to foraminal stenosis and compression of the nerve root.

Eccentric contraction theory: muscle injury

Eccentric contraction of neck muscles forms the basis of the *eccentric contraction theory*.[28–30] Under physiological circumstances, muscle contraction results in shortening of the muscle's overall length (i.e. concentric contraction). However, during eccentric contraction, muscle length increases due to an external force of greater magnitude than the contraction force. Lengthening contractions result in greater injury potential and severity to the muscle than concentric contractions.[31–33] During automotive rear-impact collisions, the anterior neck muscles are subjected to eccentric contraction during the retraction and extension phases as the relative length between muscle origin and insertion increases due to the head moving posteriorly relative to the lower cervical spine and thorax. Posterior neck muscles are subjected to eccentric contraction during the rebound phase as the head moves anteriorly. This theory was advanced in a study in which 42 human volunteers were subjected to rear-impact events at changes in velocity of 4 and 8 km/h.[28] Electromyographic (EMG) activity of the superficial neck muscles was correlated to the timing of specific rear-impact events. Based on the observation that neck muscles initiate contraction rapidly during the impact event, it was hypothesised that injury may occur to the sternocleidomastoid muscles during the retraction phase (Fig 3.3). This hypothesis is consistent with earlier findings in which injuries to the sternocleidomastoid and longus colli muscles were identified in primates, as discussed earlier.[1] As muscle injuries generally heal quickly, they may not result in chronic symptoms, reported by a considerable number of patients with WAD.

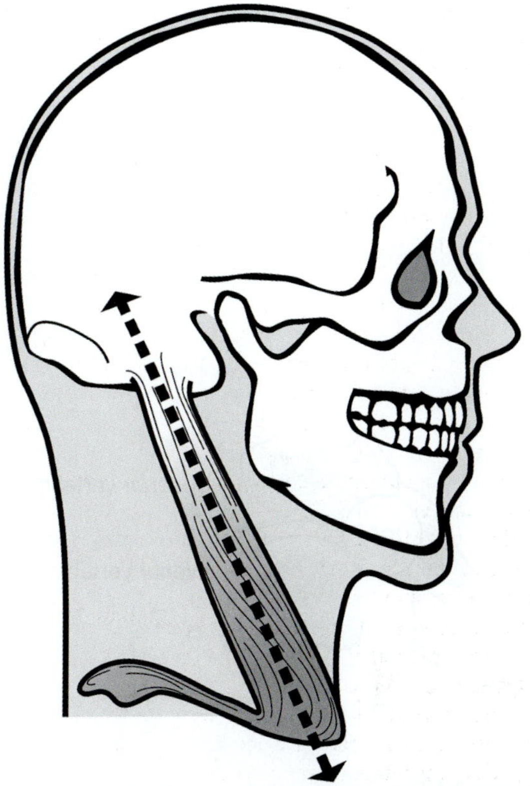

Figure 3.3 Retraction of the head relative to the thorax can lead to eccentric contraction of the anterior neck muscles.

Localised posterior joint motions: facet joint injury

Stretching of the facet joint capsule forms the basis of *the facet joint injury theory* (Fig 3.4). This theory is based on the recognition that lower cervical facet joints may be responsible for posterior neck pain, a common outcome of rear impact–induced trauma.[16, 22–24, 27, 34–39] Level-specific nerve blocks were used to determine the manifestation of facet-joint mediated pain.[40, 41] Other studies identified the presence of mechanoreceptors/nociceptors,[42–44] substance P,[45, 46] and calcitonin gene-related peptide (CGRP)[46] in facet joints. Mechanoreceptors may generate a noxious response during joint capsule stretch.[47] Substance P is responsible for the initiation of pain and CGRP is associated with the persistence of pain.[48] These anatomically and physiologically based studies have clearly identified the link between facet joint injury and neck pain. Concurrently, biomechanically based investigations were focused on defining the biomechanical role of facet joints in the injury mechanism.

Using whole-body, intact head–neck and isolated PMHS cervical spine specimens, increased and abnormal facet joint motions were reported during the retraction phase.[13, 49–51] Lower cervical facet joints demonstrated region-dependent kinematics: uniform shear motion along the joint, and distraction in ventral and compression in dorsal regions of the joint.[51] This pattern was significantly different from facet joint motions under physiological loads.[52] Excessive joint stretch can result in capsular ligament failure. The stretch theory is supported by whole-body PMHS tests that identified lower cervical joint capsule injuries following rear-impact loading.[12, 13, 53] Facet joint diastasis and capsular tear were observed in sagittal anatomical sections of the spine.[53] Using a rodent model, cervical facet joint stretch was found to be associated with allodynia.[54] Although pain symptoms were manifested in the forepaw, this study was the first to associate experimentally induced facet joint injury through joint capsule stretch with noxious response. The anatomical, physiological and biomechanical studies outlined in this section have identified a key role

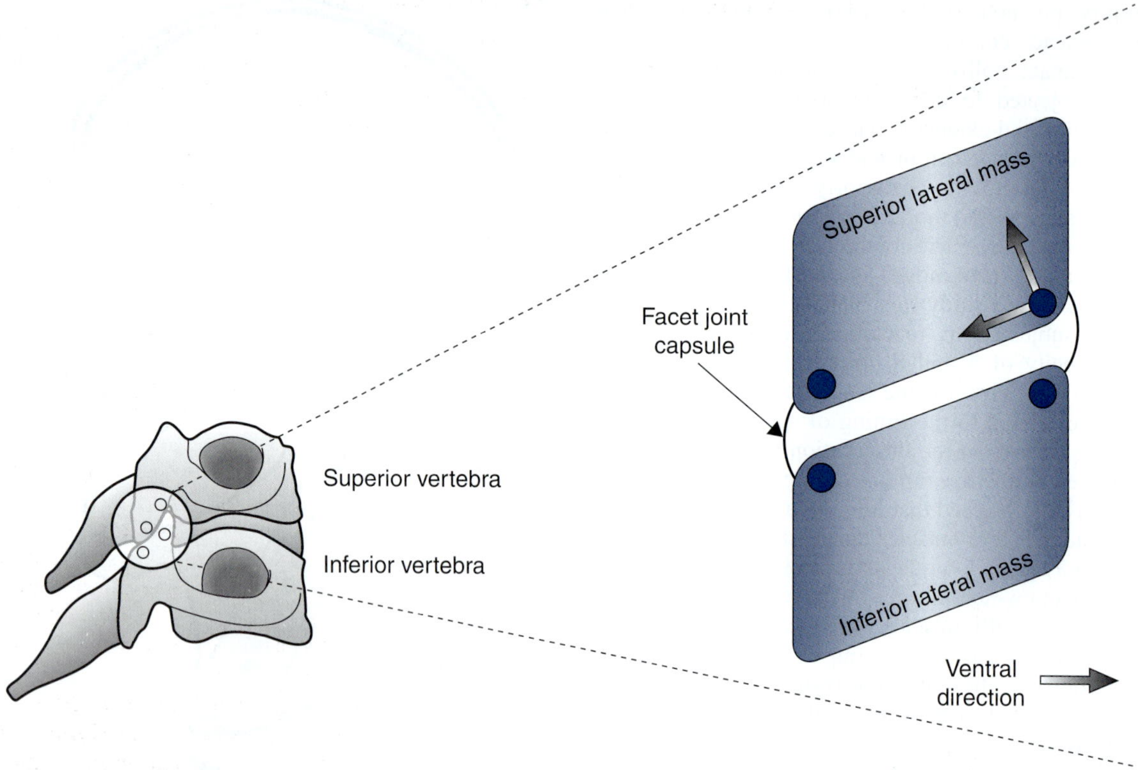

Figure 3.4 Relative ventral–dorsal displacement between adjacent lateral masses leads to tension of the facet joint capsule.

of lower cervical facet joints in the whiplash injury mechanism.

INJURY METRICS

Neck injury criterion

The *neck injury criterion* (*NIC*) is based on the spinal canal hydrodynamic theory described above.[55, 56] A mathematical model was used to predict the change in pressure within the canal at the C4 level due to changes in canal volume associated with retraction of the head relative to the thorax. Greatest pressure gradients were associated with the S-shaped curvature of the cervical spine. The mathematical equation used to predict these pressure gradients was:

$$NIC = a_{rel} \times L + v_{rel}^2 \qquad \text{(Eq. 3.1)}$$

where L is the length of the neck, and a_{rel} and v_{rel} are the relative horizontal acceleration and velocity changes between the C1 and T1 vertebrae during the retraction phase.

Because the head remains stationary during the retraction phase, a_{rel} and v_{rel} can be approximated as the acceleration and velocity of the torso, and a_{rel} and v_{rel} are derived from relative acceleration–time traces for the head and upper thorax in a dummy. Studies cited above proposed the tolerance limit at 15 m^2/s^2 for a neck length of 0.2 m. The *NIC* metric is valid when data are analysed from the time of rear impact initiation until head restraint contact.

Neck displacement criterion

The *neck displacement criterion* (*NDC*) assesses injury risk using overall head–neck rotation, anterior–posterior displacement, and vertical displacement of the occipital condyles relative to the T1 vertebra. It was developed to be used with human volunteers and dummies, including the BioRID P3 and Hybrid III,[57] and was based on data derived from human volunteer rear impact tests.[58, 59] Tolerance limits were based on linearised versions of ±2 standard deviation responses of human volunteers subjected to 9.3 km/h rear impacts. The reader is referred to the 2002 paper for the specific tolerance curves.[57]

Interaction criterion

The *interaction criterion* in its most basic form (N_{ij}) is based on the interaction of forces and moments on the cervical spine.[60] For rear impact, the criterion uses tensile force and extension moment, N_{te}. The tension intercept of 3300 N was derived from a study correlating injuries sustained in real world frontal collisions with the Hybrid III dummy responses under similar loading conditions.[61] The extension moment intercept of 57 Nm was approximated using PMHS sled test results.[62] The interaction equation is:

$$N_{te} = \frac{F_z}{F_{int}} + \frac{M_y}{M_{int}} \qquad \text{(Eq. 3.2)}$$

where F_z refers to the peak tensile force, M_y refers to the peak extension moment, and F_{int} and M_{int} refer to the respective intercepts. Values for force and moment intercepts have also been presented for different-sized occupants, such as the 95th percentile male and 5th percentile female.

Interaction criterion

The *shear-moment interaction criterion* was developed based on the argument that anterior–posterior shear forces rather than axial forces are important in cervical spine trauma induced during rear-impact collisions.[63] It also has the rationale that injuries induced in the rebound phase cannot be analysed using the *NIC* as it is only applicable to the retraction phase. Instead of the axial tensile force in the N_{te} formulation, shear force is used in the interaction equation for N_{km}:

$$N_{km} = \frac{F_x}{F_{int}} + \frac{M_y}{M_{int}} \qquad \text{(Eq. 3.3)}$$

where F_x refers to anterior–posterior shear force and M_y refers to upper neck sagittal bending moment.

Intercept limits to represent human tolerance for the Abbreviated Injury Scale (AIS) level 1 or minor injuries were: extension moment, 47.5 Nm; flexion moment, 88.1 Nm; and shear force, 845 N.[64, 65] Forty sled tests using the Hybrid III dummy with TRID neck and BioRID and production motor vehicle seats were used to validate the metric. The metric showed sensitivity to seat type, with seats equipped with a 'whiplash-protection system' resulting in lower values associated with lower injury risk.

Lower neck load

The *lower neck load* (*LNL*) criterion uses extension and lateral bending moments in conjunction with anterior–posterior and lateral shears, and tension–compression forces.[66] It is based on the assumption that the injury risk is largest with simultaneous action of forces and moments on the cervical spine. The *LNL* criterion compares lower neck moments and triaxial forces to critical intercept values:

$$LNT - index(t) = \left| \frac{\sqrt{My_{lower}(t)^2 + Mx_{lower}(t)^2}}{C_{moment}} \right| + \left| \frac{\sqrt{Fx_{lower}(t)^2 + Fy_{lower}(t)^2}}{C_{shear}} \right| + \left| \frac{Fz_{lower}(t)}{C_{tension}} \right| \qquad \text{(Eq. 3.4)}$$

where M_x and M_y refer to the lateral and flexion–extension bending moments, the C_{moment} intercept value is 15 Nm, F_x and F_y refer to anterior–posterior and lateral shear forces, the C_{shear} intercept value is 250 N, F_z refers to the axial force, and the $C_{tension}$ intercept value is 900 N.

A good correlation was found between the *LNL* determined from experiments using the Hybrid III and RID2 dummies and real-world rear impact whiplash claims data.[66] However, the response/efficacy of the BioRID dummy with the *LNL* criterion was not investigated due to a lack of a lower neck load cell in that dummy at the time of testing.

Lower neck shear force

The *lower neck shear force criterion* is based on the theory that posterior–anterior shear force at the base of the cervical spine drives the retraction phase in rear-impact collisions.[67] Other studies have indirectly supported the theory. In a study conducted to determine the effect of occupant seating posture on upper and lower neck loads, it was concluded that 'a lower neck rear impact injury criterion should be investigated'.[68] Another study investigating the influence of seating position and incorporating the BioRID concluded that 'the directly measured lower neck shear alone may be the most reliable predictor of neck injury'.[69] A third study correlating field data with seat-specific rear impact performance determined from sled tests indicated that 'real accident data correlated best with lower neck shear force for the RID3D, with R-squared values of 0.79 and 0.80 for the standard and vehicle-specific pulses'.[70]

Tolerance limits were developed by correlating lower neck loads with facet joint motions using intact head–neck PMHS specimens.[67] Lower neck shear forces had a higher correlation with facet joint motions than bending moment or axial force. The magnitude of shear force required for subcatastrophic ligamentous failure was estimated by extrapolating to the limit of facet joint motion based on the correlation slope. The tolerance limit was found to be 670 N for males and 530 N for females. These limits compared well with lower neck shear forces computed from intact PMHS sled tests, in which posterior column injuries were identified in four out of five specimens.[12, 53, 71] Shear force tolerance limits specified above would have predicted the presence or absence of posterior column injury in four out of five specimens.[72]

INFLUENCING FACTORS FOR INJURY POTENTIAL

Occupant-related factors

Gender

Clinical and epidemiological studies have shown that females are more susceptible to whiplash trauma than males.[15, 22, 24, 26, 27, 37, 39, 73–76] Females also have increased susceptibility for chronic symptoms once injured.[16, 22, 24, 73] Higher injury rates may be attributed to biomechanical, psychological, sociological or anthropometric considerations. While a definitive explanation for the gender discrepancy in whiplash injuries has been elusive, biomechanical studies discussed below have provided insight into this issue.

Two biomechanical studies exposing human volunteers to simulated rear impacts demonstrated increased overall head–neck motions in females.[77, 78] Overall, head–neck motions can be associated with localised segmental spinal kinematics. Two studies have directly measured spinal kinematics in male and female PMHS head–neck complexes. Five male and five female specimens were exposed to identical rear impacts. Segmental motions in females were greater than in males at all subaxial levels during the retraction phase, resulting in a more pronounced S-shaped curvature.[79] Shear and distraction facet joint motions in the lower cervical spine were also greater in females.[51] Greater localised and segmental motions in females identified in those studies are associated with greater soft tissue distortion and an increased injury risk.

To delineate the likely cause for increased spinal motions in females, C2–C7 vertebral geometry was analysed using computed tomography (CT) scans from 51 young and healthy male and female volunteers.[80, 81] Volunteers were size-matched based on sitting height or head circumference. Geometrical measures, including vertebral body depth and width, inter-facet width and horizontal distance from the anterior edge of the intervertebral disc to the posterior edge of the facet joints (disc-facet depth), were obtained. Additionally, the segmental support area was computed as half the disc-facet depth multiplied by inter-facet width. All geometrical measures were greater in males for both groups. Vertebral width and disc-facet depth were significantly greater in males for both groups. The support area was greater in males (significant in the circumference-matched group), indicating a more stable intervertebral coupling. Results of decreased linear and areal cervical dimensions leading to decreased cervical column stability may partially explain increased whiplash injury rates in females. Similar findings were reported in another study.[82]

Another study identified significantly greater cross-sectional areas in three superficial neck muscles in males than in females.[83] Because cross-sectional area is directly associated with maximum contractile force,[84] increased muscle areas account for increased ability to stabilise the head–neck complex during static and dynamic loading. It is generally accepted that deep neck muscles are responsible for static stabilisation, whereas superficial muscles control movement and dynamically stabilise the head–neck complex. Therefore, significantly greater cross-sectional areas in males result in a greater ability to stabilise the head–neck complex during dynamic events. Male centroid radii were also significantly longer in all the three investigated superficial muscles. As muscle moment-generating capacity is linearly proportional to the distance of the centroid from the centre of rotation, greater radii in males results in greater moment-generating capacity, greater ability to stabilise the head–neck complex and a decreased likelihood of longitudinal dysfunction than in females. Greater moment-generating capacity in males was also directly measured in human volunteers.[85]

Awareness

Clinical studies have supported the assertion that if an occupant is aware of the impending impact, some preventive action can be taken to minimise injury risk. One study reported that awareness of the impact was associated with a lower frequency of multiple symptoms and intensity of pain.[38] Another study reported that occupants who were not prepared for the impact had poorer recovery 12 weeks following the initial injury.[86] From a biomechanical perspective, pre-tension of neck muscles in occupants who were aware of the impending impact can stiffen the head–neck complex and decrease retraction phase kinematics. Neck muscle contraction has been cited as a possible protective mechanism during automotive rear-impact collisions.[87] A computational study supported this assertion by demonstrating decreased spinal kinematics with shorter neck muscle reaction times.[88] Another study using the same model demonstrated considerably decreased head–neck motions and facet-joint ligament distractions when neck muscles were contracted prior to impact.[89] Similar findings of decreased head–neck motions in aware subjects were demonstrated in volunteers exposed to very low severity simulated rear impacts.[90]

Age

Although not historically associated with higher injury risk in automotive rear-impact collisions, older age was recently identified as a significant factor in injury likelihood and chronicity. Since 2003, six articles were published associating older age with less favourable outcomes. The most recent study of 170 patients showed that older age has a significant correlation with higher pain scores and neck disability index.[91] A study of 80 patients with neck pain following impact reported that age is a significant predictor of persistent moderate-to-severe symptoms.[92] Another study found that patients older than 60 years reported at one year follow-up that their condition was slightly or significantly impaired due to the initial injury.[93] It was reported that older age was independently associated with longer recovery time.[26] Although subjective, these studies demonstrate a decreased quality of life in older occupants following relatively low severity injuries. A study of 1147 occupants in rear-impact collisions found that age independently predicts acute whiplash injuries.[75] Therefore, in addition to longer recovery times and greater morbidity, injury susceptibility may also be greater in older occupants.

Impact- and vehicle-related factors

Head restraint positioning

Head restraints were mandated in the United States in 1969 for passenger vehicles. They have reduced neck injury risk by less than 20%.[94–96] Incorrect adjustment of restraint position may account for the ineffectiveness. As many as 78% of head restraints are positioned incorrectly.[97–99] An experimental study determined that the head strikes the restraint towards the end of the retraction phase or at the beginning of the extension phase.[100] Peak facet-joint capsular strains were shown to occur prior to head restraint contact.[101] Reducing backset (horizontal head to head restraint distance) reduces head retraction and decreases injury risk. Adding 50 mm of padding to a head restraint reduced head retraction and head acceleration in volunteer tests.[102] Backset minimisation is a focus of safety engineers, evidenced by the recent development of ‘active’ head restraints, designed to dynamically reduce backset.[103–105] Motor vehicles providing decreased backset are rated higher for occupant protection.[106–108]

Impact velocity

A majority of whiplash injuries occur at velocity changes between 3 and 17 km/h.[39, 109] However, a review of human volunteer tests revealed that vehicle velocity changes less than 9 km/h are unlikely to result in significant injury.[102] Impact severity is dependent upon vehicle- and crash-related factors, such as relative velocity and seat properties. Increasing thoracic change in velocity leads to increased loading on the head–neck complex, resulting in greater relative motions between vertebrae and increased soft tissue distortion. Although greater impact velocities are generally associated with greater injury risk, an exact injury threshold has not been defined as other occupant-, vehicle- and impact-related factors may mask its effect.

Seat or occupant positioning

More vertically oriented seat or occupant positions are generally thought to increase injury risk. One study was conducted to determine the effect of occupant seating posture on neck loads.[68] Tests were conducted using the Hybrid III dummy and stock automotive seats from three different vehicles. The dummy was positioned in the normal seated position or with the torso pitched forwards such that the back of the head was 20 cm from the head restraint. Lower neck shear forces increased between 11% and 196% for tests with the occupant pitched forward, increasing injury risk in that position. Other studies incorporating full-body PMHSs also demonstrated higher injury risks for occupants seated with more vertical seatback orientations.[13, 110]

Rotated head positions may increase stretch in soft tissues and lead to greater injury risk. Clinical studies have demonstrated increased injury risk for occupants with an axially rotated head at the time of impact.[22, 38, 111] Biomechanical studies using whole PMHS cervical spine specimens or human volunteers subjected to simulated rear impacts have shown an increased risk of ganglion compression, and vertebral artery or sternocleidomastoid muscle injury when the head is rotated at the time of impact.[112–114]

SUMMARY

Whiplash injuries continue to be a burden to society, in terms of cost and human suffering. As discussed, albeit not comprehensively because of the complexity in the accurate diagnoses of the structures involved in the dysfunction at the time of the impact event, various injury theories have been proposed based on biomechanical principles. Some theories have formed a basis for the explanation of acute symptoms, while others have focused on long-term problems, the latter being critical. Continued technological advancements in clinical and experimental areas are required to determine the most optimal explanation for injury causation scenarios from a biological perspective, as both structural and psychological factors are involved in the trauma. Current biomechanical knowledge offers a fundamental platform to advance research to resolve structural issues that may be the principal cause of chronic symptoms from the rear impact event.

ACKNOWLEDGMENTS

This work was funded in part by Advancing a Healthier Wisconsin, the Medical College of Wisconsin Injury Research Center Seed Project Program, and the Department of Veterans Affairs Medical Research. The authors wish to acknowledge the contribution of Kim Chapman from the Zablocki Veterans Affairs Medical Media.

References

1. Macnab I. Acceleration injuries of the cervical spine. *J Bone Joint Surg* 1964;46A(8):1797–800.
2. Macnab I. The "whiplash syndrome". *Orthop Clin North Am* 1971;2(2):389–403.
3. Mertz HJ & Patrick LM. Investigation of the kinematics and kinetics of whiplash. In: Proceedings of the 11th Stapp Car Crash Conference, Anaheim, CA, 1967: pp 267–317.
4. Severy DM, Mathewson JH, Bechtol CO. Controlled automobile rear-end collisions, an investigation of related engineering and medical phenomena. *Can Serv Med J* 1955;11:727–59.
5. Davis SJ, Teresi LM, Bradley WG, et al. Cervical spine hyperextension injuries: MR findings. *Radiology* 1991;180(1):245–51.
6. Goldberg AC, Rothfus WE, Deeb ZL, et al. Hyperextension injuries of the cervical spine. *Skeletal Radiol* 1989;18:283–8.
7. Harris W, Hamblen D, Ojemann R. Traumatic disruption of cervical intervertebral disc from hyperextension injury. *Clin Orthop* 1968;60:163–7.
8. Johnson G. Hyperextension soft tissue injuries of the cervical spine – a review. *J Accid Emerg Med* 1996;13:3–8.
9. Kinoshita H. Pathology of hyperextension injuries of the cervical spine. *Paraplegia* 1994;32:367–74.
10. Marar BC. Hyperextension injuries of the cervical spine. *J Bone Joint Surg* 1974;56A(8):1655–62.
11. Shea M, Wittenberg RH, Edwards WT, et al. In vitro hyperextension injuries in the human cadaveric cervical spine. *J Orthop Res* 1992;10:911–16.
12. Yoganandan N, Pintar FA, Stemper BD, et al. Biomechanics of human occupants in simulated rear crashes: documentation of neck injuries and comparison of injury criteria. *Stapp Car Crash J* 2000;44:189–204.
13. Deng B, Begeman PC, Yang KY, et al. Kinematics of human cadaver cervical spine during low speed rear-end impacts. *Stapp Car Crash J* 2000;44:171–88.
14. Pettersson K, Hildingsson C, Toolanen G, et al. Disc pathology after whiplash injury. A prospective magnetic resonance imaging and clinical investigation. *Spine* 1997;22(3):283–7; discussion 8.
15. Jonsson H, Jr, Cesarini K, Sahlstedt B, et al. Findings and outcome in whiplash-type neck distortions. *Spine* 1994;19(24):2733–43.
16. Hohl M. Soft tissue injuries of the neck in automobile accidents: factors influencing prognosis. *J Bone Joint Surg* 1974;56A:1675–82.
17. Stemper BD, Yoganandan N, Pintar FA, et al. Anterior longitudinal ligament injuries in whiplash may lead to cervical instability. *Med Eng Physics* 2006;28(6):515–24.
18. Aldman B. An analytical approach to the impact biomechanics of head and neck injury. In: 30th Annual Proceedings of the American Association for Automotive Medicine, Montreal, Quebec, 1986: pp 439–54.
19. Svensson MY, Aldman B, Hansson HA, et al. Pressure effects in the spinal canal during whiplash extension motion: a possible cause of injury to the cervical spinal ganglia. In: Proceedings of the International IRCOBI Conference on the Biomechanics of Impact, Eindhoven, The Netherlands, 1993: pp 189–200.

20. Breig A. Adverse mechanical tension in the central nervous system. Stockholm: Almqvist & Wiksell Int.; 1978.
21. Hanson MR, Galvez N. Neurologic evaluation of the cervical spine. In: Clark CR, ed. The cervical spine. 4th edn. Philadelphia, PA: Lippincott Williams & Wilkins; 2005: pp 166–74.
22. Radanov BP, Sturzenegger M, Di Stefano G. Long-term outcome after whiplash injury. A 2-year follow-up considering features of injury mechanism and somatic, radiologic, and psychosocial findings. *Medicine* 1995;74(5):281–97.
23. Norris SH & Watt I. The prognosis of neck injuries resulting from rear-end vehicle collisions. *J Bone Joint Surg* 1983 Nov;65(5):608–11.
24. Cassidy JD, Carroll LJ, Côté P, et al. Effect of eliminating compensation for pain and suffering on the outcome of insurance claims for whiplash injury. *N Engl J Med* 2000;342(16):1179–86.
25. Spitzer WO, Skovron ML, Salmi LR, et al. Scientific monograph of the Quebec Task Force on Whiplash-Associated Disorders: redefining "whiplash" and its management. *Spine* 1995;20(8 Suppl):1S–73S.
26. Suissa S. Risk factors of poor prognosis after whiplash injury. *Pain Res Manage* 2003;8(2):69–75.
27. Hildingsson C, Toolanen G. Outcome after soft-tissue injury of the cervical spine. A prospective study of 93 car-accident victims. *Acta Orthop Scand* 1990;61(4):357–9.
28. Brault J, Siegmund G, Wheeler J. Cervical muscle response during whiplash: evidence of a lengthening muscle contraction. *Clin Biomech* 2000;15(6): 426–35.
29. Magnusson ML, Pope MH, Hasselquist L, et al. Cervical electromyographic activity during low-speed rear impact. *Eur Spine J* 1999;8(2):118–25.
30. Tencer AF, Mirza S, Bensel K. The response of human volunteers to rear-end impacts: the effect of head restraint properties. *Spine* 2001;26(22): 2432–40; discussion 41–2.
31. McCully KK & Faulkner JA. Injury to skeletal muscle fibers of mice following lengthening contractions. *J Appl Physiol* 1985;59(1):119–26.
32. Ogilvie RW, Armstrong RB, Baird KE, et al. Lesions in the rat soleus muscle following eccentrically biased exercise. *Am J Anatomy* 1988;182(4): 335–46.
33. Newham DJ, Mills KR, Quigley BM, et al. Pain and fatigue after concentric and eccentric muscle contractions. *Clin Sci (Lond.)* 1983;64(1):55–62.
34. Barnsley L, Lord SM, Wallis BJ, et al. The prevalence of chronic cervical zygapophyseal joint pain after whiplash. *Spine* 1995;20(1):20–6.
35. Bogduk N, Marsland A. The cervical zygapophysial joints as a source of neck pain. *Spine* 1988;13(6): 610–17.
36. Karlsborg M, Smed A, Jespersen H, et al. A prospective study of 39 patients with whiplash injury. *Acta Neurol Scand* 1997;95:65–72.
37. Mayou R, Bryant B. Outcome of 'whiplash' neck injury. *Injury* 1996;27(9):617–23.
38. Sturzenegger M, DiStefano G, Radanov BP, et al. Presenting symptoms and signs after whiplash injury: the influence of accident mechanisms. *Neurology* 1994;44:688–93.
39. Temming J, Zobel R. Neck distortion injuries in road traffic crashes (Analysis of the Volkwagen database). In: Yoganandan N, Pintar F, eds. Frontiers in whiplash trauma: clinical & biomechanical. The Netherlands: IOS Press; 2000: pp 118–33.
40. Aprill C, Dwyer A, Bogduk N. Cervical zygapophyseal joint pain patterns II: a clinical evaluation. *Spine* 1990;15(6):458–61.
41. Dwyer A, Aprill C, Bogduk N. Cervical zygapophysial joint pain patterns I: a study in normal volunteers. *Spine* 1990;15(6):453–7.
42. McLain RF. Mechanoreceptor endings in human cervical facet joints. *Spine* 1994;19(5):495–501.
43. Ohtori S, Takahashi K, Chiba T, et al. Sensory innervation of the cervical facet joints in rats. *Spine* 2001;26(2):147–50.
44. Suseki K, Takahashi Y, Takahashi K, et al. Innervation of the lumbar facet joints. *Spine* 1997;22(5):477–85.
45. Beaman DN, Graziano GP, Glover RA, et al. Substance P innervation of lumbar spine facet joints. *Spine* 1993;18(8):1044–9.
46. Kallakuri S, Singh A, Chen C, et al. Demonstration of substance P, calcitonin gene-related peptide, and protein gene product 9.5 containing nerve fibers in human cervical facet joint capsules. *Spine* 2004;29(11):1182–6.
47. Cavanaugh JM. Neurophysiology and neuroanatomy of neck pain. In: Yoganandan N, Pintar F, eds. Frontiers in whiplash trauma: clinical & biomechanical. The Netherlands: IOS Press; 2000: pp 79–98.
48. Rothman SM, Kreider RA, Winkelstein BA. Spinal neuropeptide responses in persistent and transient pain following cervical nerve root injury. *Spine* 2005;30(22):2491–6.
49. Cusick JF, Pintar FA, Yoganandan N. Whiplash syndrome: kinematic factors influencing pain patterns. *Spine* 2001;26(11):1252–8.
50. Pearson AM, Ivancic PC, Ito S, et al. Facet joint kinematics and injury mechanisms during simulated whiplash. *Spine* 2004;29(4):390–7.

51. Stemper BD, Yoganandan N, Pintar FA. Gender- and region-dependent local facet joint kinematics in rear impact: implications in whiplash injury. *Spine* 2004;29(16):1764–71.
52. Stemper BD, Yoganandan N, Gennarelli TA, et al. Localized cervical facet joint kinematics under physiological and whiplash loading. *J Neurosurg Spine* 2005;3:471–6.
53. Yoganandan N, Cusick JF, Pintar FA, et al. Whiplash injury determination with conventional spine imaging and cryomicrotomy. *Spine* 2001;26(22):2443–8.
54. Lee KE, Thinnes JH, Gokhin DS, et al. A novel rodent neck pain model of facet-mediated behavioral hypersensitivity: implications for persistent pain and whiplash injury. *J Neurosci Methods* 2004;137(2): 151–9.
55. Bostrom O, Svensson MY, Aldman B, et al. A new neck injury criterion candidate based on injury findings in the cervical spinal ganglia after experimental neck extension trauma. In: Proceedings of the International IRCOBI Conference on the Biomechanics of Impact, Dublin, Ireland, 1996: pp 123–36.
56. Bostrom O, Fredriksson R, Haland Y, et al. Comparison of car seats in low speed rear-end impacts using the BioRID dummy and the new neck injury criterion (NIC). *Accid Anal Prev* 2000;32(2):321–8.
57. Viano DC, Davidsson J. Neck displacements of volunteers, BioRID P3 and Hybrid III in rear impacts: implications to whiplash assessment by a Neck Displacement Criterion (NDC). *Traffic Inj Prev* 2002;3:105–16.
58. Ono K, Inami S, Kaneoka K, et al. Relationship between localized spine deformation and cervical vertebral motions for low speed rear impacts using human volunteers. In: Proceedings of the International IRCOBI Conference on the Biomechanics of Impact, Barcelona, Spain, 1999: pp 149–64.
59. Ono K, Kaneoka K, Inami S. Influence of seat properties on human cervical vertebral motion and head/neck/torso kinematics during rear-end impacts. In: Proceedings of the International IRCOBI Conference on the Biomechanics of Impact, Goteborg, Sweden, 1998: pp 339–56.
60. Kleinberger M, Sun E, Eppinger R, et al. Development of improved injury criteria for the assessment of advanced automotive restraint systems. Washington, DC: National Highway Traffic Safety Administration (NHTSA), 1998.
61. Nyquist GW, Begman PC, King AI, et al. Correlation of field injuries and GM hybrid III dummy responses for lap-shoulder belt restraint. *J Biomech Eng* 1980;102(2):103–9.
62. Mertz HJ & Patrick LM. Strength and response of the human neck. In: Proceedings of the Stapp Car Crash Conference, San Diego, CA, 1971.
63. Schmitt KU, Muser MH, Walz FH, et al. Nkm—a proposal for a neck protection criterion for low-speed rear-end impacts. *Traffic Inj Prev* 2002;3:117–26.
64. Goldsmith W, Ommaya AK. Head and neck injury criteria and tolerance levels. In: Aldman B, Chapon A, eds. The biomechanics of impact trauma. Amsterdam: Elsevier Science Publishers; 1984: pp 149–87.
65. Mertz H, Patrick L. Strength and response of the human neck. In: Backaitis S, ed. Biomechanics of impact injury and injury tolerance of the head-neck complex. Society of Automotive Engineers (SAE). 1993: pp 821–46.
66. Heitplatz F, Sferco R, Fay P, et al. An evaluation of existing and proposed injury criteria with various dummies to determine their ability to predict the levels of soft tissue neck injury seen in real world accidents. In: Proceedings of the 18th Technical Conference on the Enhanced Safety of Vehicles, Nagoya, Japan, 2003: pp 1–7.
67. Stemper BD, Yoganandan N, Gennarelli TA, Pintar FA. Toward a lower neck rear impact injury criterion – correlation of lower neck loads with spinal kinematics. Proceedings of the International IRCOBI Conference on the Biomechanics of Impact, Maastricht, The Netherlands, September 19–21, 2007, pp 249–60.
68. Benson BR, Smith GC, Kent RW, et al. Effect of seat stiffness in out-of-position occupant response in rear-end collisions. In: Proceedings of the 35th Stapp Car Crash Conference, San Diego, CA, 1996: pp 331–44.
69. Latchford J, Chirwa EC, Mao M. The relationship of seat backrest angle and neck injury in low-velocity rear impacts. *J Automobile Eng* 2005;219:1293–302.
70. Cappon H, Hell W, Hoschopf H, et al. Correlation of accident statistics to whiplash performance parameters using the RID3D and BioRID dummy. In: Proceedings of the International IRCOBI Conference on the Biomechanics of Impact, Prague, Czech Republic, 2005: pp 229–43.
71. Philippens M, Wismans J, Cappon J, et al. Whole body kinematics using post mortem human subjects in experimental rear impact. In: Proceedings of the International IRCOBI Conference on the Biomechanics of Impact, Montpelier, France, 2000: pp 363–78.
72. Stemper BD, Storvik SG. Lower neck shear forces in automotive rear impacts. *Traffic Inj Prev* 2010;11(3):300–8.
73. Guez M, Hildingsson C, Nilsson M, et al. The prevalence of neck pain: a population-based study from northern Sweden. *Acta Orthop Scand* 2002;73(4):455–9.

74. Côté P, Hogg-Johnson S, Cassidy JD, et al. Initial patterns of clinical care and recovery from whiplash injuries: a population-based cohort study. *Arch Int Med* 2005;165(19):2257–63.
75. Pobereskin LH. Whiplash following rear end collisions: a prospective cohort study. *J Neurol Neurosurg Psychiatry* 2005;76(8):1146–51.
76. Sterner Y, Toolanen G, Gerdle B, Hildingsson C. The incidence of whiplash trauma and the effects of different factors on recovery. *J Spinal Disord Tech* 2003;16(2):195–9.
77. Siegmund GP, King DJ, Lawrence JM, et al. Head/neck kinematic response of human subjects in low-speed rear-end collisions. In: Proceedings of the 41st Stapp Car Crash Conference, Lake Buena Vista, FL, 1997: pp 357–85.
78. van den Kroonenberg A, Philippens M, Cappon H, et al. Human head-neck response during low-speed rear end impacts. In: Proceedings of the 42nd Stapp Car Crash Conference, Tempe, AZ, 1998: pp 207–21.
79. Stemper BD, Yoganandan N, Pintar FA. Gender dependent cervical spine segmental kinematics during whiplash. *J Biomech* 2003;36(9):1281–9.
80. Stemper BD, Derosia JJ, Yoganandan N, et al. Gender dependent cervical spine anatomical differences in size-matched volunteers. *Biomed Sci Instrum* 2009;45:149–54.
81. Stemper BD, Yoganandan N, Pintar FA, et al. Anatomical gender differences in cervical vertebrae of size-matched volunteers. *Spine* 2008;33(2): E44–9.
82. Vasavada AN, Danaraj J, Siegmund GP. Head and neck anthropometry, vertebral geometry and neck strength in height-matched men and women. *J Biomech* 2008;41(1):114–21.
83. Stemper BD, Yoganandan N, Baisden JL, et al. Biomechanical implications of gender-dependent muscle locations. In: Proceedings of the ASME 2008 Summer Bioengineering Conference, Marco Island, FL, 2008.
84. Conley MS, Stone MH, Nimmons M, et al. Specificity of resistance training responses in neck muscle size and strength. *Eur J Applied Physiol Occup Physiol* 1997;75(5):443–8.
85. Vasavada AN, Li S, Delp SL. Three-dimensional isometric strength of neck muscles in humans. *Spine* 2001;26(17):1904–9.
86. Hendriks EJ, Scholten-Peeters GG, van der Windt DA, et al. Prognostic factors for poor recovery in acute whiplash patients. *Pain* 2005;114(3):408–16.
87. Awerbuch MS. Whiplash in Australia: illness or injury? *Med J Aust* 1992;157(7):502.
88. Stemper BD, Yoganandan N, Rao RD, et al. Reflex muscle contraction in the unaware occupant in whiplash injury. *Spine* 2005;30(24):2794–8; discussion 9.
89. Stemper BD, Yoganandan N, Cusick JF, et al. Stabilizing effect of precontracted neck musculature in whiplash. *Spine* 2006;31(20):E733–8.
90. Siegmund GP, Sanderson DJ, Myers BS, et al. Awareness affects the response of human subjects exposed to a single whiplash-like perturbation. *Spine* 2003;28(7):671–9.
91. Crouch R, Whitewick R, Clancy M, et al. Whiplash associated disorder: incidence and natural history over the first month for patients presenting to a UK emergency department. *Emerg Med J* 2006;23:114–18.
92. Sterling M, Jull G, Vicenzino B, et al. Physical and psychological factors predict outcome following whiplash injury. *Pain* 2005;114:1418.
93. Miettinen T, Airaksinen O, Lindgren KA, Leino E. Whiplash injuries in Finland—the possibility of some sociodemographic and psychosocial factors to predict the outcome after one year. *Disabil Rehabil* 2004;26(23):1367–72.
94. Kahane C. An evaluation of head restraints—federal motor vehicle safety standard 202. Springfield, VA: National Technical Information Service, NHTSA1982. Report no.: DOT HS-806 108.
95. O'Neill B, Haddon W, Kelley A, et al. Automobile head restraints: frequency of neck injuries insurance claims in relation to the presence of head restraints. *Am J Pub Health* 1972;62(3):569–73.
96. States JD, Balcerak JC, Williams JS. Injury frequency and head restraint effectiveness in rear-end impact accidents. In: Proceedings of the 16th Stapp Car Crash Conference, New York, NY, 1972: pp 228–57.
97. Lubin S, Sehmer J. Are automobile head restraints used effectively? *Can Fam Physician* 1993;39: 1584–8.
98. Minton R, Murray P, Stephenson W, et al. Whiplash—are current head restraints doing their job? *Accid Anal Prev* 2000;32:177–85.
99. Young AL, Ragel BT, Su E, et al. Assessing automobile head restraint positioning in Portland, Oregon. *Inj Prev* 2005;11(2):97–101.
100. Davidsson J, Deutscher C, Hell W, et al. Human volunteer kinematics in rear-end sled collisions. In: Proceedings of the International IRCOBI Conference on the Biomechanics of Impact, Goteborg, Sweden, 1998: pp 289–301.
101. Stemper BD, Yoganandan N, Pintar FA. Effect of head restraint backset on head-neck kinematics in whiplash. *Accid Anal Prev* 2006;38(2):317–23.

102. Szabo TJ & Welcher JB. Human subject kinematics and electromyographic activity during low speed rear impacts. In: Proceedings of the 40th Stapp Car Crash Conference, Albuquerque, NM, 1996: pp 295–315.
103. Tencer AF, Mirza SK, Bensel K. The response of human volunteers to rear-end impacts: the effect of head restraint properties. *Spine* 2001;26(22):2432–42.
104. Viano DC, Olsen S. The effectiveness of active head restraint in preventing whiplash. *J Trauma* 2001;51(5):959–69.
105. Wiklund K, Larsson H. Saab active head restraint (SAHR)—seat design to reduce the risk of neck injuries in rear impacts. Washington, DC: Society of Automotive Engineers, 1998. SAE paper no. 980297.
106. Estep CR, Lund AK, Vann DT. Measurement and evaluation of head restraints in 1995 vehicles. Arlington, VA: Insurance Institute for Highway Safety, 1995.
107. Morris CR, Lund AK, Vann DT. Measurement and evaluation of head restraints in 1997 vehicles. Arlington, VA: Insurance Institute for Highway Safety, 1998.
108. O'Neill B. Protection against neck injury in rear crashes. Status report. *Insurance Institute for Highway Safety* 2004;39(10).
109. Hell W & Langwieder K. Reported soft tissue neck injuries after rear-end car collisions. In: Proceedings of the International IRCOBI Conference on the Biomechanics of Impact, Goteborg, Sweden, 1998: pp 261–74.
110. Sundararajan S, Prasad P, Demetropoulos CK, et al. Effect of head-neck position on cervical facet stretch of post mortem human subjects during low speed rear end impacts. *Stapp Car Crash J* 2004;48: 331–72.
111. Jakobsson L, Isaksson-Hellman I, Lindman M. WHIPS (Volvo cars' Whiplash Protection System)—the development and real-world performance. *Traffic Inj Prev* 2008;9(6):600–5.
112. Ivancic PC, Ito S, Tominaga Y, et al. Effect of rotated head posture on dynamic vertebral artery elongation during simulated rear impact. *Clin Biomechanics* 2006;21(3):213–20.
113. Kumar S, Ferrari R, Narayan Y. The effect of trunk flexion in healthy volunteers in rear whiplash-type impacts. *Spine* 2005;30(15):1742–9.
114. Tominaga Y, Maak TG, Ivancic PC, et al. Head-turned rear impact causing dynamic cervical intervertebral foramen narrowing: implications for ganglion and nerve root injury. *J Neurosurg Spine* 2006;4(5):380–7.

CHAPTER 4
The evidence for pathoanatomical lesions

James Elliott

INTRODUCTION

There is no paucity of available information related to whiplash injury resulting from a motor vehicle crash (MVC), with well over 10,000 publications on diagnosis alone. Accurate estimates of recovery rates following whiplash have been inconsistent, likely due to the variety of outcome measures used and amount of time between follow-up.[1–3] For instance, Barnsley and colleagues originally put forth evidence to suggest that up to 40% of people with whiplash injury will, for unknown reasons, transition from acute to persistent pain.[4] However, a recent review estimates that approximately 50% of people continue to report symptoms in the long term.[5] Despite discrepancies in the reported prevalence rates for long-term symptoms, some patients, females more so than males,[6] will present acutely with a markedly complex clinical picture and a myriad of symptoms that can challenge even the most astute clinician. It is these patients who continue to report long-term symptoms.[7]

The cardinal feature of the acute and chronic condition is neck pain but can also include a variety of signs and symptoms, such as dizziness, visual and auditory disturbances, temporomandibular joint pain, photophobia, dysphonia, dysphagia, dysarthria, fatigue, cognitive difficulties (e.g. concentration and memory loss), anxiety, insomnia and even depression.[8–14] Such variability underpins the challenge of building a distinct pathoanatomical diagnosis in most cases.

Whiplash injuries from MVC are defined by energy transfer to the cervical spine resulting from acceleration–deceleration forces that typically occur with rear-end (but also frontal and side) impact MVCs (Chapter 3). Such forces can, in some cases, lead to excessive non-physiological stresses on the cervical spine,[15–17] and could result in injury to many disparate regional tissues.

Undoubtedly, the situation would benefit if there were quantitative radiological markers of the disorder; however, consistent observations of a salient structural lesion or lesions (that can be differentiated from normal variants in healthy individuals) with advanced imaging modalities in both the acute and persistent stages remains inconclusive.[18–21]

For the most part, investigations using advanced imaging (e.g. radiographic X-ray, computed tomography [CT] and magnetic resonance imaging [MRI]) have focused on various anatomical structures (e.g. osseoligamentous tissue, intervertebral discs, neural and vascular structures, and zygapophyseal [facet] joints).[18–30] However, given the infrequency of abnormalities detected, the lack of prognostic value, inaccessibility of 'clinic friendly' measures and the high cost of advanced imaging procedures, support for an evidence-based pathoanatomical model has not, in most cases, been justified.[19, 24, 25, 27, 28, 30–32] As a result, there continues to be long-standing debate about whether persistent pain is attributable to physical pathology or to mechanisms such as deliberate exaggeration and simulated gain.[33–35]

The aim of this chapter is to briefly describe the pathomechanics of the whiplash event, as well as summarise the available literature regarding the pathoanatomical features of acute and persistent whiplash-related pain and disability. The chapter is broken into a number of sections highlighting the proposed anatomical site(s) of injury (e.g. zygapophyseal joints, spinal ligaments, intervertebral discs, neural and vascular structures, and cervical muscles).[36–38]

PATHOMECHANICS OF WHIPLASH INJURY

Original observations of the whiplash mechanism detailed a rapid hyperextension of the cervical spine, which created large angular displacements in the sagittal plane.[40] On the contrary, current best evidence acknowledges that injury likely emerges from the inertial response of the body to the forces delivered to it, in which the head–neck complex undergoes displacement without being exposed to direct impact (e.g. the 'S-shaped' curve).[15, 16] The consequences of either a rear-end or frontal impact could profoundly affect the cervical spine and may injure any number of anatomical tissues, such as the intervertebral discs,[40] facet capsule,[41–44] the anterior–posterior longitudinal, supra- and interspinous ligaments,[45–47] and/or the ligamentum flavum.[47]

The preceding provides a brief overview of the pathomechanical features of the whiplash injury. For a more detailed description, the reader is referred to Chapter 3, which details the mechanisms of injury. The following sections highlight the available evidence regarding a pathoanatomical lesion, or set of lesions, in cases of acute and persistent whiplash, and how these injured anatomical sites may be responsible for the generation and maintenance of whiplash-related pain and disability.

PATHOLOGICAL LESIONS IN WHIPLASH INJURY

In a seminal study, Taylor et al. investigated cadaveric spines of individuals involved in fatal injuries compared with those who died of other natural causes.[48] They were able to demonstrate a variety of injuries involving the cervical facet joints, spinal dorsal root ganglia, intervertebral discs and ligamentous tissues. Other structures have also been implicated, including injuries of the craniocervical junction, such as fractures of the dens, laminae and articular processes,[49] vascular structures[50–55] and other soft aqueous tissues (e.g. skeletal muscle).[36, 37, 56]

Zygapophyseal (facet) joint injury

The anatomical make-up of the cervical facets from C2 to C7 consists of two adjacent synovial joint surfaces enclosed by a thin capsular ligament. This flexible ligament is not capable of influencing facet joint motion; rather, its anatomical structure is dependent on the movement of the surrounding vertebrae.[57] Extending between the margins of the articulating bony surfaces is a synovial fold of the inner facet capsule.[56, 57]

Excessive motion of articular processes, including the capsule, during whiplash loading have been identified in both cadaveric and human volunteers,[16, 42, 45] and have led to two proposed mechanisms implicating facetogenic pain:

1. excessive strain injury of the facet capsule
2. pinching of the synovial fold.[56]

A plethora of cadaveric evidence supports strain injury to the facet capsule during whiplash loads.[41, 42, 44] Normal bending of the neck joints increases capsular strain by approximately 10%, whereas whiplash loading increases peak capsule strain upwards of 40% in the lower segments (C6–C7).[17, 42] Head-turned postures, which are not uncommonly reported by patients, can double the peak capsular strain during simulated whiplash,[58] and may contribute to partial rupture of the capsule. Such partial ruptures have been observed in vitro to occur at strain levels lower than those observed in whiplash simulations,[57, 59] suggesting that elongation of capsular fibres is potentially damaging in some subjects[59] and could contribute to the transmission of pain.

Support linking facet joints in the transmission of pain following injury can be found from neuroanatomical studies that have revealed how the joints are richly innervated with Aδ- and C-fibres.[60–63] Encapsulated neurons within the joint may be sensitised or excited by a gradient change in local pressure, capsular stretching and/or in response to naturally occurring pro-inflammatory agents (e.g. substance P and phospholipase A).[64] Ohtori et al. further demonstrated that ongoing nociception can contribute to physiological changes in the sensitised dorsal root ganglion of rats,[63] suggesting that the origins of more widespread body pain may result from massive inputs of noxious stimuli following facet joint injury.

Other animal studies have demonstrated persistent afferent discharges long after the removal of abnormal facet joint loads and prolonged stretch to the facet capsule.[65, 66] Painful joint loading and capsular strain has also been shown to produce inflammatory responses in the rat spinal cord, including the development of mechanical hyperalgesia, and this cascade of events may contribute to the generation of facet-mediated pain in some following whiplash.[67, 68]

Significantly, the behavioural responses of animals are remarkably similar to those observed in the more 'complex' whiplash group, including widespread hypersensitivity,[69, 70] all of which may implicate a facetogenic cause (or at least contributor) underlying central hyperexcitability; a common feature for this complex patient group.[69, 70]

Supportive clinical evidence for a facetogenic cause (and maintenance) of persistent symptoms following whiplash is also available.[71–73] Specifically, the performance of and response to level-specific, placebo-controlled diagnostic facet joint blocks were evaluated.[72] The sample consisted of 68 consecutive patients referred for neck pain secondary to an MVC with a history of painful symptoms for more than three months. Individuals with a predominant headache underwent a third occipital nerve (TON) block and were excluded if they received pain relief, as the TON has a branch supplying the C2–C3 facet joint. Twenty-seven patients with pain from this segment were excluded from participating in the placebo-controlled study as the resultant pain response was likely due to anaesthetic blocks of the TON. Consequently, 41 patients underwent diagnostic blocks with either a short-acting or a long-acting local anaesthetic, followed by a second block with either normal saline or the other anaesthetic, followed by a third block with the remaining agent. The positive responders experienced complete relief with each anaesthetic and no relief with the normal saline. The results indicated a 60% prevalence of cervical facet joint pain after whiplash injury, and the most common levels affected were C2–C3 and C5–C6.[72] As such, the development of diagnostic facet joint blocks and subsequent management options with radiofrequency neurotomy has been shown to temporarily reduce/eliminate persistent pain.[71–73] Figure 4.1 shows a lateral radiograph and the insertion of the needle during a diagnostic facet block of the C2–C3 facet joint.

Dorsal root ganglia and nerve injury

The clinical presence of sensory disturbances, suggestive of altered pain processing, in the acute and persistent stages of whiplash, has been documented.[69, 70, 74] Changes, such as local (over the cervical spine) and remote (periphery) hypersensitivity to pressure and thermal stimuli on the skin, may be explained by augmented pain processing.[69, 70, 74–78] Such hypersensitive pain responses may signal the involvement of injured proximal structures (e.g. the dorsal root ganglion [DRG] and dorsal root). Direct trauma to the DRG may well affect the internal cell bodies connected with peripheral sensory nerves, and this may help explain many of the signs/symptoms for patients with a more complex clinical presentation. While speculative at this stage, pathoanatomical support for such a premise can be found from Taylor et al.,[48] who found a significant prevalence of cervical DRG injury in persons involved in fatal blunt trauma to the cervical spine.

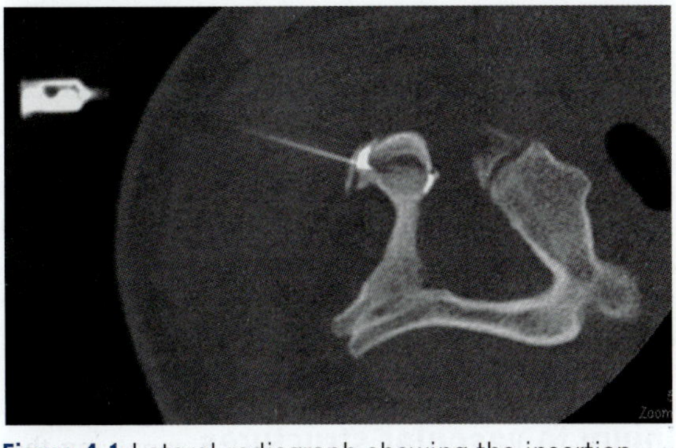

Figure 4.1 Lateral radiograph showing the insertion of the needle during a diagnostic facet block of the C2–C3 facet joint.

Animal studies also show physiological support underlying a potential DRG pain generator. For example, exposing anaesthetised pigs to whiplash conditions (extension, flexion and lateral flexion of the cervical spine) resulted in a reduced pressure inside the spinal cord.[79] Other porcine investigations demonstrated a breach in the plasma membrane of the spinal ganglia nerve cells, consistent with injury at a cellular level following an extension-type whiplash injury mechanism.[80]

The segmental DRG are comprised of distinct nerve fibres responsible for relaying specific information related to proprioception, pain and temperature.[81] Sato and Kikuchi demonstrated age-related morphological changes occurring in the cadaveric lumbar DRG.[82] While evidence suggests these changes could influence clinical symptoms in patients with lumbar spine pathology,[83–87] the impact on patients with whiplash-related pain and disability remains inconclusive.[56, 67, 80, 88, 89]

Another potential mechanism for producing persistent neck pain following whiplash injury involves the deformation of the cervical nerve roots. The cervical dorsal roots arise from the posterior and anterior surfaces of the spinal cord and travel anterolaterally, intrathecally, towards the intervertebral foramen. The anterolateral direction of the roots leaves them vulnerable to excessive stretching during rapid acceleration–deceleration (S-shaped curve) or lateral bending of the neck, as has been demonstrated in rear-end and side-vector impact whiplash. Deformation and injury of the nerve roots in response to extreme neck positions and changes in neural foramina diameters[90–92] may represent another mechanism for producing persistent pain and disability.[83, 93]

It may be that, despite a lack of radiological evidence, a minor and/or major DRG and/or nerve root injury has occurred in some patients, which may, in turn, contribute to the signs of augmented pain-processing mechanisms[69] and the development of persistent symptoms. Further work is warranted to investigate the potential mechanisms involved. This would necessitate, for example, comprehensive research on animal models, where lesions to various cervical structures could be controlled, and inflammatory markers and histological changes in nerve and muscle tissue could be manipulated and documented over time.

Disc injuries

Despite controversy, evidence suggests that one out of four patients with whiplash injury will have radicular symptoms in tandem with radiographic (MRI) documentation of cervical disc herniations and cartilaginous end-plate injuries.[40, 94, 95]

The intervertebral disc is located between adjacent vertebral bodies and consists of a central nucleus pulposus surrounded by concentric rings of annular fibres. The annular fibres are attached to the anterior–posterior longitudinal ligaments, and such an arrangement may predispose the disc to injury if the ligaments were stretched beyond their normal physiological limit, as may be the case in some whiplash events.[40, 94, 95]

The most common level of disc injury during frontal and rear-end impacts is the C5–C6 disc.[96] Subfailure injuries have also been noted in the more cephalad discs, including C2–C3. Such findings may align with recent biomechanical research showing a greater risk of low-grade spinal cord injury during whiplash in those individuals with pre-existing spinal canal narrowing at C5–C6.[96] Future research efforts should aim to correlate ligament and disc injuries for different head and neck positions, vector impact dependency and thresholds for injury before more definitive conclusions regarding the link to pain and prolonged symptoms can be drawn.

Ligament injuries

This section looks at ligamentous tissues in two parts: the middle and lower cervical spine (C3–C7); and the craniocervical junction (above C2).

Mid–lower cervical spine ligaments

Below C2 exists a network of ligamentous tissues—the anterior and posterior longitudinal, capsular, inter- and supraspinous ligaments and the ligamentum flavum. The anterior and posterior longitudinal ligaments span the entire spine, attaching directly to the anterior and posterior surfaces of the vertebral bodies, respectively. They also merge with the annulus fibrosus of each intervertebral disc and are well innervated.[97] The capsular ligaments, as described previously, envelop the facet joints.[57] The interspinous ligaments are not infrequently absent but, when present, connect between adjacent spinous processes and blend posteriorly with the supraspinous ligament.[56] The highly elastic ligamentum flavum is poorly innervated[98] and joins the adjacent lamina bilaterally.[99]

Spinal ligaments possess mechanoreceptive and nociceptive nerve endings that, if injured, may contribute to sensorimotor deficits related to abnormal neck mobility, altered proprioception and transmission of pain.[11–13, 100] However, the lack of available evidence to provide conclusive evidence linking mid–lower cervical ligament disruption and symptoms in whiplash is noted.

Upper cervical ligaments

As the craniocervical region (C0–C2) is devoid of an intervertebral disc and possesses a facet orientation perpendicular to the coronal plane, its ligaments play a key role in providing passive stability to the upper cervical region.[101] The alar and transverse ligaments have high collagen content and low elastin content, predisposing them to partial or complete rupture at low strains during high-speed elongation,[102] as is often the case in whiplash.

Radiological support for upper cervical ligamentous lesions can be found in studies using high-resolution, proton-density weighted MRI, which demonstrate increased signal intensity (indicative of damage) in both the alar and transverse ligaments and the tectorial membrane in some subjects with persistent whiplash associated disorders (WAD) (Fig 4.2).[103] Follow-up studies indicated a relationship between MRI abnormalities of the alar ligaments, head position (turned at time of impact) and neck disability index (NDI) scores.[18, 103, 104]

The detection of such lesions with MRI has been considered a potential contributor to persistent symptoms.[18, 103–109] However, the clinical value of such findings has been contested, with recent observations detailing the presence of such lesions in patients with non-traumatic neck disorders and in those with no history of neck pain.[22, 24, 110, 111] Thus, the previously reported assumption that upper cervical ligament disruption is the direct result of trauma is reported by some to be held as insufficient evidence and may, at best, only feature in a few select patients.[112] The argument of the relevance of upper cervical spine ligament disruption as measured by high-resolution MRI remains open to debate and causation will need to be evaluated in prospective studies before definitive conclusions can be drawn.[26, 113]

Injury to vascular structures

The incidence of vascular injury in those with head and neck trauma is reported to be less than 1% but

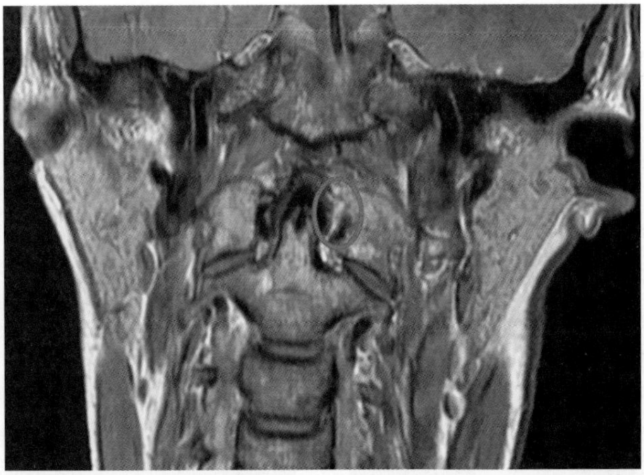

Figure 4.2 Coronal proton-density weighted MRI indicating an increased signal in the left alar ligament, suggestive of disruption (circle).

is understandably higher in those deemed to be high risk (e.g. cervical spine traumatic fracture, extreme head–neck postures and those at risk of cerebral vascular accident).[114] While the incidence of vertebral artery injury following blunt cervical spine trauma has been reported to be as high as nearly 50%, most lesions are recorded as asymptomatic.[114, 115] Despite the chance presence of symptomatic findings, normal screening is indicated following blunt cervical trauma, such as in some cases of whiplash from an MVC.[116]

The vertebral artery, which is closely adhered and fixed to adjacent structures in the fibrous osteomuscular tunnel, is the only vascular structure running through multiple bony foramina and can be impinged by uncinate and superior articular facet joints.[117] It is a viscoelastic structure and supplies the blood to the head, brain and neck tissues. Typically, the artery enters the spine at C6 and runs in cephalad fashion through the transverse foramina of each vertebra bilaterally, although anatomical anomalies cannot be dismissed. Upon exiting at C1, the vertebral artery traverses the posterior arch of C1, enters the skull via the foramen magnum and joins the contralateral vertebral artery to form the basilar artery, which supplies the brainstem and cerebellum.[118]

Nibu et al. have shown that simulated whiplash injury in cadavers can cause excessive stretch and possible damage to the tissues surrounding the artery, which could underpin a vasculogenic cause behind some of the commonly reported symptoms, including dizziness, headache and vertigo.[51] Further biomedical–mechanical research is needed to determine the influence that vector impact and head–neck postures have on injury threshold throughout the vertebral artery, and whether the injury events and the subsequent sequelae are consistent with vascular compromise.

Injury to the muscle system

The cervical spine is a region of sophisticated motor and sensory function, with well-innervated muscles that respond to mechanical and chemical irritants.[98, 119] Paraspinal muscles can understandably be a common source of tenderness and pain following whiplash.[120]

There are multiple layers of deep to superficial muscles in the cervical spine (Fig 4.3). The superficial muscles span multiple vertebrae before attaching directly to the skull and shoulder girdle, whereas the deeper muscles (e.g. the multifidus, semispinalis cervicis, scalenes, longus colli/capitis) attach to many segmental levels and thus may influence the overall control of the cervical spine. The deepest muscles, the multifidus and longus capitus/colli, are rich in muscle spindles,[121] and the multifidi are architecturally complex, attaching directly to the facet capsule.[122, 123] From a proprioceptive standpoint, the smaller, non-torque producing muscles are largely required for fine motor control, whereas muscles recruited for gross movement are comprised of comparatively smaller spindle densities.[124, 125]

While evidence for a direct muscle injury in whiplash is inconclusive, the interaction between neck muscles and the nervous system's response to ongoing pain has been documented. For example, patients with persistent neck pain demonstrate altered patterns

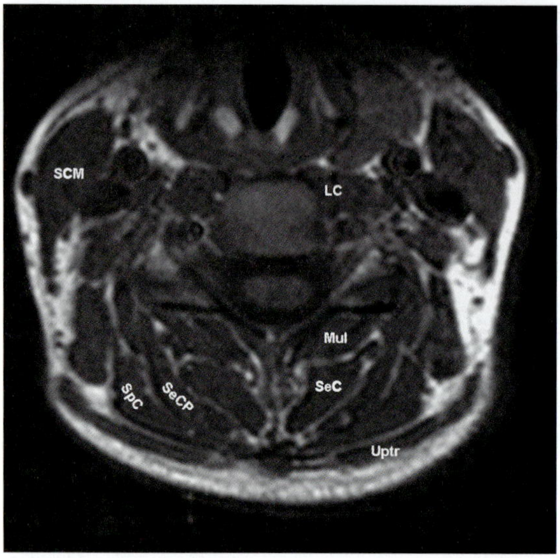

Figure 4.3 T1-weighted axial MRI at the C5 vertebral level, depicting the neck extensor and flexor muscles. (Mul, multifidus; SeC, semispinalis cervicis; SeCP, semispinalis capitis; SpC, splenius capitis; Uptr, upper trapezius; LC, longus capitis/colli; SCM, sternocleidomastoid)

of muscle activation during functional tasks,[126, 127] and these alterations could represent significant motor control impairment and/or a strategy to avoid pain with movement. However, it remains unclear whether motor deficits:

1. are the result of pain
2. help maintain painful symptoms, or
3. represent a psychological response (e.g. fear–avoidance behaviours) to ongoing pain.

In addition to motor control deficits, MRI evidence has quantified changes in the physical structure of certain muscles in cases of persistent whiplash (e.g. widespread fatty infiltrates in the neck extensors and flexors).[36, 37, 128] While widespread, the greatest changes of increased fatty infiltrates were found in all of the deep multifidus muscles, the suboccipital region, rectus capitis posterior minor/major[36] and the longus capitis/colli (Figs 4.4 and 4.5).[128] The higher levels of fatty infiltrate in these muscles are interesting and could provide data in support of the pathophysiological mechanisms underlying persistent symptoms, without assuming a pathoanatomical correlate.

Current research is investigating the temporal development of such changes to determine whether rapid alterations in muscle structure are associated with poor recovery or whether they are generic to

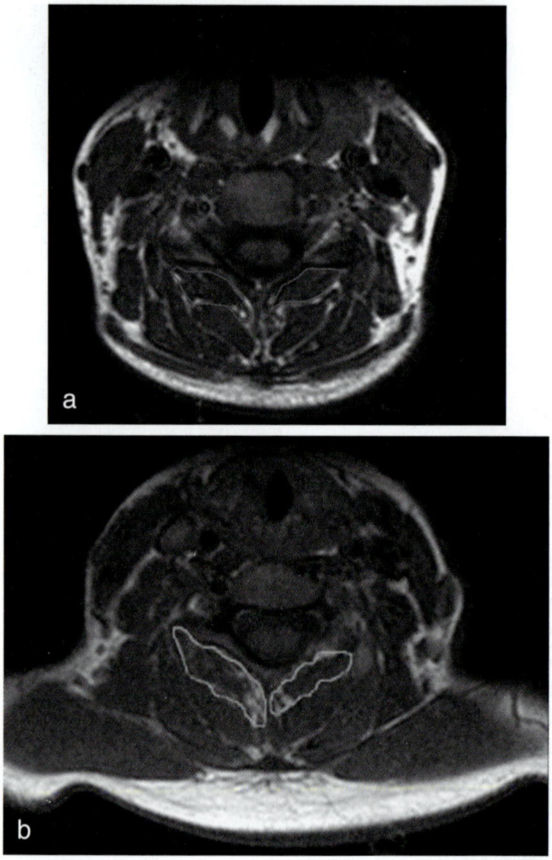

Figure 4.4 Region of interest of the right and left multifidus at C4 on axial T1-weighted MRI, showing (a) no signal change in a healthy control subject and (b) increased signal throughout the muscle, indicative of fatty infiltrates, in a subject with chronic whiplash. (Reproduced with kind permission from Lippincott, Williams and Wilkins)

all those with whiplash and occur irrespective of recovery.

Summary of pathological lesions

Several causes for symptom persistence have been suggested but the lack of diagnostic tests aimed at accurately identifying any of these proposed lesions remains commonplace. Despite this lack of gold-standard diagnostic tests, the inference could be drawn that any number of anatomical structures could be injured, but whether these injuries occur independently or in combination remains unknown. As a result, debate continues as to whether persistent pain is attributable to structural pathology or to other underlying causes.

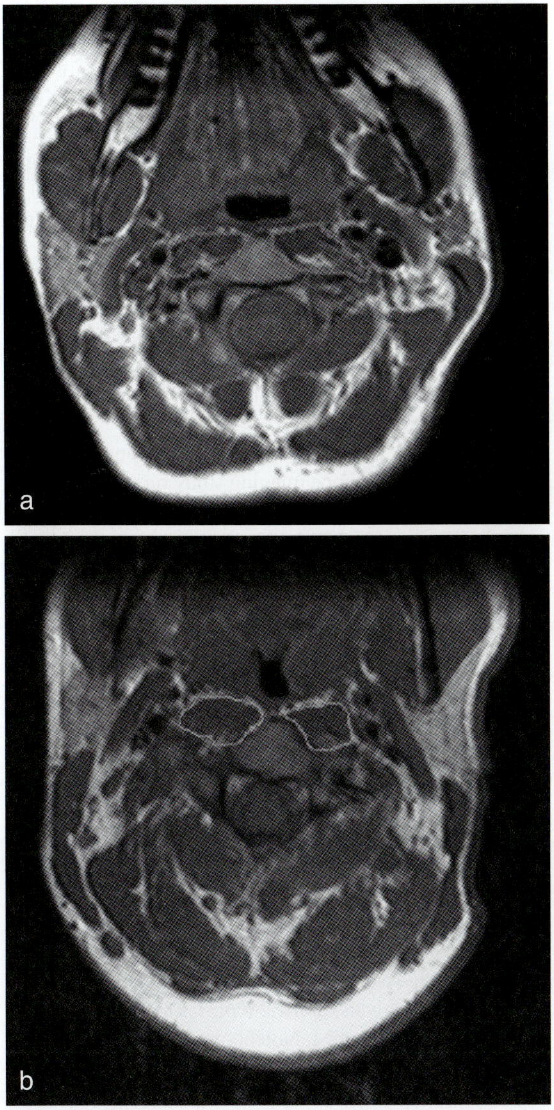

Figure 4.5 Region of interest of the right and left longus capitis/colli muscles at C2–C3 on axial T1-weighted MRI, showing (a) increased signal indicative of fatty infiltrates in a subject with chronic whiplash and (b) no such signal change in a healthy control subject. (Reproduced with kind permission from Lippincott, Williams and Wilkins)

CONCLUSION

The pathoanatomical diagnosis of the elusive whiplash injury remains a challenge but it is clear that the injury can, in some patients, trigger a cascade of events that may directly promote the development and maintenance of persistent symptoms. The possibility that injury to any number of cervical tissues has occurred in some subjects cannot be eliminated. Future research efforts should focus on:

1. higher resolution imaging techniques to consistently identify injured tissues
2. the temporal development of physiological responses to injury
3. links between biomechanical and physiological responses to injury.

References

1. Kamper SJ, Rebbeck TJ, Maher CG, et al. Course and prognostic factors of whiplash: a systematic review and meta-analysis. *Pain* 2008;138:617–29.
2. Norris SH & Watt I. The prognosis of neck injuries resulting from rear-end vehicle collisions. *J Bone Joint Surg* 1983;65:608–11.
3. Schrader H, Obelieniene D, Bovim G, et al. Natural evolution of late whiplash syndrome outside the medicolegal context. *Lancet* 1996;347:1207–11.
4. Barnsley L, Lord S, Bogduk N. Clinical review. Whiplash injury. *Pain* 1994;58:283–307.
5. Carroll LJ, Holm LW, Hogg-Johnson S, et al. Course and prognostic factors for neck pain in whiplash-associated disorders (WAD): results of the Bone and Joint Decade 2000–2010 Task Force on Neck Pain and Its Associated Disorders. *Eur Spine J* 2008;17 (Suppl 1):S83–S92.
6. Quinlan KP, Annest JL, Myers B, et al. Neck strains and sprains among motor vehicle occupants—United States, 2000. *Accid Anal Prev* 2004;36:21–7.
7. Sterling M, Jull G, Vicenzino B, et al. Physical and psychological factors predict outcome following whiplash injury. *Pain* 2005;114:141–8.
8. Provinciali L, Baroni M, Illuminati L, et al. Multimodal treatment to prevent the late whiplash syndrome. *Scand J Rehabil Med* 1996;28:105–11.
9. Stovner LJ. The nosologic status of the whiplash syndrome: a critical review based on a methodological approach. *Spine* 1996;21:2735–46.
10. Tjell C, Tenenbaum A, Sandstrom S. Smooth Pursuit Neck Torsion Test – a specific test for whiplash associated disorders? *J Whiplash and Related Disorders* 2002;1:9–24.
11. Treleaven J, Jull G, Low Choy N. The relationship of cervical joint position error to balance and eye movement disturbances in persistent whiplash. *Man Ther* 2006;11(2):99–106.
12. Treleaven J, Jull G, Low Choy N. Standing balance in persistent whiplash: a comparison between subjects with and without dizziness. *J Rehabil Med* 2005;37:224–9.

13. Treleaven J, Jull G, Sterling M. Dizziness and unsteadiness following whiplash injury: characteristic features and relationship with cervical joint position error. *J Rehabil Med* 2003;35:36–43.
14. Anagnostara A, Athanassopoulou A, Kailidou E, et al. Traumatic retropharyngeal hematoma and prevertebral edema induced by whiplash injury. *Emerg Radiol* 2005;11:145–9.
15. Grauer JN, Panjabi MM, Cholewicki J, et al. Whiplash produces an S-shaped curvature of the neck with hyperextension at lower levels. *Spine* 1997;22:2489–94.
16. Kaneoka K, Ono K, Inami S, et al. Motion analysis of cervical vertebrae during whiplash loading. *Spine* 1999;24:763–9; discussion 70.
17. Panjabi MM, Cholewicki J, Nibu K, et al. Capsular ligament stretches during in vitro whiplash simulations. *J Spinal Disord* 1998;11:227–32.
18. Kaale BR, Krakenes J, Albrektsen G, et al. Whiplash-associated disorders impairment rating: neck disability index score according to severity of MRI findings of ligaments and membranes in the upper cervical spine. *J Neurotrauma* 2005;22:466–75.
19. Pettersson K, Hildingsson C, Toolanen G, et al. MRI and neurology in acute whiplash trauma. No correlation in prospective examination of 39 cases. *Acta Orthop Scand* 1994;65:525–8.
20. Pettersson K, Hildingsson C, Toolanen G, et al. Disc pathology after whiplash injury: a prospective magnetic resonance imaging and clinical investigation. *Spine* 1997;22:283–8.
21. Riley L, Long D, Riley L. The science of whiplash. *Medicine* 1995;74:298–9.
22. Bitterling H, Stabler A, Bruckmann H. [Mystery of alar ligament rupture: value of MRI in whiplash injuries—biomechanical, anatomical and clinical studies]. *Rofo* 2007;179:1127–36.
23. Borchgrevink G, Smevik O, Haave I, et al. MRI of cerebrum and cervical column within two days after whiplash neck sprain injury. *Injury* 1997;28:331–5.
24. Borchgrevink GE, Kaasa A, McDonagh D, Stiles TC, Haraldseth O, Lereim I. Acute treatment of whiplash neck sprain injuries. A randomized trial of treatment during the first 14 days after a car accident. *Spine* 1998;23:25–31.
25. Hildingsson C, Toolanen G. Outcome after soft-tissue injury of the cervical spine. A prospective study of 93 car-accident victims. *Acta Orthop Scand* 1990;61:357–9.
26. Myran R, Kvistad KA, Nygaard OP, et al. Magnetic resonance imaging assessment of the alar ligaments in whiplash injuries: a case-control study. *Spine* 2008;33:2012–16.
27. Ronnen HR, de Korte P, Brink PR, et al. Acute whiplash injury: is there a role for MR imaging? A prospective study of 100 patients. *Radiology* 1996;Oct;201:93–6.
28. Van Goethem JWM, Biltjes I, Van den Hauwe L, et al. Whiplash injuries: is there a role for imaging? *Eur J Radiol* 1996;22:30–7.
29. Vetti N, Krakenes J, Eide GE, et al. MRI of the alar and transverse ligaments in whiplash-associated disorders (WAD) grades 1-2: high-signal changes by age, gender, event and time since trauma. *Neuroradiology* 2008;51(4):227–35.
30. Voyvodic F, Dolinis J, Moore VM, et al. MRI of car occupants with whiplash injury. *Neuroradiology* 1997;39:35–40.
31. Ichihara D, Okada E, Chiba K, et al. Longitudinal magnetic resonance imaging study on whiplash injury patients: minimum 10-year follow-up. *J Orthop Sci* 2009;14:602–10.
32. Kongsted A, Sorensen JS, Andersen H, et al. Are early MRI findings correlated with long-lasting symptoms following whiplash injury? A prospective trial with 1-year follow-up. *Eur Spine J* 2008;17:996–1005.
33. Ferrari R & Schrader H. The late whiplash syndrome: a biopsychosocial approach. *J Neurol Neurosurg Psychiatry* 2001;70:722–6.
34. Ferrari R. Epidemiology of whiplash: an international dilemma. *Ann Rheum Dis* 1999;58:1–5.
35. Joslin CC, Khan SN, Bannister GC. Long-term disability after neck injury: a comparative study. *J Bone Joint Surg [Br]* 2004;86:1032–4.
36. Elliott J, Jull G, Noteboom JT, et al. Fatty infiltration in the cervical extensor muscles in persistent whiplash-associated disorders: a magnetic resonance imaging analysis. *Spine* 2006;31:E847–55.
37. Elliott J, Sterling M, Noteboom JT, et al. Fatty infiltrate in the cervical extensor muscles is not a feature of chronic, insidious-onset neck pain. *Clin Radiol* 2008;63:681–7.
38. Elliott J, Sterling M, Noteboom JT, et al. The clinical presentation of chronic whiplash and the relationship to findings of MRI fatty infiltrates in the cervical extensor musculature: a preliminary investigation. *Eur Spine J* 2009;18(9):1371–8.
39. McNab I. Acceleration injuries of the cervical spine. *J Bone Joint Surg [Br]* 1964;46:1797–9.
40. Pettersson K, Hildingsson C, Toolanen G, et al. Disc pathology after whiplash injury. A prospective magnetic resonance imaging and clinical investigation. *Spine* 1997;22:283–7; discussion 288.
41. Luan F, Yang KH, Deng B, et al. Qualitative analysis of neck kinematics during low-speed rear-end impact. *Clin Biomech (Bristol, Avon)* 2000;15:649–57.

42. Pearson AM, Ivancic PC, Ito S, et al. Facet joint kinematics and injury mechanisms during simulated whiplash. *Spine (Phila Pa 1976)* 2004;29:390–7.
43. Yang KH & King AI. Neck kinematics in rear-end impacts. *Pain Res Manage* 2003;8:79–85.
44. Yoganandan N, Pintar F, Cusick JF. Biomechanical analyses of whiplash injuries using an experimental mode. *Accid Anal Prev* 2002;34:663–71.
45. Cusick JF, Pintar FA, Yoganandan N. Whiplash syndrome: kinematic factors influencing pain patterns. *Spine (Phila Pa 1976)* 2001;26:1252–8.
46. Ivancic PC, Pearson AM, Panjabi MM, et al. Injury of the anterior longitudinal ligament during whiplash simulation. *Eur Spine J* 2004;13:61–8.
47. Panjabi MM, Ito S, Pearson AM, et al. Injury mechanisms of the cervical intervertebral disc during simulated whiplash. *Spine* 2004;29:1217–25.
48. Taylor JR, Twomey L, Kakulas BA. Dorsal root ganglion injuries in 109 blunt trauma fatalities. *Injury* 1998;29:335–9.
49. Barnsley L, Lord S, Bogduk N. The pathophysiology of whiplash. *Spine (Phila Pa 1976)* 1998;12:209–42.
50. Chung YS, Han DH. Vertebrobasilar dissection: a possible role of whiplash injury in its pathogenesis. *Neurol Res* 2002;24:129–38.
51. Nibu K, Cholewicki J, Panjabi MM, et al. Dynamic elongation of the vertebral artery during an in vitro whiplash simulation. *Eur Spine J* 1997;6:286–9.
52. Pollanen MS, Deck JH, Blenkinsop B. Injury of the tunica media in fatal rupture of the vertebral artery. *Am J Forensic Med Pathol* 1996;17:197–201.
53. Reddy M, Reddy B, Schoggl A, et al. The complexity of trauma to the cranio-cervical junction: correlation of clinical presentation with Doppler flow velocities in the V3-segment of the vertebral arteries. *Acta Neurochir (Wien)* 2002;144:575–80; discussion 580.
54. Seric V, Blazic-Cop N, Demarin V. Haemodynamic changes in patients with whiplash injury measured by transcranial Doppler sonography (TCD). *Coll Antropol* 2000;24:197–204.
55. Taneichi H, Suda K, Kajino T, et al. Traumatically induced vertebral artery occlusion associated with cervical spine injuries: prospective study using magnetic resonance angiography. *Spine (Phila Pa 1976)* 2005;30:1955–62.
56. Siegmund GP, Winkelstein BA, Ivancic PC, et al. The anatomy and biomechanics of acute and chronic whiplash injury. *Traffic Inj Prev* 2009;10:101–12.
57. Winkelstein BA, Nightingale R, Richardson WJ, Myers BS. The cervical facet capsule and its role in whiplash injury: a biomechanical investigation. *Spine* 2000;25:1238–46.
58. Siegmund GP, Davis MB, Quinn KP, et al. Head-turned postures increase the risk of cervical facet capsule injury during whiplash. *Spine (Phila Pa 1976)* 2008;33:1643–9.
59. Siegmund GP, Myers BS, Davis MB, et al. Mechanical evidence of cervical facet capsule injury during whiplash: a cadaveric study using combined shear, compression, and extension loading. *Spine (Phila Pa 1976)* 2001;26:2095–101.
60. Inami S, Shiga T, Tsujino A, et al. Immunohistochemical demonstration of nerve fibers in the synovial fold of the human cervical facet joint. *J Orthop Res* 2001;19:593–6.
61. Kallakuri S, Singh A, Chen C, et al. Demonstration of substance P, calcitonin gene-related peptide, and protein gene product 9.5 containing nerve fibers in human cervical facet joint capsules. *Spine* 2004;29:1182–6.
62. McLain RF, Pickar JG. Mechanoreceptor endings in human thoracic and lumbar facet joints. *Spine* 1998;23:168–73.
63. Ohtori S, Takahashi K, Moriya H. Calcitonin gene-related peptide immunoreactive DRG neurons innervating the cervical facet joints show phenotypic switch in cervical facet injury in rats. *Eur Spine J* 2003;12:211–15.
64. Anderson A. Cervicogenic processes: results of injury to the cervical spine. *Pain Practitioner* 2001;11(2):9–11.
65. Lu Y, Chen C, Kallakuri S, et al. Neurophysiological and biomechanical characterization of goat cervical facet joint capsules. *J Orthop Res* 2005;23:779–87.
66. Lu Y, Chen C, Kallakuri S, et al. Development of an in vivo method to investigate biomechanical and neurophysiological properties of spine facet joint capsules. *Eur Spine J* 2005;14:565–72.
67. Lee KE, Davis MB, Winkelstein BA. Capsular ligament involvement in the development of mechanical hyperalgesia after facet joint loading: behavioral and inflammatory outcomes in a rodent model of pain. *J Neurotrauma* 2008;25:1383–93.
68. Lee KM, Kang BS, Lee HL, et al. Spinal NF-kB activation induces COX-2 upregulation and contributes to inflammatory pain hypersensitivity. *Eur J Neurosci* 2004;19:3375–81.
69. Sterling M, Jull G, Kenardy J. Physical and psychological factors maintain long-term predictive capacity post-whiplash injury. *Pain* 2006; 122(1–2):102–8.
70. Sterling M, Jull G, Vicenzio B, Kenardy J. Sensory hypersensitivity occurs soon after whiplash injury and is associated with poor recovery. *Pain* 2003;104:509–17.

71. Lord SM, Barnsley L, Bogduk N. Percutaneous radiofrequency neurotomy in the treatment of cervical zygapophysial joint pain: a caution. *Neurosurgery* 1995;36:732–9.
72. Lord SM, Barnsley L, Wallis BJ, et al. Chronic cervical zygapophysial joint pain after whiplash. A placebo-controlled prevalence study. *Spine* 1996;21:1737–44; discussion 1744–5.
73. Lord SM, Barnsley L, Wallis BJ, et al. Percutaneous radio-frequency neurotomy for chronic cervical zygapophyseal-joint pain. *N Engl J Med* 1996;335:1721–6.
74. Koelbaek Johansen M, Graven-Nielsen T, et al. Generalised muscular hyperalgesia in chronic whiplash syndrome. *Pain* 1999;83:229–34.
75. Banic B, Petersen-Felix S, Andersen OK, et al. Evidence for spinal cord hypersensitivity in chronic pain after whiplash injury and in fibromyalgia. *Pain* 2004;107:7–15.
76. Curatolo M, Petersen-Felix S, Arendt-Nielsen L, et al. Central hypersensitivity in chronic pain after whiplash injury. *Clin J Pain* 2001;17:306–15.
77. Kasch H, Stengaard-Pedersen K, Arendt-Nielsen L, et al. Pain thresholds and tenderness in neck and head following acute whiplash injury: a prospective study. *Cephalalgia* 2001;21:189–97.
78. Scott D, Jull G, Sterling M. Widespread sensory hypersensitivity is a feature of chronic whiplash-associated disorder but not chronic idiopathic neck pain. *Clin J Pain* 2005;21:175–81.
79. Svensson MY, Bostrom O, Davidsson J, et al. Neck injuries in car collisions—a review covering a possible injury mechanism and the development of a new rear-impact dummy. *Accid Anal Prev* 2000;32:167–75.
80. Ortengren T, Hansson HA, Lovsund P, et al. Membrane leakage in spinal ganglion nerve cells induced by experimental whiplash extension motion: a study in pigs. *J Neurotrauma* 1996;13:171–80.
81. Boyd-Clark LC, Briggs CA, Galea MP. Segmental degeneration in the cervical spine and associated changes in dorsal root ganglia. *Clin Anat* 2004;17:468–77.
82. Sato K, Kikuchi S. An anatomic study of foraminal nerve root lesions in the lumbar spine. *Spine (Phila Pa 1976)* 1993;18:2246–51.
83. Hasue M. Pain and the nerve root. An interdiscplinary approach. *Spine* 1993;18:2053.
84. Kobayashi S, Baba H, Uchida K, et al. Effect of mechanical compression on the lumbar nerve root: localization and changes of intraradicular inflammatory cytokines, nitric oxide, and cyclooxygenase. *Spine (Phila Pa 1976)* 2005;30:1699–705.
85. Kobayashi S, Kokubo Y, Uchida K, et al. Effect of lumbar nerve root compression on primary sensory neurons and their central branches: changes in the nociceptive neuropeptides substance P and somatostatin. *Spine (Phila Pa 1976)* 2005;30:276–82.
86. Kobayashi S, Yoshizawa H. Effect of mechanical compression on the vascular permeability of the dorsal root ganglion. *J Orthop Res* 2002;20:730–9.
87. Kobayashi S, Yoshizawa H, Yamada S. Pathology of lumbar nerve root compression. Part 2: morphological and immunohistochemical changes of dorsal root ganglion. *J Orthop Res* 2004;22:180–8.
88. Svensson MY, Aldman B, Bostrom O, et al. [Nerve cell damages in whiplash injuries. Animal experimental studies]. *Orthopade* 1998;27:820–6.
89. Tominaga Y, Maak TG, Ivancic PC, et al. Head-turned rear impact causing dynamic cervical intervertebral foramen narrowing: implications for ganglion and nerve root injury. *J Neurosurg Spine* 2006;4:380–7.
90. Carter JW, Mirza SK, Tencer AF, et al. Canal geometry changes associated with axial compressive cervical spine fracture. *Spine (Phila Pa 1976)* 2000;25:46–54.
91. Takasaki H, Hall T, Jull G, et al. The influence of cervical traction, compression, and Spurling test on cervical intervertebral foramen size. *Spine (Phila Pa 1976)* 2009;34:1658–62.
92. Yoo JU, Zou D, Edwards WT, et al. Effect of cervical spine motion on the neuroforaminal dimensions of human cervical spine. *Spine (Phila Pa 1976)* 1992;17:1131–6.
93. Loeser J. Pain due to nerve injury. *Spine* 1985;10:232.
94. Davis S, Teresi L, Bradley W, et al. Cervical spine hyperextension injuries: MR findings. *Radiology* 1991;180:245–51.
95. Jonsson H, Cesarini K, Sahlstedt B, et al. Findings and outcome in whiplash-type neck distortions. *Spine* 1991;19:2733–43.
96. Ito S, Panjabi M, Ivancic PC, Pearson AM. Spinal canal narrowing during simulated whiplash. *Spine* 2004;29:1330–9.
97. White AA & Panjabi M. Clinical biomechanics of the spine. Philadelphia: JB Lippincott Co., 1990.
98. Timothy J, Foley E, Comer C, et al. Soft tissue injuries: 3. Paraspinal. *Emerg Med J* 2008;25:514–21.
99. Yahia LH, Garzon S, Strykowski H, Rivard CH. Ultrastructure of the human interspinous ligament and ligamentum flavum. A preliminary study. *Spine (Phila Pa 1976)* 1990;15:262–8.
100. Treleaven J, Jull G, Low Choy N. Smooth-pursuit neck torsion test in whiplash-associated disorders: relationship to self-reports of neck pain and disability, dizziness and anxiety. *J Rehabil Med* 2004;36:1–5.

101. Dvorak J, Schneider E, Saldinger P, et al. Biomechanics of the craniocervical region: the alar and transverse ligaments. *J Orthop Res* 1988;6:452–61.
102. Panjabi MM, Crisco JJ, 3rd, Lydon C, et al. The mechanical properties of human alar and transverse ligaments at slow and fast extension rates. *Clin Biomech (Bristol, Avon)* 1998;13:112–20.
103. Krakenes J, Kaale BR, Moen G, et al. MRI assessment of the alar ligaments in the late stage of whiplash injury—a study of structural abnormalities and observer agreement. *Neuroradiology* 2002;44:617–24.
104. Kaale BR, Krakenes J, Albrektsen G, et al. Head position and impact direction in whiplash injuries: associations with MRI-verified lesions of ligaments and membranes in the upper cervical spine. *J Neurotrauma* 2005;22:1294–302.
105. Bogduk N. Whiplash can have lesions. *Pain Res Manage* 2006;11:155.
106. Johansson BH. Whiplash injuries can be visible by functional magnetic resonance imaging. *Pain Res Manage* 2006;11:197–9.
107. Krakenes J & Kaale BR. Magnetic resonance imaging assessment of craniovertebral ligaments and membranes after whiplash trauma. *Spine* 2006;31:2820–6.
108. Krakenes J, Kaale BR, Moen G, et al. MRI of the tectorial and posterior atlanto-occipital membranes in the late stage of whiplash injury. *Neuroradiology* 2003;45:585–91.
109. Krakenes J, Kaale BR, Nordli H, et al. MR analysis of the transverse ligament in the late stage of whiplash injury. *Acta Radiol* 2003;44:637–44.
110. Pfirrmann CW, Binkert CA, Zanetti M, et al. MR morphology of alar ligaments and occipitoatlantoaxial joints: study in 50 asymptomatic subjects. *Radiology* 2001;218:133–7.
111. Wilmink JT & Patijn J. MR imaging of alar ligament in whiplash-associated disorders: an observer study. *Neuroradiology* 2001;43:859–63.
112. Kwan O. MRI assessment of the alar ligaments in the late stage of whiplash injury. *Neuroradiology* 2003;45:195–6; author reply 197–8.
113. Roy S, Hol PK, Laerum LT, et al. Pitfalls of magnetic resonance imaging of alar ligament. *Neuroradiology* 2004;46:392–8.
114. Cothren CC, Moore EE, Biffl WL, et al. Cervical spine fracture patterns predictive of blunt vertebral artery injury. *J Trauma* 2003;55:811–13.
115. Biffl WL, Moore EE, Elliott JP, et al. The devastating potential of blunt vertebral arterial injuries. *Ann Surg* 2000;231:672–81.
116. Bagley LJ. Imaging of spinal trauma. *Radiol Clin North Am* 2006;44:1–12, vii.
117. Chopard RP, de Miranda Neto MH, Lucas GA, et al. The vertebral artery: its relationship with adjoining tissues in its course intra and inter transverse processes in man. *Rev Paul Med* 1992;110:245–50.
118. Lu J & Ebraheim NA. The vertebral artery: surgical anatomy. *Orthopedics* 1999;22:1081–5.
119. Evans WJ, Meredith CN, Cannon JG, et al. Metabolic changes following eccentric exercise in trained and untrained men. *J Appl Physiol* 1986;61:1864–8.
120. Evans RW. Some observations on whiplash injuries. *Neurol Clin* 1992;10:975–97.
121. Boyd-Clark LC, Briggs CA, Galea MP. Muscle spindle distribution, morphology, and density in longus colli and multifidus muscles of the cervical spine. *Spine* 2002;27:694–701.
122. Anderson JS, Hsu AW, Vasavada AN. Morphology, architecture, and biomechanics of human cervical multifidus. *Spine* 2005;30:E86–91.
123. Winkelstein BA, McLendon R, Barbir A, Myers BS. An anatomical investigation of the human cervical facet capsule, quantifying muscle insertion area. *J Anat* 2001;198:455–61.
124. Cooper S & Daniel PM. Human muscle spindles. *J Physiol* 1956;133:1–3P.
125. Peck D, Buxton D, Nitz A. A comparison of spindle concentrations in large and small muscles acting in parallel combinations. *J Morphol* 1984;180:243–52.
126. Falla D, Bilenkij G, Jull G. Patients with chronic neck pain demonstrate altered patterns of muscle activation during performance of a functional upper limb task. *Spine* 2004;29:1436–40.
127. Nederhand MJ, Hermens HJ, IJzerman MJ, et al. Cervical muscle dysfunction in chronic whiplash-associated disorder grade 2: the relevance of the trauma. *Spine* 2002;27:1056–61.
128. Elliott JM, O'Leary S, Sterling M, et al. Magnetic resonance imaging findings of fatty infiltrate in the cervical flexors in chronic whiplash. *Spine (Phila Pa 1976)* 2010;35(9):948–54.

CHAPTER 5
Pain-processing mechanisms in whiplash associated disorders

Michele Curatolo and Michele Sterling

INTRODUCTION

It is now generally acknowledged that an initial peripheral injury of some kind occurs to the neck following whiplash injury,[1] although the specific injured structure in individual patients is difficult to clinically identify with current imaging techniques.[2] Regardless of the specific structures involved, following injury and ensuing inflammation, a cascade of events occurs in the periphery, spinal cord and supraspinal nervous centres leading to upregulation of nociceptive processes. These changes have the potential to amplify the individual's pain experience.

Even if identification of injured peripheral (neck) structures was easily achieved, it remains unclear whether it would improve management directions and outcomes, as the correlation between objective findings and pain and disability is well known to be equivocal in patients with whiplash.[3, 4] Rather, recent calls have been made for greater consideration of underlying pain processes that contribute to the condition in question, as this may enable the direction of the most appropriate intervention strategies.[5] Research has now demonstrated indirect evidence, via sensory testing and other methods, of altered pain processes as contributing factors to the clinical presentation, outcome and response to treatment of whiplash associated disorders (WAD).

This chapter outlines the mechanisms that occur in the peripheral and central nervous systems (CNS) following injury, and discusses the evidence for altered pain-processing mechanisms in acute and chronic whiplash, as well as the implications for management of this condition.

MECHANISMS FOR POST-INJURY CENTRAL HYPEREXCITABILITY

Peripheral mechanisms

Tissue injury leads to an inflammatory response, with the release of different mediators, such as potassium ions, substance P, bradykinin and prostaglandins.[6] These substances may induce a sensitisation of peripheral receptors, with changes in the response characteristics of primary afferent fibres.[7] They may also activate normally inactive or 'silent' nociceptors.[8] Furthermore, the inflammatory response induces a gene expression in the dorsal root ganglion, resulting in an increased synthesis of peripheral receptors, which contributes to the increased sensitivity of the nociceptor.[9] Long-lasting nociceptive stimulation may lead to a modification in the peripheral fibres: A_β-fibres may start synthesising receptors that are normally found only in C-fibres, with the A_β-fibre adopting C-fibre characteristics.[10]

These sensitising events mediate primary hyperalgesia,[11] in which a reduced threshold for eliciting pain and enhanced pain to supra-threshold stimuli within the injured area can be recorded. Peripheral sensitisation ultimately results in an increased nociceptive input to the spinal cord.

Spinal cord plasticity

Afferent nociceptive input induces an increase in the excitability of central sensory neurons,[12] which is mediated by the *N*-methyl-D-aspartate (NMDA) receptor.[13, 14] The expression of the isoenzyme cyclooxygenase-2 (COX-2) in the spinal cord is also involved in spinal cord hyperexcitability.[15] Importantly, COX-2 expression is not confined to the neural structures connected to the site of inflammation, but involves the whole spinal cord and the supraspinal centres.[16] This phenomenon may be responsible, at least in part, for a generalised hypersensitivity to peripheral stimulation, such as the one evoked after stimulation of tissues that are a distance from the site of injury.

In animal models using direct neuronal measurements, peripheral tissue or nerve damage induced an expansion of receptive fields on individual dorsal horn neurons.[17] This phenomenon represents an important manifestation of central sensitisation, leading to increased nociceptive input into the CNS and expansion of areas of referred pain and hyperalgesia.

Inflammation and nerve injury also produce depression of the inhibitory mechanisms within the spinal cord, with consequent amplification of the nociceptive signal being transmitted to higher centres.[18] An important substrate of such disinhibition is the loss of inhibitory control of GABAergic (gamma-aminobutyric acid) and glycinergic spinal cord neurons that follows inflammation and nerve injury.[19] Furthermore, nerve damage leads to destruction of inhibitory interneurons, which contributes to hyperexcitability.[20]

Endogenous modulation

Spinal cord hyperexcitability elicited by trauma or inflammation is influenced by descending facilitatory and inhibitory pathways.[21] Opioidergic,[22] serotonergic[23] and noradrenergic systems[23] are involved in descending inhibition.

Pathways that excite 5-hydroxytryptamine-3 (5-HT-3) receptors in the whole spinal cord after regional peripheral damage are involved in descending facilitation.[24] Their activity could be driven by anxiety and fear, which are common features in patients with pain.[25] These data provide an additional explanation for the widespread pain hypersensitivity following a peripheral lesion, a common phenomenon in patients with chronic pain.[26] They may also represent a physiological basis for an amplification of the pain experience in patients with psychological distress.

The efficiency of the endogenous modulatory system can be tested in humans by diffuse noxious inhibitory control (DNIC), whereby a conditioning painful stimulus is expected to attenuate the response to an additional test stimulus. DNIC has been found to be altered in different pain syndromes, such as fibromyalgia,[27] osteoarthritis of the hip[28] and irritable bowel syndrome.[29] Alteration in DNIC before surgery has been found to be a predictor of chronic post-thoracotomy pain.[30]

Brain plasticity

Several clinical studies have revealed that the brain is capable of substantial plastic changes. Using equal levels of sensory stimulation in patients with chronic low back pain and pain-free controls, patients with chronic low back pain showed not only more pain than healthy controls, but also more extensive patterns of neuronal activation in pain-related cortical areas.[31] This confirmed the occurrence of enhanced central pain processing.

Patients with various chronic pain syndromes, such as phantom limb pain, low back pain and complex regional pain syndrome (CRPS), display substantial cortical reorganisation, whereby the representation of the different body areas is altered.[32–34]

Using magnetic resonance imaging (MRI), patients with chronic low back pain were found to have 5–11% less neocortical grey matter volume than control subjects.[35] The decreased volume was related to the pain duration, indicating a 1.3 cm^3 loss of grey matter for every year of chronic pain. These concerning findings indicate that chronic low back pain is accompanied by brain atrophy, although the clinical implications remain unclear.

Summary

There is clear evidence that tissue trauma leads to structural changes in the CNS, mostly resulting in hyperexcitability. Potentially irreversible changes have been documented. These alterations may be partly responsible for persisting pain after injury.

EVIDENCE FOR CENTRAL HYPEREXCITABILITY IN CHRONIC WAD

In a first investigation comparing whiplash patients with healthy controls, patients displayed lower pain detection and tolerance thresholds after cutaneous electrical stimulation of the neck.[36] The absence of tissue damage at the site of testing suggested that a central sensitisation of nociceptive pathways was the cause of the pain hypersensitivity.

This finding has been confirmed by a study testing muscle pain sensibility after injection of hypertonic saline into the supraspinatus and tibialis anterior muscle.[37] Patients with whiplash displayed higher pain scores, longer duration of pain and larger areas of local and referred pain after intramuscular injection of hypertonic saline, compared with healthy controls. In particular, the areas of referred pain were impressively larger in patients than in controls, at both the neck and leg. Several patients reported pain spreading to the whole leg and on the contralateral side, which was not the case in healthy subjects. These data suggest that pain hypersensitivity is not limited to the injured and surrounding areas (primary and secondary hyperalgesia), but may be generalised to the whole CNS. The impressive spread of referred pain is strongly suggestive of central hyperexcitability, possibly involving disinhibitory processes and expansion of receptive fields.

In a following investigation, pain thresholds to electrical and heat stimulation, applied at the skin and muscles of both the neck and a lower limb, were measured.[26] Patients displayed lower pain thresholds with both cutaneous and muscular electrical stimulation, applied at both the neck and the lower limb, compared with a group of healthy subjects. This confirmed the previous findings of generalised central hypersensitivity. Infiltration of a local anaesthetic into the painful and tender muscles did not reduce either neck pain or pain thresholds. This indicates that the source of pain was not located in the infiltrated muscles and central hypersensitivity was not maintained by a nociceptive input arising from these muscles.

A study that analysed responses to a variety of non-painful stimuli in whiplash patients and healthy controls found that 65% of patients, but no control subject, reported pain after vibration stimulus.[38] Patients reacted with more pain to heat and cold stimulation than healthy subjects. Because sensory stimuli were applied to non-damaged tissues, the results of this study provided additional evidence for the presence of central hyperexcitability in whiplash patients.

In a study that analysed spinal hyperexcitability using the nociceptive withdrawal reflex, patients with whiplash injury and patients with fibromyalgia displayed lower reflex thresholds than healthy subjects.[39] These findings provide objective electrophysiological evidence for generalised spinal cord hyperexcitability.

A recent study addressed the question of the relationship between parameters of central hypersensitivity and psychological factors.[40] While there was a weak correlation between catastrophising and cold pain thresholds, spinal excitability as assessed by the nociceptive withdrawal reflex did not correlate significantly with either catastrophising or psychological distress. A more recent investigation on 300 healthy volunteers found no impact of depression, anxiety and catastrophising on the nociceptive withdrawal reflex, indicating that spinal cord excitability is little or not affected by descending psychological influences.[41]

In summary, there is consistent evidence that patients with chronic pain after whiplash injury display pain hypersensitivity after sensory stimulation of healthy tissues. This is strongly suggestive of an alteration in the central processing of the sensory input. Importantly, these central alterations are not only regional, but also generalised.

It is important to recognise that central hypersensitivity is not specific for patients with whiplash, but has been observed in different chronic pain syndromes, such as endometriosis,[42] fibromyalgia,[43] osteoarthritis,[44] tension-type headache,[45] temporomandibular joint pain[46] and post-mastectomy pain.[47]

EVIDENCE FOR CENTRAL HYPEREXCITABILITY IN ACUTE WAD AND IN THE TRANSITION TO CHRONICITY

Most investigations of the nociceptive processes involved in WAD have focused on the chronic stage of the condition. However, recent data demonstrate that sensory disturbances observed in patients with chronic WAD are, in fact, present from soon after injury. In the acute phase post injury, local cervical mechanical hyperalgesia (decreased pressure pain thresholds) is found in individuals with both lower and higher levels of pain and disability.[48, 49] This local hyperalgesia tends to resolve within a few months in individuals with good and fair recovery but persists unchanged in those who report ongoing moderate-to-severe symptom levels six months to two to three years post accident.[50] Mechanical hyperalgesia is also found at sites away from the site of injury, including the upper and lower limbs.[48, 49] The absence of tissue damage at the site of testing suggests the involvement of central sensitisation of nociceptive pathways. In contrast to local hyperalgesia, which occurs irrespective of pain and disability levels, the presence of generalised hyperalgesia has been shown to be more apparent in those individuals reporting higher pain and disability,[49] and subsequent poor recovery.[50] In addition to mechanical hyperalgesia, both cold and heat hyperalgesia have also been found to be features of individuals with higher symptom levels and poor functional recovery (Fig 5.1).[50]

Most studies have explored the presence of positive sensory signs or sensory hypersensitivity. Recently, the presence of negative sensory responses or widespread hypoaesthesia (or elevated detection thresholds) occurring concurrently with hypersensitivity has also been found in patients with acute WAD.[51] Similar to findings of sensory hypersensitivity, the hypoaesthetic changes were widespread and occurred in response to a variety of stimuli, including vibration (Fig 5.2), and thermal and electrical stimulation.[51] While they occurred in the majority of participants in the acute injury stage (three to four weeks), the hypoaesthesia persisted only in those who were initially classified as at high risk of poor recovery (higher pain and disability and sensory hypersensitivity).[52] Consideration of these findings of both positive and negative sensory changes to various stimuli, which are widespread and generalised throughout various body locations, infers that disturbances in both excitatory and inhibitory CNS processes are at play.

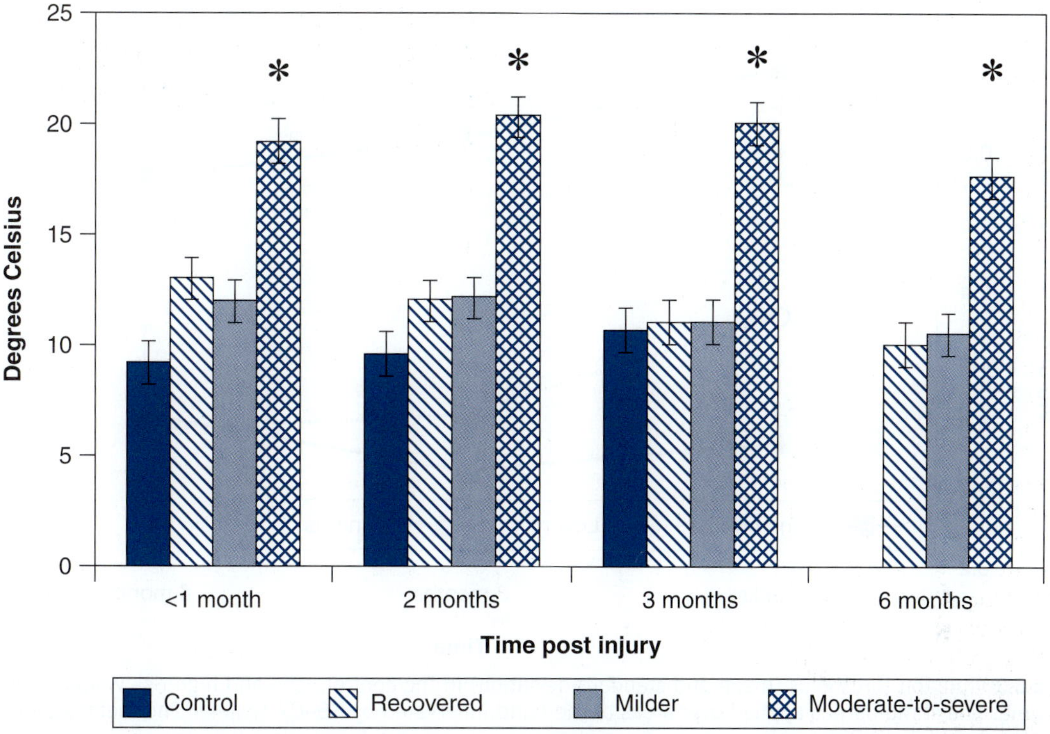

Figure 5.1 Cold pain thresholds (measured over the cervical spine) in controls (1–3 months) and three whiplash groups classified at six months post injury (recovered: nerve disability index [NDI] <8; milder symptoms: NDI: 10–28; and moderate-to-severe symptoms: NDI: >30) at 1, 2, 3 and 6 months post injury.[50] The whiplash group with persistent moderate-to-severe symptoms demonstrates cold hyperalgesia from within a month of injury that does not resolve. * = $P < 0.05$. (Adapted from Sterling et al.[50])

Importantly, some of the sensory phenomena demonstrate an ability to predict individuals at risk of poor recovery. In particular, the early presence of cold hyperalgesia is emerging as a consistent prognostic factor. Initial studies demonstrated that in addition to initial moderate pain, decreased neck movement, older age and post-traumatic stress symptoms, cold hyperalgesia predicted higher levels of pain and disability at both six months and two to three years post injury.[53, 54] Cold pain tolerance measured using the cold pressor test has also shown predictive capacity.[55] More recently, it has been shown that when injured people are classified based on the presence of moderate or greater initial pain and sensory hypersensitivity, 86% of those deemed at high risk of poor recovery did indeed develop persistent symptoms at six months post injury.[52] Further research using trajectory modelling has validated cold hyperalgesia as a predictor of a clinical pathway to chronicity.[56]

While sensory hypersensitivity is thought to reflect augmented central pain processes, the precise underlying mechanisms are not clear. A recent prospective study investigating the nociceptive withdrawal reflex in patients progressing from acute to chronic WAD showed a different picture to what is seen for sensory hypersensitivity.[57] Lowered reflex thresholds indicative of spinal cord hyperexcitability were found to be present at three weeks post injury in all whiplash subgroups, irrespective of the extent of recovery. However, by six months post injury, lowered reflex thresholds persisted only in those with moderate-to-severe symptoms, having resolved in those who recovered or reported lesser symptoms at this point in time. In contrast, generalised sensory hypersensitivity (pressure and cold) was only ever present in those with persistent moderate-to-severe symptoms and remained unchanged throughout the study period. This suggests different mechanisms underlie sensory hypersensitivity and nociceptive flexion responses (NFRs), or at least that sensory hypersensitivity does not appear to be solely due to spinal processes.

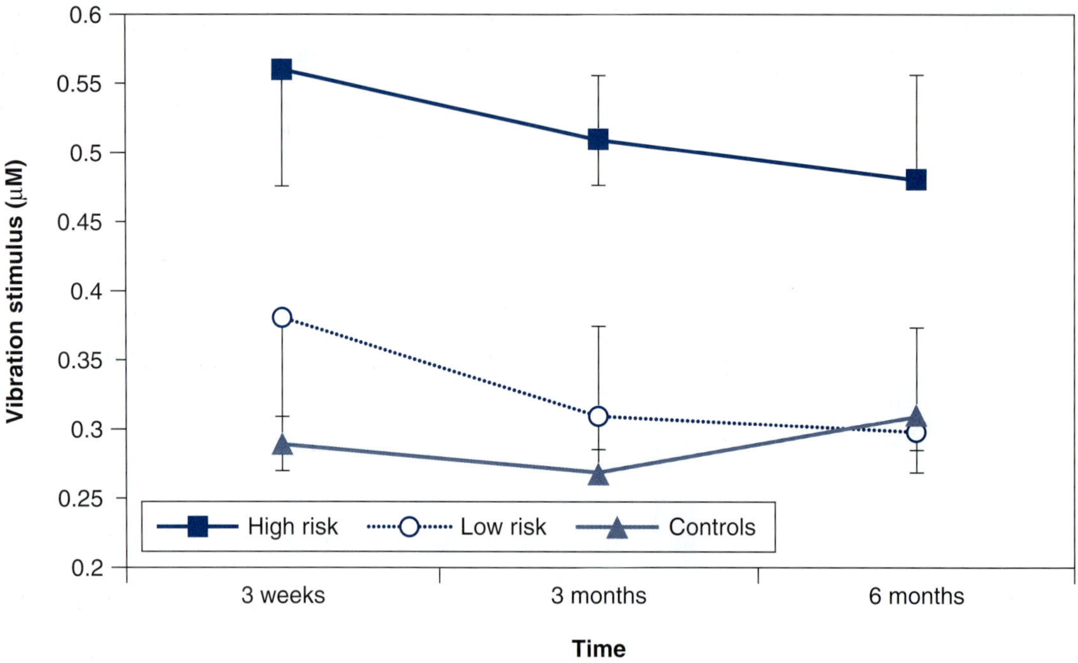

Figure 5.2 Vibration thresholds (mean and standard deviation) in the control, low- and high-risk whiplash groups over time. The stimulus was applied over areas of the hand innervated by C6–C7 (palmar 2nd metacarpal) dermatomes.[52] ($P < 0.05$)

In summary, current evidence would suggest that some CNS pain processes are augmented from soon after injury in those individuals who do not recover but develop chronic moderate-to-severe pain and disability. The reasons as to why this group manifests more profound changes in pain processes is not clear but there are numerous possibilities, including but not limited to: the nature, extent and duration of the original injury providing peripheral nociceptive input to the CNS;[6] stress-related responses;[58] psychological augmentation;[59] poorer health prior to the injury;[60] or a genetic predisposition.[61] Irrespective of the cause of the changes, the data indicate that consideration of these processes in the early management of WAD will be required.

RELATIONSHIPS BETWEEN SENSORY HYPERSENSITIVITY AND PSYCHOLOGICAL DISTRESS

Sensory hypersensitivity and psychological distress coexist in individuals with whiplash, particularly in those with moderate-to-severe symptoms.[54] For this reason, some have argued that the sensory changes may reflect psychological factors and their associated influence on nociceptive processing.[59] It would be worthwhile to have some idea of these relationships as this may provide information on how best to target or integrate different management approaches.

There does appear to be some relationship between psychological factors and sensory disturbance. Sterling et al. demonstrated moderate associations between pain thresholds (pressure and cold) at some sites, particularly at more remote sites, such as in the lower limb, and both psychological distress (GHQ-28) and catastrophisation (Pain Catastrophising Scale, PCS) in individuals with chronic WAD.[40] Similar results have been found in patients with acute WAD, where cold pain threshold and catastrophisation show moderate correlations.[62] Notably, there appears to be no relationship between psychological factors and the intensity of electrical stimulation required to elicit a flexor withdrawal response in biceps femoris in patients with chronic whiplash,[40] nor in healthy controls.[41] These findings indicate that psychological factors may play a role in central hyperexcitability. However, they do not support the assumption that psychological factors are the only or main factors responsible for central hyperexcitability in whiplash patients. In particular, spinal cord hyperexcitability appears not to be affected, at least significantly, by psychological factors.

The relationships between sensory changes and post-traumatic stress symptoms have also been explored. Sterling and Kenardy showed that the early presence of sensory hypersensitivity (mechanical and cold hyperalgesia) was associated with persistent post-traumatic stress symptoms but that this relationship was mediated by initial pain and disability levels (in this case, neck disability index [NDI] scores).[63] These findings suggest that the link between sensory hypersensitivity and post-traumatic stress symptoms is influenced by the level of pain and disability. The relationships between sensory hypersensitivity, pain and disability and post-traumatic stress has been corroborated in a recent study. Using trajectory modelling analyses, distinct trajectories or clinical pathways for both pain and disability and post-traumatic stress disorder (PTSD) symptoms were identified.[64] Interestingly, cold hyperalgesia (cold pain thresholds of less than 13°C) predicted inclusion in both more severe pain and disability trajectories and PTSD trajectories.[56] This suggests common mechanisms may underlie the development of chronic pain and PTSD symptoms following whiplash injury. Additionally, dual analyses revealed that the developmental trajectories of pain and disability and PTSD were mostly in synchrony. For example, individuals are more likely to show higher pain/disability and higher PTSD symptoms or low pain/disability and low PTSD symptoms rather than contradictory inclusion in, say, low pain/disability and high PTSD trajectories.[56] Together, the findings of these studies suggest close relationships between reported pain/disability levels, PTSD symptoms and the sensory presentation of WAD, and that all factors should be considered in the assessment and management of WAD.

Thus, it appears that psychological factors, such as distress, catastrophisation and post-traumatic stress symptoms, show some association with sensory hypersensitivity in cases of chronic whiplash. However, this relationship is not consistent for all modalities, measures or at all body sites tested, and may be mediated by levels of pain and disability. This would suggest that psychological factors are not the only or main factors responsible for central hyperexcitability in whiplash patients. Central hyperexcitability after whiplash is, therefore, a complex phenomenon that probably involves both neurobiological changes as well as psychological factors.

Recent models have been put forward in an attempt to provide a basis for the complex interrelationships between physical and psychological aspects of the whiplash condition. It has been suggested that the dysregulation of neurobiological pain processing is related to the stress response and/or sympathetic activation in the early stages following injury, and that this interaction may be a critical step in the development of persistent pain.[58, 65] These aspects are discussed in Chapter 9.

IMPLICATIONS FOR CLINICAL MANAGEMENT OF WHIPLASH

Assessment of the patient with whiplash

From the data presented in this chapter, it is clear that the identification of sensory hypersensitivity in patients with WAD is important for several reasons, including: the prognostic capacity of some sensory measures;[54] as a potential indicator of non-responsiveness to physical treatment approaches;[66] and as a possible indicator for alternative treatment approaches, such as medication.

As outlined, recent calls have been made to direct clinical examination towards the recognition and identification of mechanisms involved in the patient's pain syndrome.[67] At present, sensory examination, such as that required to detect the variety of sensory disturbances outlined above, is rarely performed and, if it is performed, is usually limited to rudimentary assessment of muscle power, deep tendon reflexes and light touch sensation. More detailed assessment of sensory changes in patients with neck pain is necessary. The first stage of this assessment would be a thorough recording of the patient's symptoms, including the nature of the pain. Although the usefulness of symptom classification as a way of clarifying pain mechanisms is debatable, it is a necessary part of the patient's assessment.[68] In recent times, questionnaires have been developed that aim to specifically identify neuropathic-like pain. Using one of these tools, the S-LANSS questionnaire,[69] it was shown that 30% of an acute whiplash cohort most likely have a predominantly neuropathic pain condition, with certain items being particularly associated with higher levels of pain and disability.[70] These items were 'electric shock' type pain that comes in bursts, burning pain in the neck and hyperalgesia to manual pressure. Inclusion of this questionnaire with particular attention to these items may be a useful addition to the clinical assessment of patients with acute WAD.

Quantitative sensory testing can also be utilised. This could include the measurement of mechanical pain thresholds with pressure algometry and determination of the presence of allodynia with light tactile stimulation. Cold hyperalgesia is emerging as an important factor both in the prediction of outcome[54] and for gauging treatment responsiveness.[66] It is more difficult to measure clinically, but options may include the use of thermorollers set at predetermined temperatures[68] or the time taken to reach pain threshold following the application of ice.[71]

The development of the most appropriate sensory examination of whiplash-injured patients is at an early stage, and moves towards further development into clinically valid and useful measures is of vital importance. Advances have been made in the development of clinical approaches to identify pain processes and these will, no doubt, assist in the future assessment of the whiplash condition.[72]

Drug management and other interventions

In the frame of translation of basic knowledge into clinical practice, a number of issues need to be addressed. Central hyperexcitability is now recognised as being present in patients with whiplash. However, this knowledge applies to the comparison of groups of patients with groups of healthy volunteers. Within patients, a high variability of measures of central hypersensitivity is usually observed. This means that different patients probably display different degrees of altered central pain processing. Furthermore, it is possible that not all patients are characterised by central hypersensitivity, as suggested by the overlap of pain thresholds between patients and controls.[39] In this respect, an essential step is the identification and validation of methods to assess and quantify central hypersensitivity in individual patients. Data on large samples that define the reference values of measures of pain sensitivity are becoming available.[41, 72] This information may soon provide the clinician with comparative data to explore a patient's nociceptive system on an individual basis.

A further aspect is the identification of treatments that attenuate central hypersensitivity. Possibly, interventions aiming at treating tissue damage or preventing nociceptive impulses from arriving at the spinal cord could also produce resolution of central hypersensitivity. However, there is no way of providing a long-lasting block of peripheral nociceptive afferents in most chronic pain conditions. One of the few exceptions is the use of radiofrequency neurotomy to treat whiplash pain arising from the zygapophyseal joints.[73, 74] Pharmacological interventions that affect the encoding and transmission of nociceptive signals at the CNS may provide unspecific attenuation of central hyperexcitability. COX-2 inhibitors and opioids belong to this category. There is a lack of controlled data on the efficacy of these interventions in patients with whiplash, but clinical experience shows, at best, modest results.

Modulatory mechanisms at the CNS can be affected by antidepressants via their effect on the monoaminergic system that is involved in endogenous modulation. Anticonvulsants may also have efficacy in attenuating central hyperexcitability. Indeed, both antidepressants and anticonvulsants are effective in pain syndromes characterised by central hyperexcitability, such as fibromyalgia.[75, 76]

GABA agonists have potential usefulness for the reversion of the disinhibitory processes described above. However, sedation strongly limits the clinical usefulness of GABAergic drugs for pain management. Subtype-selective compounds targeting alpha-2 and/or alpha-3 subunit-containing $GABA_A$ receptors produce antinociception and antihyperalgesia in mice and rats without sedation and without tolerance induction.[77] Such compounds may become available for clinical trials in pain management and could give new perspectives for a more selective targeting of pain pathways with GABAergic drugs.

A general major problem is the untargeted use of interventions. To date, 'classes' of drugs are given to 'classes' of patients (e.g. whiplash), although the mechanisms that are responsible for the pain conditions are probably highly variable within the same 'class' of patients. The progresses in the elucidation of altered pain mechanisms in single patients may lead, in the future, to a more targeted therapeutic approach. The perspective is that drugs acting on specific pain mechanisms would be given to those patients in which alterations in that mechanism are detected. So far, such an approach still needs to be subjected to intensive translational pain research.

Physical interventions

Clinical guidelines for the management of acute and chronic WAD promote education, assurance to the patient, the maintenance of activity levels, general and specific exercises, simple analgesics and encouragement of coping strategies.[78–80] Some recent clinical guidelines have recognised the complex presentation of some individuals with whiplash and have attempted to include recommendations for the identification of factors such as sensory disturbance and psychological distress.[79]

While the resumption of activity is almost universally recommended, the case for the avoidance of pain provocation may be an important aim of any physical intervention for patients demonstrating features of central hyperexcitability. The application of non-judicious, physical, mechanically stimulating treatments may serve to maintain and prolong this hypersensitivity and have a deleterious effect on the patient's long-term outcome.[81] It is not suggested that these patients avoid activity, as the maintenance of activity levels opposed to rest and the use of a collar has been shown to be important in the management of acute whiplash.[82] Recently, it has been shown that immobilisation in asymptomatic individuals can lead to sensory disturbances similar to those seen in WAD, indicating that this approach may have a detrimental effect on outcomes.[83] Certainly, studies investigating fibromyalgia, a condition also proposed to have disturbed central pain-processing mechanisms, have shown that sensory hypersensitivity increases following some forms of exercise, including isometric and submaximal aerobic exercise.[84] While similar investigations have not yet been conducted in patients with WAD, it would seem prudent that care is taken with the physical rehabilitation and exercise prescription for individuals with WAD and sensory hypersensitivity.

This is not to suggest that exercise and movement approaches are not indicated for individuals with whiplash. A combined specific exercise and manual therapy approach has demonstrated efficacy in the management of cervicogenic headache (idiopathic neck pain),[85] and this treatment approach has shown to decrease pain and disability in patients with chronic whiplash *without* the presence of mechanical and cold hyperalgesia—signs of central hyperexcitability.[66] It may be that such an approach has a greater role in patients in these subgroups of neck pain. However, it is apparent that it will be important to identify those patients with the presence of sensory hypersensitivity (and psychological distress, particularly post-traumatic stress) such that additional or alternative management can be provided. The difficulty at present is knowing what the best management approaches are for this more complex patient.

Theoretically, physical interventions such as transcutaneous electrical nerve stimulation (TENS) and acupuncture may be useful in modulating sensory hypersensitivity but these have not been specifically investigated in patients with WAD. A recent pilot study showed that cervical manual therapy (lateral glide technique) modulated spinal hyperexcitability measured via nociceptive withdrawal thresholds in the lower limb but had no effect on sensory hypersensitivity immediately post-treatment in participants with chronic WAD, indicating that different mechanisms may underlie nociceptive withdrawal responses and sensory hypersensitivity.[86] While more long-term effects on pain processing of this form of treatment are unknown, and the authors were not advocating the use of spinal manual therapy as a monotherapy for whiplash,[86] nevertheless it may indicate that combinations of treatment approaches targeted at different mechanisms may be beneficial. Intuitively, innovative interventions, such as sensory discrimination training[87] or motor imagery[88] shown to decrease pain in complex regional pain syndrome, may be helpful for whiplash management but such approaches have not been investigated for whiplash.

Psychological interventions with respect to central hyperexcitability

The relationships between pain and disability, sensory characteristics and psychological features of the whiplash condition suggest that psychologically based interventions may influence both former manifestations. Cognitive approaches, including education in various forms, have been shown to be effective in reducing pain and disability in acute whiplash when compared to usual care,[89] as well as influencing pain cognitions in low back pain.[90] Such approaches may also have the capacity to decrease central hyperexcitability via descending supraspinal influences. While evidence in this regard is at present scant, some preliminary data indicate some promise in this regard. Wiech et al. demonstrated the modulation of pain-related activity in the brain (using functional MRI) and hyperalgesia in an experimental pain model following a cognitive task.[91] In a single case study, Moseley showed reduced pain-related brain activity in a person with chronic low back pain following an educational intervention.[92] Other cognitive approaches, including progressive muscle relaxation and hypnosis, have shown a capacity to modulate spinal hyperexcitability via measurement of nociceptive withdrawal reflex responses.[93, 94]

Further studies are required investigating the influence of educational approaches and psychological interventions on central hyperexcitability and health outcomes following whiplash injury.

CONCLUSION

The identification of a peripheral structural lesion following whiplash injury has been only partially successful and, instead, focus has shifted towards the identification of processes that underlie pain and disability associated with the whiplash condition. The presence of sensory features indicative of augmented central pain-processing mechanisms is a characteristic of some whiplash-injured individuals, in both the acute and chronic stages of the condition. Sensory hypersensitivity shows the capacity both to predict those individuals at risk of poor functional recovery and to identify those who may not respond well to standard physical rehabilitation approaches. For these reasons, it is important that the clinical assessment of the patient with whiplash includes sensory evaluation. Intuitively, it would seem that drug management may be a treatment option to attenuate CNS changes but there is a lack of controlled data on the efficacy of these interventions in patients with whiplash. Physical treatment approaches, while important, will need to be undertaken with care in order to avoid amplifying central augmentation. The modulating effects of physical and psychological interventions on central hyperexcitability require further investigation.

References

1. Siegmund G, Winkelstein B, Ivancic P, et al. The anatomy and biomechanics of acute and chronic whiplash injury. *Traffic Inj Prev* 2009;10(2):101–12.
2. Haldeman S, Carroll L, Cassidy D, et al. The Bone and Joint Decade 2000–2010 Task Force on Neck Pain and Its Associated Disorders Executive Summary. *Spine* 2008;33(4s):S5–S7.
3. Elliott J, Sterling M, Noteboom T, et al. The clinical presentation of chronic whiplash and the relationship to findings of MRI fatty infiltrates in the cervical extensor musculature: a preliminary investigation. *Eur Spine J* 2009;18(9):1371–8.
4. Ichihara D, Okado E, Chiba K, et al. Longitudinal magnetic resonance imaging study on whiplash injury patients: minimum 10-year follow-up. *J Orthop Sci* 2009;14(5):602–10.
5. Haanpaa M, Backonja M, Bennett M, et al. Assessment of neuropathic pain in primary care. *Am J Med* 2009;122(10S):S13–21.
6. Rang H, Bevan S, Dray A. Chemical activation of nociceptive peripheral neurones. *Br Med Bull* 1991;47: 534–48.
7. Treede R, Meyer R, Raja S, Campbell J. Peripheral and central mechanisms of cutaneous hyperalgesia. *Prog Neurobiol* 1992;38:397–421.
8. Schmidt R, Schmelz M, Forster C, et al. Novel classes of responsive and unresponsive C nociceptors in human skin. *J Neurosci* 1995;15(1):333–41.
9. Michael G & Priestly J. Differential expression of the mRNA for the vanilloid receptor subtype 1 in cells of the adult rat dorsal root and nodose ganglia and its downregulation by axotomy. *J Neurosci* 1999;19(5):1844–54.
10. Neumann S, Doubell T, Leslie T, Woolf C. Inflammatory pain hypersensitivity mediated by phenotypic switch in myelinated primary sensory neurons. *Nature* 1996;384:360–4.
11. LaMotte R, Thalhammer J, Torebjork H, Robinson C. Peripheral neural mechanisms of cutaneous hyperalgesia following mild injury by heat. *J Neurosci* 1982;2(6):765–81.
12. Woolf C & Salter M. Neuronal plasticity: increasing the gain in pain. *Science* 2000;288:1765–9.
13. Woolf C & Thompson S. The induction and maintenance of central sensitization is dependent on N-methyl-D-aspartic acid receptor activation; implications for the treatment of post-injury pain hypersensitivity states. *Pain* 1991;44(3):293–9.
14. Dickenson A & Sullivan A. Evidence for a role of the NMDA receptor in the frequency dependent potentiation of deep rat dorsal horn nociceptive neurones following C fibre stimulation. *Neuropharmacology* 1987;26(8):1235–8.
15. McCrory C, Diviney D, Moriarty J, et al. Comparison between repeat bolus intrathecal morphine and an epidurally delivered bupivacaine and fentanyl combination in the management of post-thoracotomy pain with or without cyclooxygenase inhibition. *J Cardiothorac Vasc Anesth* 2002;16(5):607–11.
16. Samad T & Abdi S. Cyclooxygenase-2 and antagonists in pain management. *Curr Opinion Anaesthesiol* 2001;14(5):527–32.
17. Hoheisel U, Mense S, Simons D, Yu X. Appearance of new receptive fields in rat dorsal horn neurons following noxius stimulation of skeletal muscle – a model for referral of muscle pain. *Neurosci Lett* 1993;153(1):9–12.
18. Woolf C & Mannion R. Neuropathic pain: aetiology, symptoms, mechanisms and management. *Lancet* 1999;353:1959–64.
19. Zeilhofer H & Zeilhofer U. Spinal dis-inhibition in inflammatory pain. *Neurosci Lett* 2008;437(3):170–4.
20. Scholz J, Broom D, Youn D, et al. Blocking caspase activity prevents transsynaptic neuronal apoptosis and the loss of inhibition in lamina II of the dorsal horn after peripheral nerve injury. *J Neurosci* 2005;25(32): 7317–23.
21. Dubner R & Ren K. Endogenous mechanisms of sensory modulation. *Pain* 1999;Suppl 6:S45–S53.
22. Yu L & Han J. Habenula as a relay in the descending pathway from nucleus accumbens to periaqueductal grey subserving antinociception. *Int J Neurosci* 1990;54(3–4):245–51.
23. Li P & Zhuo M. Cholinergic, noradrenergic, and serotonergic inhibition of fast synaptic transmission in spinal lumbar dorsal horn of rat. *Brain Res Bull* 2001;54(6):639–47.

24. Green G, Scarth J, Dickenson A. An excitatory role for 5-HT in spinal inflammatory nociceptive transmission; state-dependent actions via dorsal horn 5-HT(3) receptors in the anaesthetized rat. *Pain* 2000;89(1):81–8.
25. Suzuki R & Dickenson A. Neuropharmacologic targets and agents in fibromyalgia. *Curr Pain Headache Rep* 2002;6(4):267–73.
26. Curatolo M, Petersen-Felix S, Arendt-Nielsen L, et al. Central hypersensitivity in chronic pain after whiplash injury. *Clin J Pain* 2001;17(4):306–15.
27. Kosek E, Ekholm J, Hansson P. Sensory dysfunction in fibromyalgia patients with implications for pathogenic mechanisms. *Pain* 1996;68:375–83.
28. Kosek E & Ordeberg G. Abnormalities of somatosensory perception in patients with painful osteoarthritis normalize following successful treatment. *Eur J Pain* 2000;4:228–38.
29. Song G, Venkatraman V, Ho K, et al. Cortical effects of anticipation and endogenous modulation of visceral pain assessed by functional brain MRI in irritable bowel syndrome patients and healthy controls. *Pain* 2006;126(1–3):79–90.
30. Yarnitsky D, Crispel Y, Eisenberg E, et al. Prediction of chronic post-operative pain: Pre-operative DNIC testing identifies patients at risk. *Pain* 2008;138:22–8.
31. Giesecke T, Graceley R, Grant M, et al. Evidence of augmented central pain processing in idiopathic chronic low back pain. *Arthritis Rheum* 2004;50(2):613–23.
32. Flor H, Elbert T, Knecht S, et al. Phantom-limb pain as a perceptual correlate of cortical reorganization following arm amputation. *Nature* 1995;375(6351):482–4.
33. Maihofer C, Handwerker H, Neundorfer B, Birklein F. Cortical reorganization during recovery from complex regional pain syndrome. *Neurology* 2004;63(4):693–701.
34. Flor H, Knost B, Birbaumer N. Processing of pain- and body-related verbal material in chronic pain patients: central and peripheral correlates. *Pain* 1997;73(3):413–21.
35. Apkarian A, Sosa Y, Sonty S, et al. Chronic back pain is associated with decreased prefrontal and thalamic gray matter density. *J Neurosci* 2004;24(46):104–5.
36. Sheather-Reid R & Cohen M. Psychophysical evidence for a neuropathic component of chronic neck pain. *Pain* 1998;75:341–7.
37. Koelbaek-Johansen M, Graven-Nielsen T, Schou-Olesen A, Arendt-Nielsen L. Muscular hyperalgesia and referred pain in chronic whiplash syndrome. *Pain* 1999;83:229–34.
38. Moog M, Quintner J, Hall T, Zusman M. The late whiplash syndrome: a psychophysical study. *Eur J Pain* 2002;6(4):283–94.
39. Banic B, Petersen-Felix S, Andersen O, et al. Evidence for spinal cord hypersensitivity in chronic pain after whiplash injury and in fibromyalgia. *Pain* 2004;107 (1–2):7–15.
40. Sterling M, Pettiford C, Hodkinson E, Curatolo M. Psychological factors are related to some sensory pain thresholds but not nociceptive flexion reflex threshold in chronic whiplash. *Clin J Pain* 2008;24(2):124–30.
41. Neziri A, Andersen O, Petersen-Felix S, et al. The nociceptive withdrawal reflex: normative values of thresholds and reflex receptive fields. *Eur J Pain* 2010;14(2):134–41.
42. Bajaj P, Bajaj P, Madsen H, Arendt-Nielsen L. Endometriosis is associated with central sensitization: a psychophysical controlled study. *J Pain* 2003;4(7):372–80.
43. Sorensen J, Graven-Nielsen T, Henriksson K, et al. Hyperexcitability in fibromyalgia. *J Rheumatol* 1998; 25(1):152–5.
44. Bajaj P, Bajaj P, Graven-Nielsen T, Arendt-Nielsen L. Osteoarthritis and its association with muscle hyperalgesia: an experimental controlled study. *Pain* 2001;93(2):107–14.
45. Bendtsen L, Jensen R, Olesen J. Decreased pain detection and tolerance thresholds in chronic tension-type headache. *Arch Neurol* 1996;53(4):373–6.
46. Ayesh E, Jensen T, Svensson P. Hypersensitivity to mechanical and intra-articular electrical stimuli in persons with painful temporomandibular joints. *J Dental Res* 2007;86(12):1187–92.
47. Gottrup H, Andersen J, Arendt-Nielsen L, Jensen T. Psychophysical examination in patients with post-mastectomy pain. *Pain* 2000;87(3):275–84.
48. Kasch H, Stengaard-Pedersen K, Arendt-Nielsen L, Staehelin Jensen T. Pain thresholds and tenderness in neck and head following acute whiplash injury: a prospective study. *Cephalalgia* 2001;21:189–97.
49. Sterling M, Jull G, Vicenzino B, Kenardy J. Characterisation of acute whiplash associated disorders. *Spine* 2004;29(2):182–8.
50. Sterling M, Jull G, Vicenzino B, Kenardy J. Sensory hypersensitivity occurs soon after whiplash injury and is associated with poor recovery. *Pain* 2003;104:509–17.
51. Chien A, Eliav E, Sterling M. Hypoaesthesia occurs in acute whiplash irrespective of pain and disability levels and the presence of sensory hypersensitivity. *Clin J Pain* 2008;24(9):759–66.
52. Chien A, Eliav E, Sterling M. The development of sensory hypoaesthesia after whiplash injury. *Clin J Pain* 2010;26(8):722–8.
53. Sterling M, Jull G, Kenardy J. Physical and psychological predictors of outcome following whiplash injury maintain predictive capacity at long term follow-up. *Pain* 2006;122:102–8.

54. Sterling M, Jull G, Vicenzino B, et al. Physical and psychological factors predict outcome following whiplash injury. *Pain* 2005;114:141–8.
55. Kasch H, Qerama E, Bach F, Jensen T. Reduced cold pressor pain tolerance in non-recovered whiplash patients: a 1 year prospective study. *Eur J Pain* 2005;9(5):561–9.
56. Sterling M, Hendrikz J, Kenardy J. Developmental trajectories of pain and disability and posttraumatic stress symptoms following whiplash injury. In: Williamson O (ed.). Australian Spine Society Annual Meeting. Brisbane, 2009.
57. Sterling M. Differential development of sensory hypersensitivity and a measure of spinal cord hyperexcitability following whiplash injury. *Pain* 2010;150:501–6.
58. McLean S, Clauw D, Abelson J, Liberzon I. The development of persistent pain and psychological morbidity after motor vehicle collision: integrating the potential role of stress response systems into a biopsychosocial model. *Psychosom Med* 2005;67: 783–90.
59. Wand B, O'Connell N, Parkitny L. Letter to the editor: Depression may contribute to the sensory changes in whiplash patients? *Man Ther* 2010;15(3):e1.
60. Wynne-Jones G, Jones G, Wiles N, et al. Predicting new onset of widespread pain following a motor vehicle collision. *J Rheumatol* 2006;33:968–74.
61. Hocking L, Smith B, Jones G, et al. Genetic variation in the beta2-adrenergic receptor but not catecholamine-O-methyltransferase predisposes to chronic pain: results from the 1958 British Birth Cohort Study. *Pain* 2010;149(1):143–51.
62. Rivest K, Cote J, Dumas J-P, et al. Relationships between pain thresholds, catastrophizing and gender in acute whiplash injury. *Man Ther* 2010;15:154–9.
63. Sterling M & Kenardy J. The relationship between sensory and sympathetic nervous system changes and acute posttraumatic stress following whiplash injury – a prospective study. *J Psychosom Res* 2006;60: 387–93.
64. Sterling M, Hendrikz J, Kenardy J. Developmental trajectories of pain/disability and PTSD symptoms following whiplash injury. *Pain* 2010;in press.
65. Passatore M & Roatta S. Influence of sympathetic nervous system on sensorimotor function: whiplash associated disorders (WAD) as a model. *Eur J Appl Physiol* 2006;98(5):423–49.
66. Jull G, Sterling M, Kenardy J, Beller E. Does the presence of sensory hypersensitivity influence outcomes of physical rehabilitation for chronic whiplash? A preliminary RCT. *Pain* 2007;129(2): 28–34.
67. Max M. Is mechanism-based pain treatment attainable? Clinical trial issues. *J Pain* 2000;1(3): 2–9.
68. Jensen T & Baron R. Translation of symptoms and signs into mechanisms in neuropathic pain. *Pain* 2003;102(2):1–8.
69. Bennett M, Smith B, Torrance N, Potter J. The S-LANSS score for identifiying pain of predominantly neuropathic origin: validation for use in clinical and postal research. *J Pain* 2005;6(3):149–58.
70. Sterling M & Pedler A. A neuropathic pain component is common in acute whiplash and associated with a more complex clinical presentation. *Man Ther* 2009;14(2):173–9.
71. Cathcart S & Pritchard D. Relability of pain threshold measurement in young adults. *J Headache Pain* 2006;7:21–6.
72. Rolke R, Magerl W, Cambell K, et al. Quantitative sensory testing: a comprehensive protocol for clinical trials. *Eur J Pain* 2006;10:77–88.
73. Lord S, Barnsley L, Wallis B, et al. Percutaneous radiofrequency neurotomy for chronic cervical zygapophyseal joint pain. *N Engl J Med* 1996;335(23):1721–6.
74. Barnsley L. Percutaneous radiofrequency neurotomy for chronic neck pain: outcomes in a series of consecutive patients. *Pain Med* 2005;6(4):282–6.
75. Hauser W, Bernardy K, Uceyler N, Sommer C. Treatment of fibromyalgia syndrome with gabapentin and pregabalin–a meta-analysis of randomized controlled trials. *Pain* 2009;145(1–2):69–81.
76. Rao S. Current progress in the pharmacological therapy of fibromyalgia. *Expert Opin Investig Drugs* 2009;18(10):1479–93.
77. Knabl J, Witschi R, Hosl K, et al. Reversal of pathological pain through specific spinal GABAA receptor subtypes. *Nature* 2008;451(7176): 330–4.
78. Scholten-Peeters G, Bekkering G, Verhagen A, et al. Clinical practice guideline for the physiotherapy of patients with whiplash associated disorders. *Spine* 2002;27(4):412–22.
79. Motor Accident Authority (MAA). Guidelines for the management of whiplash associated disorders. Sydney: MAA (NSW), 2007.
80. South Australian Centre for Trauma and Injury Recovery. A clinical pathway for best practice management of acute and chronic whiplash-associated disorders. Adelaide: TRACsa, 2008.
81. Sterling M & Kenardy J. Physical and psychological aspects of whiplash: important considerations for primary care assessment. *Man Ther* 2008;13(2): 93–102.

82. Rosenfeld M, Seferiadis A, Carllson J, Gunnarsson R. Active intervention in patients with whiplash associated disorders improves long-term prognosis: a randomised controlled clinical trial. *Spine* 2003;28(22):2491–8.
83. Terkelsen A, Bach F, Jensen T. Experimental forearm immobilisation in humans induces cold and mechanical hyperalgesia. *Anesthesiology* 2008;109(2):297–307.
84. Vierck C. Mechanisms underlying development of spatially distributed chronic pain (fibromyalgia). *Pain* 2006;124:242–63.
85. Jull G, Trott P, Potter H, et al. A randomised controlled trial of physiotherapy management for cervicogenic headache. *Spine* 2002;27(17):1835–43.
86. Sterling M, Pedler A, Chan C, et al. Cervical lateral glide increases nociceptive flexion reflex but not pressure or thermal pain thresholds in chronic whiplash associated disorders. *Man Ther* 2010;15(2):149–53.
87. Moseley G & Wiech K. The effect of tactile discrimination training is enhanced when patients watch the reflected image of their unaffected limb during training. *Pain* 2009;144(3):314–19.
88. Daly E & Bialocerkowski A. Does evidence support physiotherapy management of adult complex regional pain syndrome type one? A systematic review. *Eur J Pain* 2009;13(4):339–53.
89. Oliveira A, Gevirtz R, Hubbard R. A psycho-educational video used in the emergency department provides effective treatment for whiplash injuries. *Spine* 2006;31(15):1652–7.
90. Moseley G, Nicholas M, Hodges P. A randomised controlled trial of intensive neurophysiology education in chronic low back pain. *Clin J Pain* 2004;20(5): 324–30.
91. Wiech K, Seymour B, Kalisch R, et al. Modulation of pain processing in hyperalgesia by cognitive demand. *Neuroimage* 2005;27:59–69.
92. Moseley G. Widespread brain activity during an abdominal task markedly reduced after pain physiology education: *f*MRI evaluation of a single patient with chronic low back pain. *Aust J Physiother* 2005;51:49–52.
93. Emery C, France C, Harris J, et al. Effects of progressive muscle relaxation training on nociceotive flexion reflex threshold in healthy young adults: a randomised trial. *Pain* 2008;138(2):375–9.
94. Kiernan B, Dane J, Phillips L, Proce D. Hypnotic analgesia reduces the R-III nociceptive reflex: further evidence concerning the multifactorial nature of hypnotic analgesia. *Pain* 1995;60:39–47.

CHAPTER 6
Neuromuscular dysfunction in whiplash associated disorders

Deborah Falla, James Elliott, Gwendolen Jull

The pain and trauma of a whiplash injury cause changes in muscle properties and in neuromuscular function. This chapter explores what is known of these reactions and their potential interactions with other features associated with a whiplash injury. Such knowledge underpins a research-informed rationale and approach to rehabilitation of neuromuscular dysfunction.

CHANGES IN THE PROPERTIES OF THE CERVICAL MUSCLES

Imaging studies (e.g. ultrasound and magnetic resonance imaging [MRI]) have shown alterations in the physical characteristics (i.e. fatty infiltrates, changes in cross-sectional area) in the cervical extensor and flexor muscles in patients with chronic whiplash-related neck pain.[1–3] These changes are present in both the neck extensors and flexors,[2, 3] and are most notable in muscles that possess a larger proportion of type I, slow-oxidative fibres and a higher density of muscle spindles (e.g. the deep longus colli/capitis, suboccipital muscles and multifidus) (Fig 6.1).[4, 5]

In relation to fatty infiltrates, the mechanism(s) of the traumatic whiplash injury event itself may underlie the changes in the muscles in some patients. The fatty replacement in the cervical extensor muscles was present in those with persistent symptoms following whiplash but not in individuals with persistent insidious-onset neck pain or in those without neck pain.[2, 6, 7] The degree of fatty infiltrate was not associated with age, body mass index, the duration of the disorder or compensation status, suggesting that the traumatic event may be a potential trigger for the changes.

While trauma may be a trigger, a preliminary investigation has shown that sensory, physical, kinaesthetic and psychological features all contribute to some extent to explain the varying levels of fatty infiltrate in muscle tissue.[8] These features characterise a complex, non-resolving injury and some are prognostic of non-recovery.[9] Of note, regression analysis determined that decreased cold pain threshold was a significant factor in the predictive model ($r^2 = 0.28$; $P = 0.02$), and this may provide new insights into the clinical presentation of the chronic condition. Hyperalgesia to cold stimuli, which has been identified in several investigations of WAD, may relate to alterations in the central nervous system's processing of pain.[10–13] These centrally driven changes, possibly indicative of neuropathic pain, may be potentially irreversible.[14] Thus, identifying quantifiable MRI changes in muscle properties and relating them to prognostic clinical measures in the chronic state could provide some plausible clinical hypotheses for possible pathophysiological processes of recalcitrant WAD.

A number of potential mechanisms could explain the changes in muscle structure and subsequent alterations in neuromuscular behaviour. Such factors include, but are not limited to: generalised disuse,[15] chronic denervation,[16, 17] systemic or inflammatory

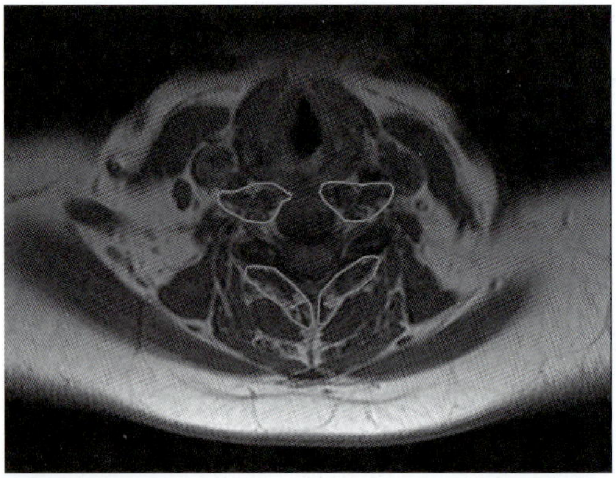

Figure 6.1 T1-weighted axial magnetic resonance image at the C6 vertebral level demonstrating outlined regions of interest for the right and left longus colli and the right and left posterior cervical multifidus. Increased signal, indicative of fatty infiltration, is noted in both sets of muscles in a person with chronic whiplash associated disorders (WAD).

myopathy following trauma[18, 19] or involvement of the sympathetic nervous system.[20]

Disuse

With disuse, morphometric changes in muscles are not uniform. For example, greater changes have been shown in muscles with more type I, slow-oxidative fibres.[21–24] This could account for the larger fat infiltration in the deep cervical muscles,[6, 8] which feature a greater density of type I fibres.[5] Disuse is, thus, a plausible hypothesis for muscle degeneration in whiplash-injured people with a long duration of symptoms. Nevertheless, recent evidence may refute disuse as the primary mechanism for long-term muscle alterations, as patients with chronic non-traumatic neck pain, despite having a greater mean duration of pain than those in a chronic whiplash group, showed values of fatty infiltrate that mirrored those with no history of neck pain.[6] Nevertheless, disuse may be more closely related to higher levels of pain rather than duration of symptoms. Pain levels may profoundly affect activity levels and, thus, muscle composition. Further investigations of people with pain and disability levels comparable to chronic whiplash are required to draw more definitive conclusions.

Response to trauma

The fatty changes observed in muscle may be adipoplastic or myoblastic in origin.[16] In particular, fibroblasts and pre-adipocytes are present in the perimuscular connective tissue and these precursor cells can differentiate into adipose tissue in response to traumatically induced local inflammation.[25, 26] Such a hypothesis follows the results of investigations in animals by Gradl et al.[27, 28] Profound changes in muscle tissue, including myocyte apoptosis, were observed in animals with a more severe injury and subsequently greater inflammatory reactions.[27, 28] Animals with a lesser injury did not exhibit such muscle changes. It is plausible that the changes (fatty infiltrates) in the neck muscles of patients with chronic whiplash may represent a more severe injury with greater motor impairments.

Muscular response to nerve injury

Until recently, it has been difficult to explain the specific mechanisms by which injury to different anatomical tissues in the spine alters the composition of the paraspinal muscles. Hodges et al.[29] demonstrated differential and rapid muscular changes within three days following experimental nerve and disc lesions. Specifically, this study demonstrated rapid ipsilesional and monosegmental atrophy and fat proliferation in the porcine lumbar multifidus with a disc lesion. In contrast, with injury to the medial branch of the third lumbar dorsal ramus, rapid atrophy and fat tissue were observed bilaterally and in multisegments of the multifidus muscle. These results provide evidence of rapid and differential alterations to the lumbar paraspinal muscles following induced injury to different anatomical tissues. It is possible that similar time frames and patterns for fat development occur in some patients following traumatic whiplash injury and, as such, could implicate specific anatomical tissues.

The segmental posterior cervical muscles receive their nerve supply from dorsal branches that are most proximal to the spinal nerve root.[30, 31] Thus, injury that is proximal to the origin of the dorsal branch may denervate the posterior paraspinal muscles. However, denervation of these muscles is unlikely if the injury is distal to the origin of the dorsal branch.[30, 31] An interesting aspect of the study by Hayashi et al.[30] was that abnormal MRI enhancement of the multifidus muscle did not occur without abnormal findings in the more superficial paraspinal muscles and without root avulsion. The pattern of fatty infiltrate in a chronic whiplash cohort (greater muscle changes in the deep multifidi compared to the superficial muscles[2]) reflects that of Hayashi et al.[30] While the cause of symptoms in whiplash is not likely to be due to nerve root avulsion, the multisegmental paraspinal fatty infiltrates in the multifidi together with the presence of altered pain processing in some subjects with chronic symptoms may implicate a lesser injury that was either proximal or just distal to the dorsal root ganglion prior to the 'take-off' of the medial branch of the dorsal ramus. Animal studies are required to test this hypothesis, whereby lesions can be made to specific anatomical structures and their effects on the muscular system can be controlled.

The possible diverse mechanisms for muscular alterations highlight a potentially confusing pathological presentation. The relationship between neck muscle degeneration, pain and disability levels and clinical features in the acute whiplash state must be confirmed or refuted before drawing strong clinical conclusions. Current and future research with advanced imaging should not assume a direct pathoanatomical correlate with symptoms. Rather, efforts should be placed on establishing whether the temporal development and the magnitude and location of neck muscle changes are related to clinical features (i.e. range of movements and neuromuscular functioning) and varying levels of pain and disability.

ALTERED NEUROMUSCULAR CONTROL IN WAD

In addition to changes in muscle properties, changes occur in neuromuscular control. Individuals who have experienced a whiplash injury are known to have impaired neck strength, which is apparent around all axes.[32] Furthermore, they show an impaired ability to maintain a steady neck contraction around a target force value.[33] Reduced force steadiness in patients with whiplash has been attributed to alterations in group Ia afferent input as these patients show greater power in the low frequency band of the force signal compared to asymptomatic subjects (Fig 6.2). Altered cervical afferent input may result from damaged or functionally impaired neck mechanoreceptors,[34] sensitisation of mechanoreceptors from pain,[35] decreased central inhibition[14] and sympathetic effects on muscle spindle sensitivity.[20] Accordingly, short-term vibration of the neck, which stimulates group Ia afferent input, increases force steadiness in women with whiplash-induced neck pain.[33]

Changes in motor output are accompanied by alterations in muscle strategies. Evidence suggests that neck pain may alter the task-related modulation of neck muscle activity so that motor control of the cervical spine is solved by alternative, presumably less efficient, combinations of muscle synergistic activities. As an example, impaired performance on a task of craniocervical flexion (anatomical action of the deep longus colli and longus capitis) has been shown to be a feature of whiplash-induced neck pain[36–38] and is present in other neck pain disorders, such as idiopathic neck pain,[39] work-related neck pain[40] and cervicogenic headache.[41] Reduced activation of the deep cervical flexors is associated with increased activation of the superficial neck muscles in patients with neck pain,[39] which is known

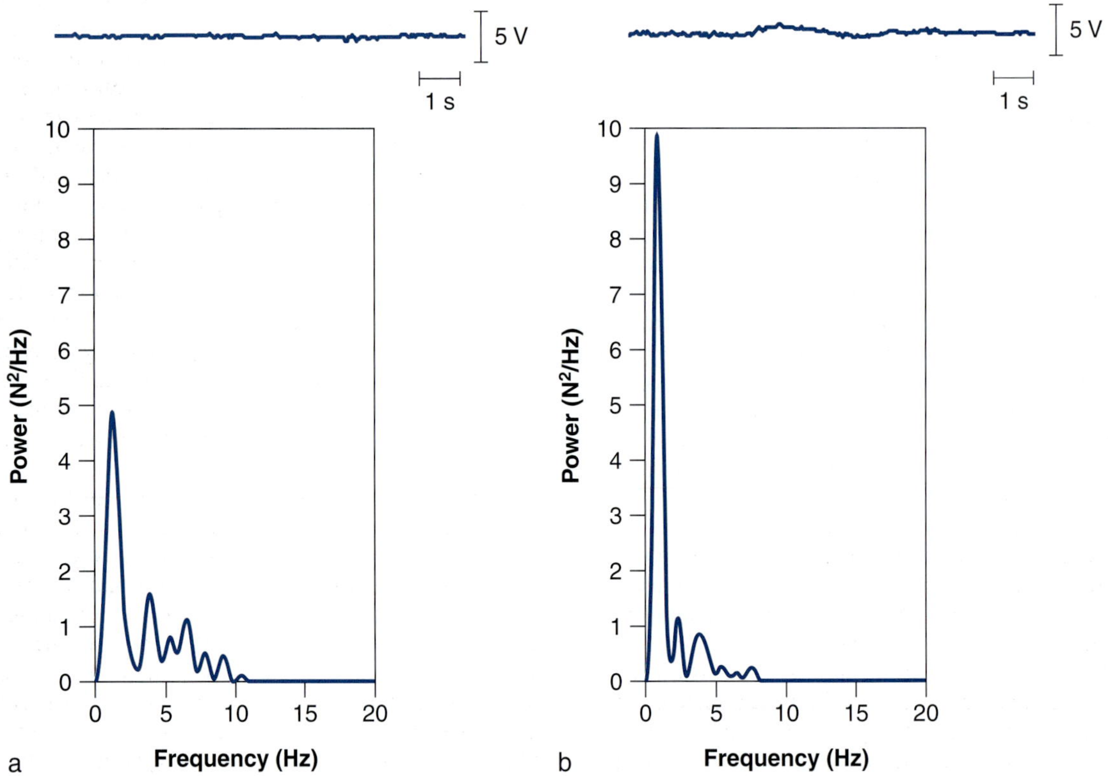

Figure 6.2 Representative force traces (top panel) obtained for (a) a control subject and (b) a patient with chronic neck pain patient during a 10-s isometric cervical flexion at 25% of maximal force. The bottom panel presents the power of the force signal in various frequency ranges (highlighted in grey). Note the increased power of the force signal in the low frequency band for the patient data. This is attributed to alterations in group Ia afferent input. (Reprinted with permission from Muceli et al.[33])

to occur within the first four weeks of a whiplash injury.[36]

A recent study showed that when women with either whiplash-induced or idiopathic neck pain performed isometric circular contractions of their neck at a fixed force level but with changes in force direction in the range 0–360° (Figs 6.3a, b), they displayed reduced specificity of sternocleidomastoid muscle activation with respect to asymptomatic individuals.[42] In particular, increased activation of the sternocleidomastoid muscle was evident when the muscle acted as an antagonist (Figs 6.3c, d). This observation indicates that the augmented activity of the superficial muscles in patients with neck pain reflects a loss of the predefined patterns of muscle activation and supports the consistent finding of augmented activity of the sternocleidomastoid muscle in such patients, regardless of the task examined; for example, cervical flexion,[43] craniocervical flexion[39, 44] and movements of the upper limb.[40, 45]

Reduced specificity of sternocleidomastoid muscle activity in patients with whiplash is associated with impaired neck flexion strength, which suggests that reduced strength is partially due to increased coactivation of their neck muscles.[32] Likewise, increased coactivation of the splenius capitis muscle during isometric cervical flexion (Fig 6.4) is inversely correlated with total neck strength and positively correlated with the patient's reported pain and perceived disability (Fig 6.5).[32] The strategy adopted by the patients, despite being inefficient, may reflect an attempt to voluntarily increase the stability of the head for the fear of performing potentially painful movements or the need to compensate for decreased activity of the deep cervical muscles.[39]

Direct recordings of single motor unit activity have been performed in order to better understand the mechanisms underlying augmented superficial neck muscle activity associated with neck pain. A recent study investigated the discharge rate of sternocleidomastoid motor units during brief isometric contractions performed in multiple directions of force in the horizontal plane.[42] The discharge rates of active motor units during a task will depend on the net excitatory input to the motor neuron pool and the intrinsic excitability of the motor neurons. Thus, it is expected that the excitatory input changes with direction of force with a consistent modulation that reflects the biomechanical efficiency in force production. Observations of motor unit behaviour in asymptomatic individuals confirm this hypothesis by revealing a consistent modulation in discharge of motor units depending on the direction of force (Fig 6.6). In contrast, women with neck pain display the same neural drive to the sternocleidomastoid muscle regardless of the direction of force. This result additionally explains the consistent finding of increased activity of this muscle in patients with neck pain. Furthermore, the patient group, but not controls, showed prolonged motor unit activity in their neck muscles following a contraction (Fig 6.7),[42] which confirms the reduced ability to relax muscles previously shown in surface EMG studies.[45, 46] Taken together, reduced modulation of neural drive to the muscle and prolonged motor unit activity following a contraction may indicate a potential change in motor neuron excitability due to pain and/or sympathetic activity (discussed below).

In addition to their role in neck movement and stability, the neck muscles are involved in proprioception and reflexes controlling postural orientation and stability.[47–49] Not surprisingly, whiplash-induced pain is also associated with impaired proprioception, reduced postural stability and reduced smoothness of eye movements. Alterations in proprioception may reflect abnormal spindle afferent discharge due to activation of chemoreceptive and nociceptive sensory afferent input,[50–53] direct trauma to cervical structures, or increased sympathetic drive,[54] resulting in a conflict of inputs from visual, vestibular and somatosensory sources; this may underlie the sensation of unsteadiness and dizziness frequently reported in whiplash patients.[55] Although greater errors in positioning the head following voluntary movement have been shown in persons with neck pain of both insidious[56] and traumatic onset,[57–59] proprioceptive acuity appears to be more affected in people with chronic whiplash,[58] especially in those reporting higher pain and disability[36, 60] and dizziness.[55] In addition to greater repositioning errors with head movement, people with whiplash show reduced proprioception at the shoulder and elbow.[61, 62]

Disturbed postural stability is also a feature of whiplash,[63–65] which includes larger postural trunk sway in both stance tasks and complex tasks, such as walking up and down stairs,[64, 66, 67] and reduced head stability in response to predictable and unpredictable postural perturbations.[64] Although balance disturbances have been reported in both traumatic and non-traumatic neck pain disorders, consistent with observations for head relocation, people with whiplash-induced pain generally show greater disturbances,[68] and postural instability is positively associated with the symptom of dizziness.[69] Disturbances of postural control are also thought to reflect disruption of cervical somatosensory input and a mismatch between somatosensory, visual and vestibular inputs.

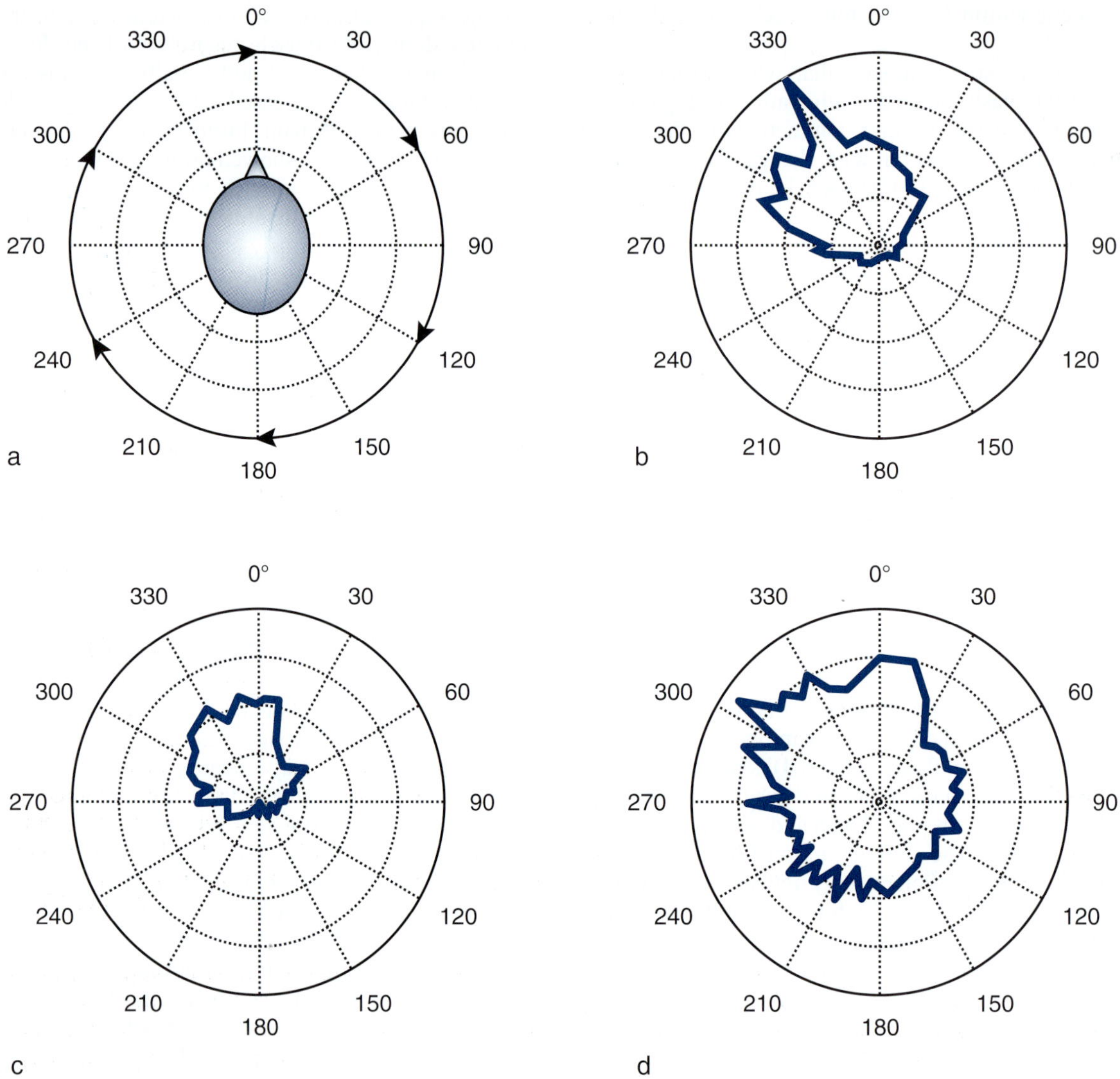

Figure 6.3 (a) Patients with chronic neck pain and control subjects performed isometric circular contractions at 15 N of force with change in force direction between 0° and 360°. (b) Surface electromyogram (EMG) was obtained from the sternocleidomastoid muscle and directional activation curves were calculated. The directional activation curve represents the modulation in intensity of muscle activity with the direction of force exertion. Representative directional activation curves are presented for the left sternocleidomastoid muscle for a (c) control subject and (d) patient. In this example, the control subject presents with defined activation of the sternocleidomastoid muscle with the highest amplitude of activity towards the ipsilateral anterolateral flexion direction. The sternocleidomastoid muscle is minimally active during extension or posterolateral extension, as expected. Conversely, the sternocleidomastoid directional activation curves for the representative patient indicate more even activation levels of the sternocleidomastoid muscle for all directions. (Reprinted with permission from Falla et al.[39])

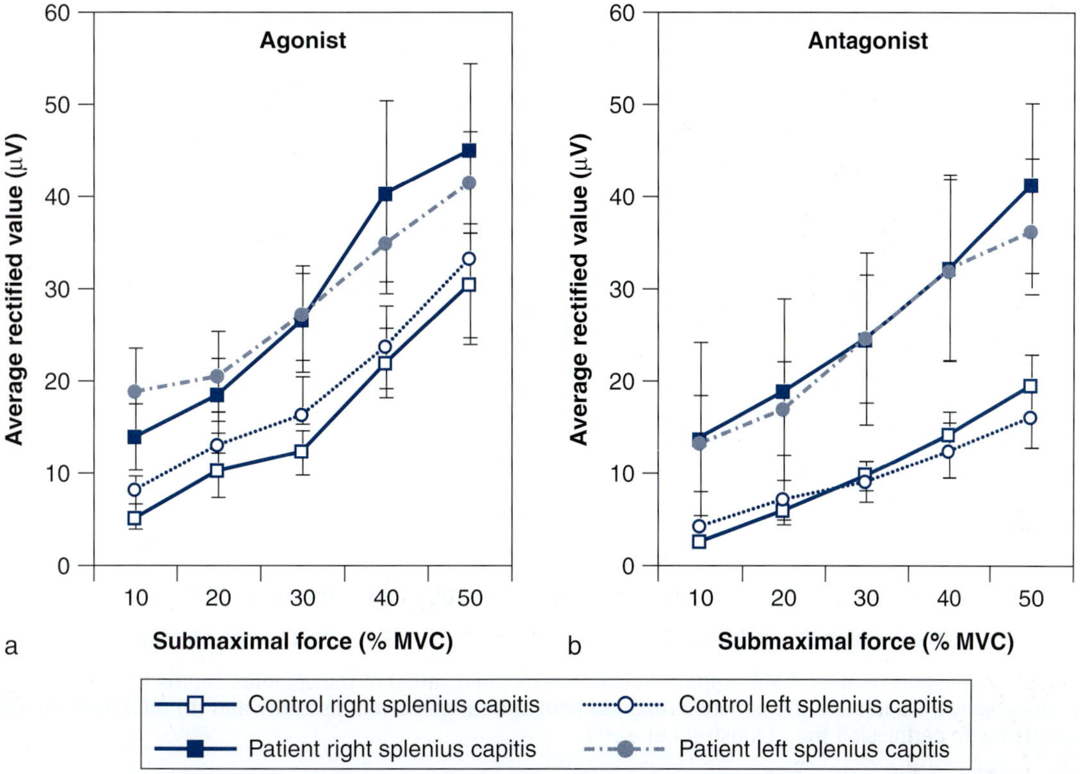

Figure 6.4 Mean and standard error of electromyographic (EMG) amplitude (average rectified value) recorded from the splenius capitis muscle bilaterally in a group of patients with chronic neck pain and control subjects. Subjects performed ramped contractions from 0% to 50% of their maximal force in both (a) cervical extension and (b) flexion. Note the elevated EMG amplitude of the splenius capitis muscle for the patient group, particularly when the muscle is acting as an antagonist. (Reprinted with permission from Lindstrøm et al.[32])

Consistent with this hypothesis, changes in oculomotor control have also been demonstrated in people with whiplash, which is suggestive of disturbances in the cervicocollic and cervico-ocular reflexes.[70–73]

Nociceptive effects on sensorimotor function

Group III and IV muscle afferent receptors are sensitive to nociceptive stimuli[74] and this can be experimentally elicited in humans using various exogenous or endogenous methods, including intramuscular injection of hypertonic saline.[75] Experimental neck pain models provide a means to increase our understanding of the basic mechanisms underlying alterations of muscle activity in people with whiplash since injection of hypertonic saline produces a deep pain similar in quality to clinical pain.[76]

At rest, only a small and transient increase in postural electromyographic (EMG) activity has been observed in response to deep noxious stimulation of cervical muscles.[77, 78] However, experimental pain research has demonstrated convincingly that nociception substantially alters the load sharing among muscles during activity, which may lead to subsequent muscle overuse or disuse in functional activities. Evidence for an altered motor strategy has been provided at levels ranging from the motor unit[79] and motor unit pool[80] to a reorganisation of activity among agonist, synergist and antagonist muscles,[81, 82] and is known to occur immediately after the onset of pain.

As an example, hypertonic saline-evoked unilateral upper trapezius muscle pain induces an immediate bilateral reorganisation in the coordinated activity of the three subdivisions of the trapezius muscle during a dynamic task of the upper limb.[82] Overall, the results of experimental studies suggest that pain induces a dynamic reorganisation of the coordination among muscles in order to minimise the use of the

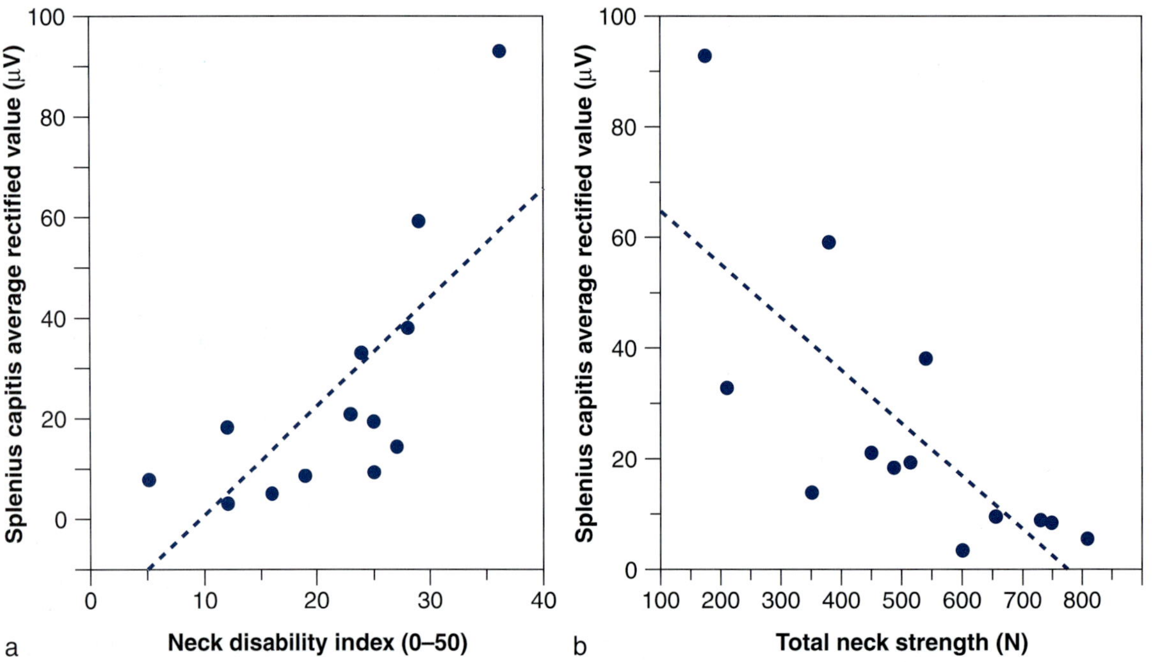

Figure 6.5 Correlation between EMG amplitude (average rectified value) of the splenius capitis muscle during isometric cervical flexion and the patient's reported pain and (a) perceived disability and (b) total neck strength. (Reprinted with permission from Lindstrøm et al.[32])

painful muscle with minimal disruption to the task. The reorganisation of motor strategy may be mediated by spinal (reflex) and supraspinal (cortical motor drive) mechanisms.

Although a reorganisation of neck muscle activity may have benefits in the short-term for reducing the load on the painful region, in the long term, pain-induced altered neural control may dispose some muscles to overload and, as a consequence, injury to other muscles due to reduced activity, with consequent atrophy of specific fibre types. Thus, long-term alterations in motor control may partially explain the morphological and histological changes documented in the cervical muscles in people with neck pain.[83]

Experimental studies also show that activation of nociceptive afferent fibres from neck muscles and joints affects the proprioceptive activity of muscle spindle afferent fibres[50–52] which may partially explain impaired proprioception in patients with whiplash. Furthermore, preliminary findings suggest that activation of the sympathetic nervous system via the cold pressor test is sufficient to induce altered neck proprioception (unpublished observations).

Sympathetic effects on sensorimotor function

Whiplash is frequently associated with psychosocial stress, which implies sympathetic nervous system activation,[9, 84] and impaired sympathetic vasoconstriction has demonstrated some prognostic capacity for poor outcome following a whiplash injury.[9] Sympathetic activity, which is influenced by pain,[85] affects muscle function and motor control by modulating local muscle blood flow, muscle contractility and proprioceptive activity from muscle spindle afferent input (see Passatore and Roatta for review[20]). These actions, together with the sympathetic control of other organ systems, support motor activity. However, some sympathetic actions on skeletal muscles may not always be functionally advantageous.

Adrenaline exerts a weakening effect on slow-twitch muscle fibres due to shortening of the muscle fibre twitch force, resulting in decreased development of force during subtetanic contractions.[86, 87] This effect is particularly relevant in postural muscles, including the neck muscles, which are composed of a high proportion of slow-twitch muscle fibres. A sympathetically mediated muscle weakening implies that the neural

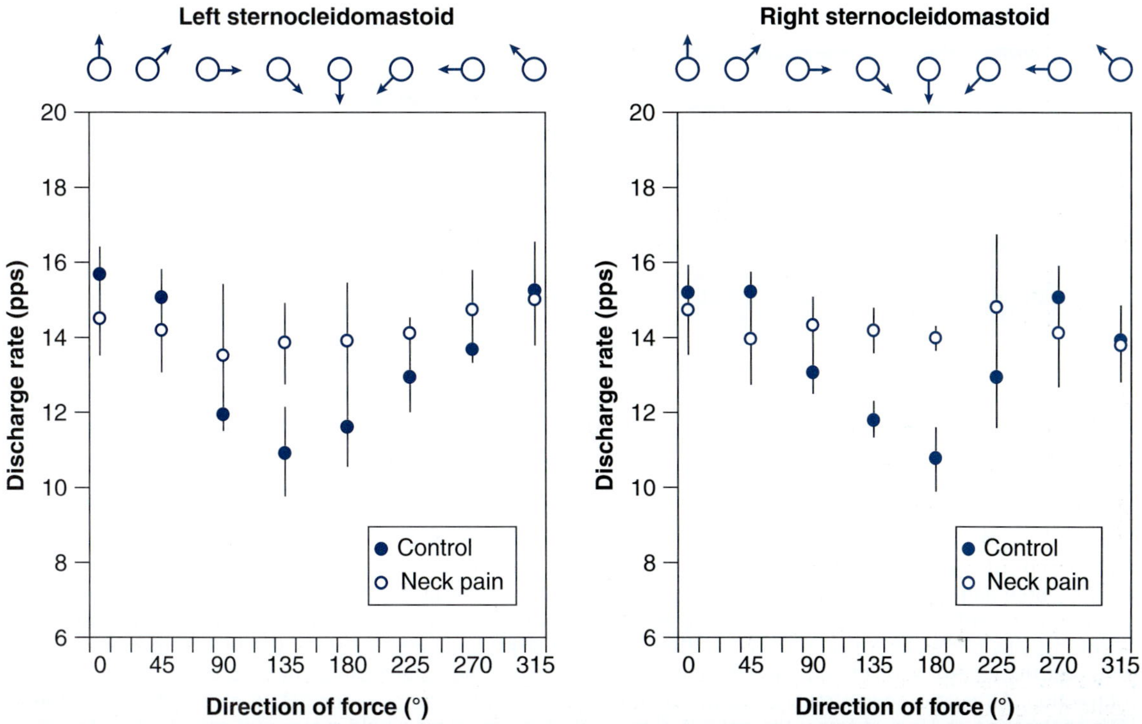

Figure 6.6 Mean and standard deviation of left and right sternocleidomastoid motor unit discharge rate (pps: pulses per second) for a group of control subjects and patients with chronic neck pain during 10-s contractions performed at 15 N of force in eight directions (45° intervals from 0° to 360°) in the horizontal plane. The symbols at the top of the image illustrate the directions of force. The control subjects display a consistent modulation in discharge of motor units depending on the direction of force. In contrast, the patient group displayed the same neural drive to the sternocleidomastoid muscle for all force directions. (Reprinted with lpermission from Falla et al.[42])

drive to motor neurons innervating slow-twitch muscle fibres should be increased in order to produce the same motor output.[87] Reduced maximal force and increased surface EMG amplitude of the superficial neck muscles in patients with whiplash are consistent with this effect.

In addition to influencing fibre contractility, the sympathetic nervous system is known to modulate the discharge of muscle spindles through an action exerted either on the receptors themselves or on their first neurons (see Akoev for review[88]). Sympathetic activation reduces the sensitivity of muscle spindles to muscle length changes, especially in jaw and neck muscles.[54, 89–91] This implies that the quality of proprioceptive information on muscle length changes is reduced, which should negatively impact on feedback correction of movements, as well as on the ability of the motor system to correct perturbations. As previously reviewed, whiplash patients show greater errors in positioning the head,[57–59] shoulder[61, 62] and elbow,[61, 62] disturbed postural stability,[63–65] and reduced head stability in response to predictable and unpredictable postural perturbations,[64] findings which may partially reflect sympathetic-induced changes in sensorimotor control.

The increased neural drive to the sternocleidomastoid muscle, which has been observed in whiplash patients, may also reflect an attempt to enhance kinaesthetic sense by muscular contraction, since increased muscle activity can enhance the acuity of movement detection.[92] This interpretation is also supported by the observation that stress increases the amplitude of muscle activation and results in increased co-contraction of the forearm muscles during typing or repetitive finger movement tasks.[93, 94]

Increased sympatho-adrenal outflow may also induce changes in the input–output relationships for motor neurons by providing metabotropic input. Noradrenaline is known to facilitate the generation of persistent inward currents in spinal motor neurons, which affects their excitability.[95] Increased motor neuron excitability produces higher motor unit discharge rates with similar excitatory input, which is in agreement with the observed higher activity of

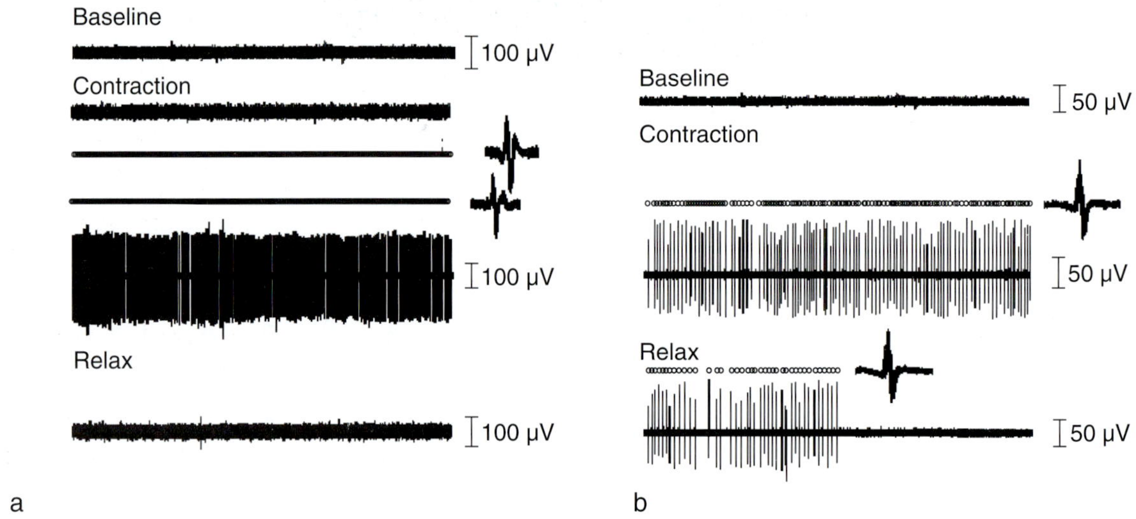

Figure 6.7 Representative single motor unit recordings from the sternocleidomastoid muscle of (a) one control subject and (b) one patient with neck pain obtained at rest, during a 10-s cervical flexion contraction at 15 N of force and immediately following the contraction when the subjects were asked to relax completely. Ten-second recordings of intramuscular EMG signals are presented, with the identified motor unit discharges represented by circles above each trace together with the corresponding template of the identified motor units. Note that the control subject and patient were able to fully relax their sternocleidomastoid muscle prior to contraction. Although the control subject was able to fully relax the sternocleidomastoid muscle following the 10-s contraction at 15 N of force, the patient data illustrates persistent single motor unit activity despite the instruction to fully relax. (Reprinted with permission from Falla et al.[42])

antagonist muscles in patients with neck pain.[32, 42] A further characteristic feature of neck pain is a reduced ability to relax the neck muscles following contractions. For example, persistent motor unit activity has been observed in patients with neck pain despite the instruction to fully relax their muscles.[42] This observation supports the possibility of persistent inward currents to neck motor neurons since, during relaxation, the input to motor neurons should be null. This interpretation is supported by the observations that the patients can voluntarily relax before a contraction but not immediately after a contraction, and is in agreement with the presence of activity-induced persistent inward currents.[96] Thus, stress and physiological distress can play a role in facilitating the development of altered muscle behaviour in chronic pain states and in maintaining chronic pain syndromes following a whiplash injury (Fig 6.8).

IMPLICATIONS FOR THE MANAGEMENT OF THE PATIENT WITH WHIPLASH

The evidence indicates that pain, the tissue injury and their various sequelae induce changes in cervical muscle function in patients with acute and chronic WAD. As has been discussed, clinical and experimental studies indicate that the dysfunction is characterised by a complex set of cervical neuromuscular adaptations, in both cervical motor control and the muscles' morphology. The changes in muscle behaviour appear early and persist in the long term.[36, 38, 97] Some evidence suggests that even with a reduction in symptoms, the altered muscle behaviour does not necessarily automatically reverse with time.[36] This enforces the need for high-quality and specific rehabilitation, especially if the altered patterns of muscle use involve less efficient combinations of muscle synergies, which may increase the vulnerability of the cervical region to strain and further pain.

Based on the evidence which has been presented in this chapter, the patient with WAD can present with several features of impaired motor control, including: loss of predefined patterns of muscle activation; increased coactivation of the neck flexors and extensors; increased activity but reduced specificity and efficiency of contraction in the superficial neck muscles; and impaired feed-forward and feedback control which, with other factors, contributes to reductions in strength and endurance. Changes in the properties in the neck flexor and extensor muscles affect the deep muscles to a larger extent than the superficial muscles.

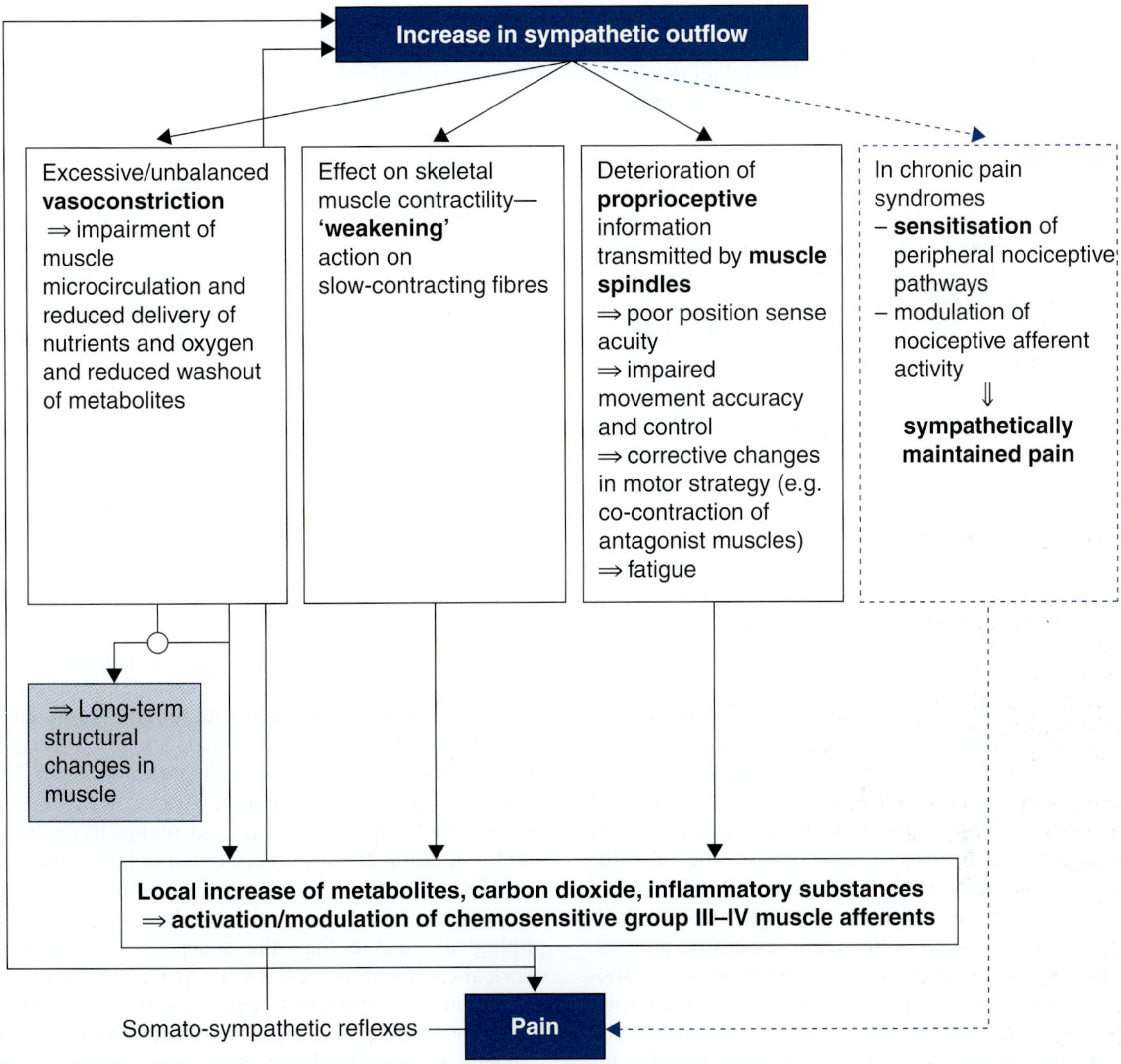

Figure 6.8 Actions of the sympathetic system on muscle function, which may play a role in the development and maintenance of chronic muscle pain states. From the left, continuous line boxes list physiological actions that may account for the development of chronic pain. Each factor contributes to an increase in the local concentration of metabolites, thus activating group III and IV afferent input. These, in turn, further activate the sympathetic system via somato-sympathetic reflexes, thus potentially establishing multiple positive feedback loops, which may maintain the pain state. On the right, the dashed box illustrates that sympathetic action in chronic pain states may increase pain sensation and, consequently, further increase sympathetic activity (pain-mediated vicious circle). (Reprinted with permission from Passatore and Roatta[20])

The magnitude of change varies between patients, as reflected in the variability between individuals observed in any experiment measuring muscle behaviour or properties in a whiplash group. This variability probably relates to interactions between the nature and extent of the injury, the magnitude of pain and disability and the presence and magnitude of attendant stress reactions. Thus, any exercise program is prescribed on the basis of the assessment of the individual patient.

Rehabilitation of patients with WAD

The nature and extent of the neuromuscular dysfunction informs a rehabilitation approach that sequentially addresses the impaired functions.[98]

Not unexpectedly, evidence is emerging that specific exercise strategies that address the precise impairments are more effective in reducing altered neuromuscular control of the neck than general exercise.[99–102] This research-informed exercise approach is partitioned into two phases. Phase 1 is concerned with rehabilitation of the aspects of motor and sensorimotor control. Phase 2 consists of a muscle strengthening and endurance program, and is introduced once the disturbed sensorimotor behaviours have been adequately addressed.[98]

Phase 1 is a motor learning program. It is designed to focus on motor control and aims to improve the activation and control of the deep cervical flexor and extensor muscles and the axioscapular muscles. Attention is given to training the coordination between the layers of the neck and axioscapular muscles for their appropriate patterns of activation in functional and work activities. Precise, low-load exercise is used in this phase, using specific movement strategies to target the deep muscles, to train the coordination between the layers of the neck muscles and to reduce any unwanted activity or co-contraction of the superficial muscles.

The principles of motor relearning are used,[103] namely: segmentation—the task is broken into smaller parts and practised as independent units, which are then integrated progressively to practise the complete skill; simplification—the movement is simplified to increase the ease of performance; and provision of augmented feedback. For example, the rehabilitation of the deep neck flexors for their function of control of posture and angle of the cervical curve[104] follows several steps in the motor relearning process. The first control exercise for the deep cervical flexors (the longus capitis and longus colli) is simplified by positioning the patient in supine lying, where the gravitational load is reduced, making it simpler for the patient to perform a craniocervical flexion exercise (the anatomical action of these muscles) in a precise manner.[98] The absence of load (as would occur in a head lift exercise) is a predetermined strategy to reduce activity in the often overactive superficial flexors towards training the coordination between the neck flexor synergists. Feedback on the correct sagittal rotation action is attained by patients feeling the back of their head slide on the supporting surface as they perform cranial flexion. Feedback of the quality of the deep muscle contraction is provided indirectly to patients via an air-filled pressure sensor inserted behind the neck, which monitors the slight flattening of the cervical curve that occurs with the contraction of the longus colli. In tandem, patients palpate the sternocleidomastoid and anterior scalene muscles and learn to perform craniocervical flexion without overt activity in these muscles. This helps train the appropriate coordination between the deep and superficial neck muscles, as well as assisting patients to learn the sensation of relaxation in the superficial muscles immediately on completion of the task. Repetition is a key component of the motor relearning process. The endurance of the deep neck flexors is trained under these low-load, controlled conditions in line with their functional requirements of support of head and neck posture and in response to the evidence of deficits in their endurance capacity at low loads.[105]

The principles of motor relearning are likewise employed in the first phase of exercise for the cervical extensors. Training is commenced with the patient either prone, propped on elbows or in four-point kneeling with a neutral spine position.[98] The deep suboccipital muscles are targeted with craniocervical extension and craniocervical rotation exercises. These muscles are vital for normal cervical somatosensory function and contain high proportions of muscle spindles,[106] but they demonstrate some of the greatest morphological changes in patients with chronic whiplash.[2] The exercises to target the suboccipital extensors, rectus capitis minor and major, and the suboccipital rotators, obliquus capitis superior and inferior are performed with precision, with an emphasis on movement quality. Active head extension is practised with the cervical region in neutral, and the rotation exercise is restricted to head rotation only. For the deep cervical extensors (multifidus and semispinalis cervicis), which also show greater morphological change than the superficial extensors,[2] cervical extension is performed with the craniocervical region maintained in a neutral position to initially lessen the contribution of the superficial extensors.

There is some evidence of a direct translation of effects of this specific muscle training into function via improvement in control of the upright posture of the head and neck[100] and improvement in the feed-forward responses of the neck flexors.[102] In the motor learning process, the work of, for example, the deep neck flexors is then integrated progressively in the practice of functional skills. Practice that involves facilitation of a neutral spinal posture will activate the deep neck flexors.[107] This contraction can be augmented by an active neck-lengthening manoeuvre by visualising lifting the base of the skull off the top of the neck,[108] with a focus on relaxation of the superficial neck flexors in this task.[42] Practice that involves eccentric and concentric control of the correct pattern of head and neck extension trains the appropriate synergistic action between the superficial and deep neck flexors.

The specific muscle training in this motor learning phase also improves the feedback responses required for proprioception.[101] Training of the suboccipital and deep neck extensors and flexors is an integral component of a multimodal program to address deficits in proprioception, postural orientation and stability and eye movement control, as determined to be present in the individual patient.

Similar principles and strategies for motor relearning are used to train changes found in the assessment of axioscapular muscle function. The activation and endurance of target muscles is first trained with simple and specific exercise tasks. The training is then integrated progressively in the practice of functional skills, relevant to the individual's work and recreational needs, ensuring that appropriate muscle synergies are employed.

Phase 2 of the program is commenced once the disturbed pattern of neck muscle activation has been addressed in the motor learning process and as the individual's pain level permits. This phase aims to improve the muscles' strength and endurance capacity to meet the patient's functional recreational and work demands. Endurance needs to be trained at low, moderate and maximal loads as relevant to the individual to address the impairments shown at these different contraction intensities.[105] The strengthening program follows the principles of progressive resisted exercise.[109] While the program will include formal strength training exercise for the neck flexor and extensor and axioscapular muscles, it must expand to train strength and control in tasks relevant to the individual patient. Throughout this phase, particular attention is given to the quality and control of the movement and the pattern of muscle activity to ensure appropriate patterns of activation between antagonist muscles and no inappropriate increase in coactivation between neck flexors and extensors. Quality and control of movement remain premier goals in this phase of the rehabilitation program.

Neuromuscular rehabilitation in context

As discussed, many factors can contribute to disturbed motor activity in the whiplash-injured patient, including the nature of injury, pain and associated psychological distress. These factors not only contribute to the responses in the neuromuscular system but they can moderate the effect of exercise.

There is ample evidence that exercise can reduce pain in many individuals, but exercises that cause pain can, counterproductively, reinforce altered motor behaviours and, importantly, inhibit the process of motor relearning.[110] Thus, exercises in either phase of the rehabilitation program should not provoke neck pain. The potential physiological mechanisms underlying the individual whiplash patient's pain also appear to moderate the effect of exercise. This was revealed in a clinical trial testing the effect of this rehabilitation program on individuals with chronic WAD.[38] Persons with initial higher levels of pain and disability in association with widespread mechanical and cold hyperalgesia (suggesting the presence of augmented central pain processing mechanisms, loss of descending inhibition or a neuropathic pain state) were not as responsive to the rehabilitation program in terms of reduction in pain and disability and improvement in motor control. In contrast, individuals presenting with widespread mechanical hyperalgesia only or without abnormal sensory features were more responsive to the exercise program.

Rehabilitation of neuromuscular control is a key component of the management program for the whiplash-injured individual, but as the outcomes of clinical trials reveal, it is not the sole answer for all individuals.[38, 111, 112] Further research may inform more effective exercise strategies. Nevertheless, the challenge in rehabilitation is the management of the more than 50% of individuals who transition into a chronic state.[9, 113] Many of these individuals have quite complex clinical presentations, and more effective management of the initial injury, the pain and any psychological mediators may enhance the effect of neuromuscular rehabilitation. Certainly, current evidence points to the need for multimodal management, particularly for the individuals at risk of transition to chronicity.

CONCLUSION

The whiplash injury can result in complex changes in neuromuscular function, as well as changes in muscle properties. Current research informs the rehabilitation approach, with directions to include specific therapeutic exercise that focuses on motor relearning prior to strengthening as a component of multimodal interventions. The exercise program should be based on a detailed assessment of the individual and the exercises should be designed to address the specific changes identified in muscle function. Precision in exercise is emphasised in the motor learning process. The muscles are trained specifically and within the functional and task-specific context of the individual patient. Repetition is essential in the learning process to establish or re-establish appropriate movement and muscle control. The program should be commenced early in the rehabilitation process, but exercise should not provoke neck pain. Importantly, patients must understand the rationale underpinning the various components and phases of the exercise approach. Their compliance with the exercise program is critical to the learning process and the success of the program.

References

1. Kristjansson E. Reliability of ultrasonography for the cervical multifidus muscle in asymptomatic and symptomatic subjects. *Man Ther* 2004;9:83–8.
2. Elliott J, Jull G, Noteboom JT, et al. Fatty infiltration in the cervical extensor muscles in persistent whiplash-associated disorders: a magnetic resonance imaging analysis. *Spine* 2006;31(22):847–55.
3. Elliott J, O'Leary S, Sterling M, et al. Magnetic resonance imaging findings of fatty infiltrate in the cervical flexors in chronic whiplash. *Spine* 2010;35(9):948–54.
4. Boyd Clark LC, Briggs CA, Galea MP. Comparative histochemical composition of muscle fibres in a pre- and a postvertebral muscle of the cervical spine. *J Anat* 2001;199:709–16.
5. Boyd Clark LC, Briggs CA, Galea MP. Muscle spindle distribution, morphology, and density in longus colli and multifidus muscles of the cervical spine. *Spine* 2002;27:694–701.
6. Elliott J, Sterling M, Noteboom JT, et al. Fatty infiltrate in the cervical extensor muscles is not a feature of chronic, insidious-onset neck pain. *Clin Radiol* 2008;63:681–7.
7. De Loose V, van den Oord M, Keser I, et al. MRI study of the morphometry of the cervical musculature in F-16 pilots. *Aviat Space Environ Med* 2009;80:727–31.
8. Elliott J, Noteboom JT, Sterling M, et al. The clinical presentation of chronic whiplash and the relationship to findings of MRI fatty infiltrate in the cervical extensor musculature. *Eur Spine J* 2009;18:1371–8.
9. Sterling M, Jull G, Vicenzino B. Physical and psychological factors predict outcome following whiplash injury. *Pain* 2005;114:141–8.
10. de Medinaceli L, Hurpeau J, Merle M, Begorre H. Cold and post-traumatic pain: modeling of the peripheral nerve message. *Biosystems* 1997;43:145–67.
11. Sterling M, Jull G, Vicenzino B, Kenardy J. Sensory hypersensitivity occurs soon after whiplash injury and is associated with poor recovery. *Pain* 2003;104:509–17.
12. Banic B, Petersen-Felix S, Andersen OK, et al. Evidence for spinal cord hypersensitivity in chronic pain after whiplash injury and in fibromyalgia. *Pain* 2004;107:7–15.
13. Kasch H, Qerama E, Bach FW, Jensen TS. Reduced cold pressor pain tolerance in non-recovered whiplash patients: a 1-year prospective study. *Eur J Pain* 2005;9:561–9.
14. Curatolo M, Petersen-Felix S, Arendt-Nielsen L, et al. Central hypersensitivity in chronic pain after whiplash injury. *Clin J Pain* 2001;17:306–15.
15. Hides JA, Stokes MJ, Saide M, et al. Evidence of lumbar multifidus muscle wasting ipsilateral to symptoms in patients with acute/subacute low back pain. *Spine* 1994;19(2):165–72.
16. Dulor JP, Cambon B, Vigneron P, et al. Expression of specific white adipose tissue genes in denervation-induced skeletal muscle fatty degeneration. *FEBS Lett* 1998;439:89–92.
17. Fleckenstein JL, Conner KE, Ezaki M, et al. Denervated human skeletal muscle: MR imaging evaluation. *Radiology* 1993;187:213–18.
18. Krssak M, Falk Petersen K, Dresner A, et al. Intramyocellular lipid concentrations are correlated with insulin sensitivity in humans: a 1H NMR spectroscopy study. *Diabetologia* 1999;42:113–16.
19. Lovitt S, Moore SL, Marden FA. The use of MRI in the evaluation of myopathy. *Clin Neurophysiol* 2006;117:486–95.
20. Passatore M & Roatta S. Influence of sympathetic nervous system on sensorimotor function: whiplash associated disorders (WAD) as a model. *Eur J Appl Physiol* 2006;98:423–49.
21. Fitts RH, Riley DR, Widrick JJ. Physiology of a microgravity environment invited review: microgravity and skeletal muscle. *J Appl Physiol* 2000;89:823–39.
22. Haggmark T, Jansson E, Eriksson E. Fiber type area and metabolic potential of the thigh muscle in man after knee surgery and immobilization. *Int J Sports Med* 1981;2:12–17.
23. Jiang B, Ohira Y, Roy RR, et al. Adaptation of fibers in fast-twitch muscles of rats to spaceflight and hindlimb suspension. *J Appl Physiol* 1992;73: 58S–65S.
24. Meyer DC, Pirkl C, Pfirrmann CW, et al. Asymmetric atrophy of the supraspinatus muscle following tendon tear. *J Orthop Res* 2005;23:254–8.
25. Floss T, Arnold HH, Braun T. A role for FGF-6 in skeletal muscle regeneration. *Genes Dev* 1997;11:2040–51.
26. Lefaucheur JP, Gjata B, Lafont H, Sebille A. Angiogenic and inflammatory responses following skeletal muscle injury are altered by immune neutralization of endogenous basic fibroblast growth factor, insulin-like growth factor-1 and transforming growth factor-beta 1. *J Neuroimmunol* 1996;70:37–44.

27. Gradl G, Gaida S, Finke B, et al. Exaggeration of tissue trauma induces signs and symptoms of acute CRPS I, however displays distinct differences to experimental CRPS II. *Neurosci Lett* 2006;402: 267–72.
28. Gradl G, Gaida S, Gierer P, et al. In vivo evidence for apoptosis, but not inflammation in the hindlimb muscle of neuropathic rats. *Pain* 2004;112:121–30.
29. Hodges P, Holm AK, Hansson T, Holm S. Rapid atrophy of the lumbar multifidus follows experimental disc or nerve root injury. *Spine* 2006;31:2926–33.
30. Hayashi N, Matsumoto T, Abe O, et al. Accuracy of abnormal paraspinal muscle findings on contrast-enhanced MR images as indirect signs of unilateral cervical root-avulsion injury. *Radiology* 2002;223:397–402.
31. Uetani M, Hayashi K, Hashmi R, et al. Traction injuries of the brachial plexus: signal intensity changes of the posterior cervical paraspinal muscles on MRI. *J Comput Assist Tomogr* 1997;21:790–5.
32. Lindstrøm R, Schomacher J, Farina D, et al. Association between neck muscle coactivation, pain, and strength in women with neck pain. *Man Ther* 2010 [Epub ahead of print].
33. Muceli S, Farina D, Kirkesola G, et al. Force steadiness in women with neck pain and the effect of short term vibration. *J Electromyogr Kinesiol* 2010; in press.
34. Lu Y, Chen C, Kallakuri S, et al. Neural response of cervical facet joint capsule to stretch: a study of whiplash pain mechanism. *Stapp Car Crash J* 2005;49:49–65.
35. Seaman D. Dysafferentation: a novel term to describe the neuropathological effects of joint complex dysfunction. A look at likely mechanisms of symptom generation. *J Manipulative Physiol Ther* 1999;22:493–4.
36. Sterling M, Jull G, Vicenzino B, et al. Development of motor dysfunction following whiplash injury. *Pain* 2003;103:65–73.
37. Jull GA. Deep cervical flexor muscle dysfunction in whiplash. *J Musculoskeletal Pain* 2000;8:143–54.
38. Jull G, Sterling M, Kenardy J, Beller E. Does the presence of sensory hypersensitivity influence outcomes of physical rehabilitation for chronic whiplash? A preliminary RCT. *Pain* 2007;129: 28–34.
39. Falla D, Jull G, Hodges PW. Patients with neck pain demonstrate reduced electromyographic activity of the deep cervical flexor muscles during performance of the craniocervical flexion test. *Spine* 2004;29:2108–14.
40. Johnston V, Jull G, Souvlis T, Jimmieson NL. Neck movement and muscle activity characteristics in female office workers with neck pain. *Spine* 2008;33:555–63.
41. Jull G, Barrett C, Magee R, Ho P. Further clinical clarification of the muscle dysfunction in cervical headache. *Cephalalgia* 1999;19:179–85.
42. Falla D, Lindstrøm R, Rechter L, Farina D. Effect of pain on the modulation in discharge rate of sternocleidomastoid motor units with force direction. *Clin Neurophysiol* 2010;121(5):744–53.
43. Falla D, Jull G, Edwards S, et al. Neuromuscular efficiency of the sternocleidomastoid and anterior scalene muscles in patients with chronic neck pain. *Disabil Rehabil* 2004;26:712–17.
44. Jull G, Kristjansson E, Dall'Alba P. Impairment in the cervical flexors: a comparison of whiplash and insidious onset neck pain patients. *Man Ther* 2004;9:89–94.
45. Falla D, Bilenkij G, Jull G. Patients with chronic neck pain demonstrate altered patterns of muscle activation during performance of a functional upper limb task. *Spine* 2004;29:1436–40.
46. Barton PM, Hayes KC. Neck flexor muscle strength, efficiency, and relaxation times in normal subjects and subjects with unilateral neck pain and headache. *Arch Phys Med Rehabil* 1996;77:680–7.
47. Roberts TDM. Neurophysiology of postural mechanisms. London: Butterworths, 1978.
48. Taylor JL, McCloskey DI. Proprioception in the neck. *Exp Brain Res* 1988;70:351–60.
49. Dutia MB. The muscles and joints of the neck: their specialisation and role in head movement. *Prog Neurobiol* 1991;37:165–78.
50. Pedersen J, Sjolander P, Wenngren BI, Johansson H. Increased intramuscular concentration of bradykinin increases the static fusimotor drive to muscle spindles in neck muscles of the cat. *Pain* 1997;70:83–91.
51. Thunberg J, Hellstrom F, Sjolander P, et al. Influences on the fusimotor-muscle spindle system from chemosensitive nerve endings in cervical facet joints in the cat: possible implications for whiplash induced disorders. *Pain* 2001;91:15–22.
52. Hellstrom F, Thunberg J, Bergenheim M, et al. Increased intra-articular concentration of bradykinin in the temporomandibular joint changes the sensitivity of muscle spindles in dorsal neck muscles in the cat. *Neurosci Res* 2002;42:91–9.
53. Wenngren BJ, Pederson J, Sjolander P, et al. Bradykinin and muscle stretch alter contralateral cat neck muscle spindle output. *Neurosci Res* 1998;32:119–29.

54. Roatta S, Windhorst U, Ljubisavljevic M, et al. Sympathetic modulation of muscle spindle afferent sensitivity to stretch in rabbit jaw closing muscles. *J Physiol (Lond.)* 2002;540:237–48.
55. Treleaven J, Jull G, Sterling M. Dizziness and unsteadiness following whiplash injury: characteristic features and relationship with cervical joint position error. *J Rehabil Med* 2003;35:36–43.
56. Revel M, Andre Deshays C, Minguet M. Cervicocephalic kinesthetic sensibility in patients with cervical pain. *Arch Phys Med Rehabil* 1991;72:288–91.
57. Heikkila H, Astrom P. Cervicocephalic kinesthetic sensibility in patients with whiplash injury. *J Rehab Med* 1996;28:133–8.
58. Kristjansson E, Dall'Alba P, Jull G. A study of five cervicocephalic relocation tests in three different subject groups. *Clin Rehabil* 2003;17:768–74.
59. Treleaven J, Jull G, Low Choy N. The relationship of cervical joint position error to balance and eye movement disturbances in persistent whiplash. *Man Ther* 2006;11:99–106.
60. Feipel V, Salvia P, Klein H, Rooze M. Head repositioning accuracy in patients with whiplash-associated disorders. *Spine* 2006;31:E51–E58.
61. Knox J, Beilstein DJ, Charles SD, et al. Changes in head and neck position have a greater effect on elbow joint position sense in people with whiplash-associated disorders. *Clin J Pain* 2006;22:512–18.
62. Sandlund J, Djupsjobacka M, Ryhed B, et al. Predictive and discriminative value of shoulder proprioception tests for patients with whiplash-associated disorders. *J Rehab Med* 2006;38:44–9.
63. McPartland JM, Brodeur RR, Hallgren RC. Chronic neck pain, standing balance, and suboccipital muscle atrophy—a pilot study. *J Manipulative Physiol Ther* 1997;20:24–9.
64. Michaelson P, Michaelson M, Jaric S, et al. Vertical posture and head stability in patients with chronic neck pain. *J Rehabil Med* 2003;35:229–35.
65. Karlberg M, Persson L, Magnusson M. Impaired postural control in patients with cervico-brachial pain. *Acta Otolaryngol Suppl* 1995;520:440–2.
66. Sjostrom H, Allum JH, Carpenter DM, et al. Trunk sway measures of postural stability during clinical balance tests in patients with chronic whiplash injury symptoms. *Spine* 2003;28:1725–34.
67. Madeleine P, Prietzel H, Svarrer H, Arendt-Nielsen L. Quantitative posturography in altered sensory conditions: a way to assess balance instability in patients with chronic whiplash injury. *Arch Phys Med Rehabil* 2004;85:432–8.
68. Field S, Treleaven J, Jull G. Standing balance: a comparison between idiopathic and whiplash-induced neck pain. *Man Ther* 2008;13:183–91.
69. Treleaven J, Jull G, Low Choy N. Standing balance in persistent whiplash: a comparison between subjects with and without dizziness. *J Rehabil Med* 2005;37:224–9.
70. Heikkila HV & Wenngren B. Cervicocephalic kinesthetic sensibility, active range of cervical motion, and oculomotor function in patients with whiplash injury. *Arch Phys Med Rehabil* 1998;79:1089–94.
71. Tjell C & Rosenhall U. Smooth pursuit neck torsion test: a specific test for cervical dizziness. *Am J Otol* 1998;19:76–81.
72. Treleaven J, Jull G, Low Choy N. Smooth pursuit neck torsion test in whiplash-associated disorders: relationship to self-reports of neck pain and disability, dizziness and anxiety. *J Rehabil Med* 2005;37:219–23.
73. Wenngren BI, Pettersson K, Lowenheilm G, Hildingsson C. Eye motility and auditory brainstem response dysfunction after whiplash injury. *Acta Otolaryngol* 2002;122:276–83.
74. Mense S & Meyer H. Different types of slowly conductive afferent units in cat skeletal muscle and tendon. *J Physiol* 1985;363:403–17.
75. Graven-Nielsen T, Arendt-Nielsen L, Svensson P, Jensen TS. Experimental muscle pain: a quantitative study of local and referred pain in humans following injection of hypertonic saline. *J Musculoskel Pain* 1997;5:49–69.
76. Madeleine P, Lundager B, Voigt M, Arendt-Nielsen L. Sensory manifestations in experimental and work-related chronic neck-shoulder pain. *Euro J Pain* 1998;2:251–60.
77. Ashton Miller JA, McGlashen KM, Herzenberg JE, Stohler CS. Cervical muscle myoelectric response to acute experimental sternocleidomastoid pain. *Spine* 1990;15:1006–12.
78. Svensson P, Wang K, Sessle BJ, Arendt-Nielsen L. Associations between pain and neuromuscular activity in the human jaw and neck muscles. *Pain* 2004;109:225–32.
79. Farina D, Arendt-Nielsen L, Merletti R, Graven-Nielsen T. Effect of experimental muscle pain on motor unit firing rate and conduction velocity. *J Neurophysiol* 2004;91:1250–9.
80. Falla D, Arendt-Nielsen L, Farina D. Gender-specific adaptations of upper trapezius muscle activity to acute nociceptive stimulation. *Pain* 2008;138:217–25.

81. Falla D, Farina D, Kanstrup Dahl M, Graven-Nielsen T. Muscle pain induces task-dependent changes in cervical agonist/antagonist activity. *J Appl Physiol* 2007;102:601–9.
82. Falla D, Farina D, Graven-Nielsen T. Experimental muscle pain results in reorganization of coordination among trapezius muscle subdivisions during repetitive shoulder flexion. *Exp Brain Res* 2007;178: 385–93.
83. Falla D & Farina D. Neural and muscular factors associated with motor impairment in neck pain. *Curr Rheumatol Rep* 2007;9:497–502.
84. Holm LW, Carroll LJ, Cassidy JD, Ahlbom A. Factors influencing neck pain intensity in whiplash-associated disorders. *Spine* 2006;31:E98–E104.
85. Janig W. Systemic and specific autonomic reactions in pain: efferent, afferent and endocrine components. *Eur J Anaesthesiol* 1985;2:319–46.
86. Bowman WC. Prejunctional and postjunctional cholinoceptors at the neuromuscular junction. *Anesth Analg* 1980;59:935–43.
87. Roatta S, Arendt-Nielsen L, Farina D. Sympathetic-induced changes in discharge rate and spike-triggered average twitch torque of low-threshold motor units in humans. *J Physiol* 2008;586:5561–74.
88. Akoev GN. Catecholamines, acetylcholine and excitability of mechanoreceptors. *Prog Neurobiol* 1981;15:269–94.
89. Hunt CC. The effect of sympathetic stimulation on mammalian muscle spindles. *J Physiol (Lond.)* 1960;151:332–41.
90. Matsuo R, Ikehara A, Nokubi T, Morimoto T. Inhibitory effect of sympathetic stimulation on activities of masseter muscle spindles and the jaw jerk reflex in rats. *J Physiol (Lond.)* 1995;483:239–50.
91. Hellstrom F, Roatta S, Thunberg J, et al. Responses of muscle spindles in feline dorsal neck muscles to electrical stimulation of the cervical sympathetic nerve. *Exp Brain Res* 2005;165:328–42.
92. Gandevia SC, McCloskey DI, Burke D. Kinaesthetic signals and muscle contraction. *Trends Neurosci* 1992;15:62–5.
93. Finsen L, Sogaard K, Jensen C, et al. Muscle activity and cardiovascular response during computer-mouse work with and without memory demands. *Ergonomics* 2001;44:1312–29.
94. Van Galen GP, Muller ML, Meulenbroek RG, Van Germmert AW. Forearm EMG response activity during motor performance in individuals prone to increased stress reactivity. *Am J Ind Med* 2002;41:406–19.
95. Lee RH & Heckman CJ. Enhancement of bistability in spinal motoneurons in vivo by the noradrenergic alpha1 agonist methoxamine. *J Neurophysiol* 1999;81:2164–74.
96. Heckman CJ, Johnson M, Mottram C, Schuster J. Persistent inward currents in spinal motoneurons and their influence on human motoneuron firing patterns. *Neuroscientist* 2008;14:264–75.
97. Sterling M, Jull G, Vicenzino B, Kenardy J. Characterization of acute whiplash-associated disorders. *Spine* 2004;29:182–8.
98. Jull G, Sterling M, Falla D, et al. Whiplash, headache and neck pain: research based directions for physical therapies. Edinburgh: Churchill Livingstone, 2008.
99. Falla D, Jull G, Hodges P, Vicenzino B. An endurance-strength training regime is effective in reducing myoelectric manifestations of cervical flexor muscle fatigue in females with chronic neck pain. *Clin Neurophysiol* 2006;117:828–37.
100. Falla D, Jull G, Russell T, et al. Effect of neck exercise on sitting posture in patients with chronic neck pain. *Phys Ther* 2007;87:408–17.
101. Jull G, Falla D, Treleaven J, et al. Retraining cervical joint position sense: the effect of two exercise regimes. *J Orthop Res* 2007;25:404–12.
102. Jull G, Falla D, Vicenzino B, Hodges PW. The effect of therapeutic exercise on activation of the deep cervical flexor muscles in people with chronic neck pain. *Man Ther* 2009;14:696–701.
103. Magill RA. Motor learning: concepts and applications. 6th edn. New York: McGraw-Hill, 2001.
104. Mayoux-Benhamou MA, Revel M, Vallee C, et al. Longus colli has a postural function on cervical curvature. *Surg Radiol Anat* 1994;16:367–71.
105. O'Leary S, Jull G, Kim M, Vicenzino B. Cranio-cervical flexor muscle impairment at maximal, moderate, and low loads is a feature of neck pain. *Man Ther* 2007;12:34–9.
106. Liu JX, Thornell LE, Pedrosa-Domellof F. Muscle spindles in the deep muscles of the human neck: a morphological and immunocytochemical study. *J Histochem Cytochem* 2003;51:175–86.
107. Falla D, O'Leary S, Fagan A, Jull G. Recruitment of the deep cervical flexor muscles during a postural-correction exercise performed in sitting. *Man Ther* 2007;12:139–43.
108. Fountain FP, Minear WL, Allison RD. Function of longus colli and longissimus cervicis muscles in man. *Arch Phys Med Rehabil* 1966;47:665–9.
109. McArdle W, Katch F, Katch V. Exercise physiology. Baltimore: Williams Wilkins, 1996.

110. Boudreau S, Romaniello A, Wang K, et al. The effects of intra-oral pain on motor cortex neuroplasticity associated with short-term novel tongue-protrusion training in humans. *Pain* 2009;132:169–78.
111. Provinciali L, Baroni M, Illuminati L, Ceravolo MG. Multimodal treatment to prevent the late whiplash syndrome. *Scand J Rehabil Med* 2009;28:105–11.
112. Stewart MJ, Maher C, Refshauge KM, et al. Randomized controlled trial of exercise for chronic whiplash associated disorders. *Pain* 2007; 128: 59–68.
113. Scholten-Peeters GG, Verhagen AP, Bekkering GE, et al. Prognostic factors of whiplash-associated disorders: a systematic review of prospective cohort studies. *Pain* 2003;104:303–22.

CHAPTER 7
Dizziness, visual and sensorimotor control disturbances following whiplash injury

Julia Treleaven

After pain, symptoms of dizziness, unsteadiness and visual disturbances are some of the next most frequent complaints, with between 40% and 75% of those with persistent whiplash reporting these symptoms.[1] In addition, altered head position and movement sense, problems in maintaining and performing postural stability tasks,[1–4] and deficits in eye movement control[5–7] have also been demonstrated in individuals with chronic whiplash. A better understanding of the causes and relationships of such persistent problems following a whiplash injury is vital to establish appropriate diagnostic measures and relevant rehabilitation.

AETIOLOGY OF DIZZINESS, VISUAL DISTURBANCES AND SENSORIMOTOR CONTROL DISTURBANCES IN WHIPLASH ASSOCIATED DISORDERS

A myriad of causes have been suggested to underlie the symptoms of dizziness and visual disturbances in whiplash associated disorders (WAD). Anxiety, malingering and medication use have been raised as factors contributing to the persistence of these symptoms.[8] However, disturbances to the sensorimotor control system appear to be the most likely causative factors of these symptoms, due to traumatic damage to one or more of the three main systems providing input to the sensorimotor control system: vestibular, visual or neck receptors, or damage directly to the central nervous system (CNS).[9, 10] Structural damage to the vertebral artery is also possible following a whiplash injury.[11] Nevertheless, in those with a pure whiplash injury (i.e. no head injury), there is reasonable evidence to suggest that the disturbances are primarily of a cervical origin from both damaged or functionally impaired neck joint and muscle receptors. Secondary vestibular hypo- or hyperfunction may also occur due to disturbed cervical afferents.[9, 10, 12] Thus, the focus of this chapter is on cervical-related causes of such disturbances. Nevertheless, as people with persistent whiplash may be taking medications, anxious or seeking compensation, may or may not have had a mild head injury, may have had some peripheral vestibular or vertebral artery damage, and have neck pain and associated musculoskeletal damage, each of these factors should be considered in the differential diagnosis (Fig 7.1).

Anxiety

Elevated levels of anxiety have been recorded in subjects with persistent whiplash.[13] Anxiety is well recognised as a cause of dizziness[14] and has been implicated in balance disturbance, with some evidence for a neurological relationship between anxiety and the vestibular apparatus.[15] Interestingly, it has also been suggested that a causal or perpetuating link may exist between anxiety and associated increased muscle tension and neck-related causes of dizziness.[16] Stress may also influence cervical muscle spindle sensitivity via activation of the sympathetic nervous system.[17]

However, a series of studies have found no differences in anxiety levels between participants with whiplash who did and did not complain of dizziness. In addition, both general anxiety levels and anxiety at the time of testing did not appear to influence between group differences of the sensorimotor deficits.[1, 5, 18] However, it is possible that anxiety may play a secondary or exacerbating role in the production of these symptoms and signs in some with persistent WAD.

Secondary gain

Assertions that people are exaggerating symptoms for secondary gain have, for many years, been a common thread in the literature related to persistent complaints of symptoms, such as pain and dizziness, following a whiplash injury.[19] Despite this, there is no evidence to demonstrate significant differences in symptomatic complaints, or response to treatment between patients who are or are not involved in compensation claims.[20] In recent studies, there was also no evidence that compensation status was associated with complaints of dizziness and/or any of the deficits seen in sensorimotor control in individuals with persistent whiplash.[1, 5, 18] In addition, in a recent study, the pattern of balance disturbances in asymptomatic

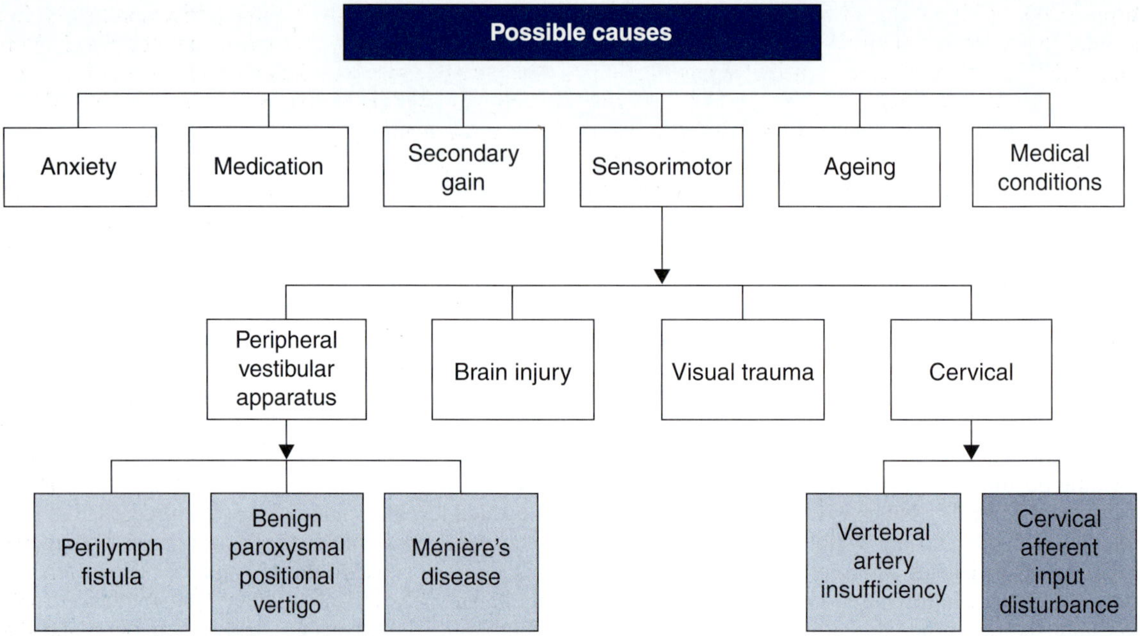

Figure 7.1 Possible causes of dizziness and unsteadiness following a whiplash injury.

people instructed to feign balance deficits was found to be significantly more exaggerated when compared to disturbances seen in those with whiplash.[21]

Medications

Medications, such as anti-inflammatory, antipsychotic and narcotic drugs, are commonly prescribed to patients with persistent whiplash, and may adversely affect postural sway.[22] Similarly, antidepressants, muscle relaxants or vestibular depressants may create gaze-evoked nystagmus and influence oculomotor function.[22] Thus, some of the signs and symptoms seen in whiplash could also be a side-effect of these medications. Despite this occurrence, recent studies have found no evidence that medications were associated with whiplash symptoms. The results indicated no differences in either the frequency of dizziness and/or deficits in balance, head or eye movement control in participants who were routinely taking medication up to 24 hours prior to testing, compared to those not taking these medications.[1, 5, 18]

Vertebral artery insufficiency

Vertebral artery insufficiency is another possible cause of dizziness and visual disturbances following a whiplash injury. It is possible that cervical trauma may result in damage to the vertebral vessels,[23] but the evidence suggests that this rarely occurs (0.5–4%) in survivors of blunt cervical or head trauma.[24] This would suggest that the incidence of vertebral artery injury following a whiplash injury is low, albeit possible.[25] Isolated case reports have been identified, with symptoms usually occurring within a few minutes of the injury,[26, 27] although longer delays have been reported.[28]

Only one study has looked specifically at vertebral blood flow in patients following a whiplash injury.[29] Few patients in this study reported vascular symptoms, despite a relatively high incidence of abnormal vertebral artery blood flow.[29] Evidence from studies of those with traumatic vertebral artery dissection post cervical fracture would also suggest that, in the majority of cases, there are minimal clinical signs and symptoms,[23] and the symptom of dizziness is uncommon.[30] It is unlikely that in people with persistent signs and symptoms following a whiplash injury, the symptom of dizziness is due to trauma to the vertebral artery. However, owing to the considerable danger such an event poses, it should be noted as a possibility and should always be considered in the differential diagnosis.

Disturbances to structures influencing sensorimotor control

The forces generated during a whiplash injury can potentially cause definitive damage to many neck structures,[31] and thus be a primary source of altered proprioceptive input to the sensorimotor control system.[32] The forces may also be sufficient to produce CNS and/or peripheral vestibular dysfunction. Relatively slow crash speeds, of up to 15 kilometres per hour, have been shown to generate 8*g* of force on the head and neck.[33] In a controlled study involving primates, the forces that were artificially reproduced resulted in cerebral concussion, and brainstem and cranial nerve stretch in 50% of the cases.[34] However, in other crash testing, humans have been exposed to 10*g* without apparent effects on the CNS or peripheral vestibular apparatus.[35] It is thought that higher forces of up to 25*g* are necessary to cause damage to these structures in humans.[36] Thus, disturbance of the cervical afferents is considered the most likely primary source of dizziness, visual disturbances and sensorimotor control disturbances, particularly in slow-speed, impact collisions that cause a whiplash injury.

Brain injury

A brain injury may occur concomitantly with a whiplash injury, especially when the forces are strong and result in a direct blow to the head. However, it is generally felt that brain injury is unlikely with a pure whiplash injury.[37] Studies using various technologies have been relatively unsuccessful in identifying the presence of brain injury in people with whiplash not reporting an associated mild head injury.[10, 37–39] Although some correlations between cognitive deficits, anxiety and pain have been demonstrated, no actual deficits in neuropsychological testing relating to altered brain function have been substantiated.[39] Gimse et al.[40] demonstrated reading difficulties in patients with whiplash without any evidence of brain injury, and concluded that cognitive and reading problems were likely to be due to abnormal afferent input from the cervical spine rather than a brain injury. Wenngren et al.[41] investigated the prevalence of brain/brainstem dysfunction following a whiplash injury and concluded that in only a small proportion of patients with very severe symptoms could these be explained by lesions to the brain/brainstem.

Damage to the peripheral vestibular apparatus

Forces generated during a whiplash injury, especially when there is concomitant mild head injury, could result in at least three possible peripheral vestibular causes of dizziness and disturbances to postural control: benign paroxysmal positional vertigo (BPPV), damage to the endolymphatic sac which could cause hydrops (Ménière's disease), or rupture of the otic capsule window resulting in a perilymph fistula. In a retrospective review,[36] it was estimated that 35% of people had some combination of these conditions as a consequence of inner ear concussion associated with a whiplash injury.

Debate continues as to the frequency of vestibular disorders following a whiplash injury. High percentages (up to 85%) of peripheral vestibular dysfunction have been reported.[42] However, these studies often lacked control groups and the conclusion that vestibular dysfunction was the cause was based on clinical patterns rather than definitive objective measures. In studies where objective measures have been used, reports of BPPV and perilymph fistula have been suggested to occur in as little as 5% to in as much as 25% of patients.[43] Isolated reports of acute vestibular pathology occurring shortly after a pure whiplash injury have also been documented.[44]

Fischer et al.[12] reported normal vestibular test results in most of their subjects with whiplash, although vestibular hyperactivity was seen in 53% of subjects. They proposed that this could be due to limited neck movement, secondary to neck pain, with subsequent vestibular–ocular reflex enhancement. Fischer et al.[45] also found that 38% of subjects hyperventilated, suggesting a possible relationship between stress, anxiety and vestibular findings. Solarino et al.[46] recently suggested that increased latency in vestibular evoked potentials in those with a whiplash injury may be a result of a primary disorder of the vestibulocollic reflex rather than actual peripheral vestibular dysfunction.

Recent studies have also compared symptoms and sensorimotor deficits in those with whiplash compared to those with a discrete unilateral peripheral vestibular dysfunction and demonstrated that subjects with whiplash had differences in performance in both balance tests and eye movement tests. Additionally, they reported different characteristics of dizziness.[47] Secondary adaptive changes in the vestibular system are possible, but these findings suggest that these are not the primary cause of the deficits in patients following a whiplash injury.

Damage to vision—post-trauma visual syndrome

Damage to the ambient visual system has also been suggested as a possibility following a whiplash injury.[48] The ambient visual system is important for knowledge of where you are in space rather than what you are looking at (focal vision) and provides general information needed for balance, movement, coordination and posture. Photophobia, convergence insufficiency, accommodation insufficiency and eye alignment malfunctions, such as cross eyes, rotation and one eye up one down, are thought to be due to altered ambient vision and have been demonstrated in some people following a whiplash injury.[49, 50] Together these symptoms have been labelled as *post-trauma visual syndrome*, which is thought to result in symptomatic complaints of dizziness, visual disturbances and alterations in head and eye movement and postural stability.[48] Research into this area is in its infancy and currently lies in the domain of behavioural optometry.

Damage to cervical afferents

Afferent input from nociceptors and mechanoreceptors in the cervical region, as with those throughout the body, mediates pain, temperature, pressure, touch and proprioceptive information to the nervous system. The abundant cervical receptors in the muscles and joints of the cervical spine, as well as their central and reflex connections to the vestibular, visual and postural control systems, suggest that these receptors have an important role in providing information for general sensorimotor control affecting balance, and head and eye movement control.[51, 52] Conflict between the converging input from the different sensory systems or a sensory mismatch is the mechanism thought to be responsible for disturbances in sensorimotor control following interference to the cervical afferents, such as could occur following a whiplash injury.

Cervical receptors

Cervical receptors are important for sensorimotor control. Muscle receptors, particularly muscle spindles, are considered to be of most significance as they are found in high densities in the cervical region. Muscle spindle density is highest in the muscles of the suboccipital region, particularly in the deeper part of these muscles, with up to 240 muscle spindles per gram of muscle.[53, 54] In a study of human neck muscles, distinct morphological features and the composition of the muscle spindles in the deep neck muscles were considered to demonstrate their influence on both movement precision and proprioceptive information for the control of head position and eye–head coordination.[55] Others also believe that these small deep muscles may not function as traditional muscles but rather as monitors of proprioceptive function.[53]

While there are higher numbers of mechanoreceptors in the upper cervical compared to the lower cervical joints, their numbers are much lower in comparison to those in the muscles, and it has been suggested that joint receptors only supplement information from the abundant muscle spindles.[56] Nevertheless, joint and ligament receptors are thought to be important for control of feed-forward muscle activity, by way of complex sensory feedback mechanisms involving both ascending pathways and reflex activity via the gamma muscle spindle system.[57] Thus, joint and ligament receptors are likely to impact on sensorimotor control through their influence on the muscle spindle system.[58]

Reflex and central connections

The neck is not unique in having central connections that contribute to local proprioception and neuromuscular control but, compared to other areas of the body, the receptors also play an important role in the mediation of postural reflex responses and the subsequent connections between the visual and vestibular apparatus. Neck afferents have been shown to project to the medial and lateral vestibular nuclei[59] and the superior colliculus, a reflex centre for coordination between the ambient visual system and neck movement.[60] It has been suggested that cervical afferents can also influence the sympathetic system via beta receptors in the cervical muscles and vice versa.[61] Recently, this link between the cervical afferents and the sympathetic nervous system suggests an association between elevated psychological stress and altered sensorimotor control.[17]

Synaptic connections from the cervical receptors to other areas also play an important role in neck reflex activity. The neck afferents are involved in three posturally related reflexes influencing head and eye movement and postural stability, the cervicocollic reflex (CCR), the cervico-ocular reflex (COR) and the tonic neck reflex (TNR). These reflexes work in conjunction with other reflexes acting on the neck and eye musculature, stimulated by vestibular and visual input, for coordinated stability of the head and eyes (Fig 7.2).

The CCR causes reflex activation of neck muscles when the muscles are stretched with movement of the head in relation to the body. The CCR integrates with the vestibular system via the vestibulocollic reflex (VCR) to assist in the maintenance of head position and minimise head rotation.[62]

The COR works together with the vestibular ocular reflex (VOR) and optokinetic reflex (OKR) to act on the extraocular muscles (via the extraocular nuclei) and assist in maintaining eye position, such that head

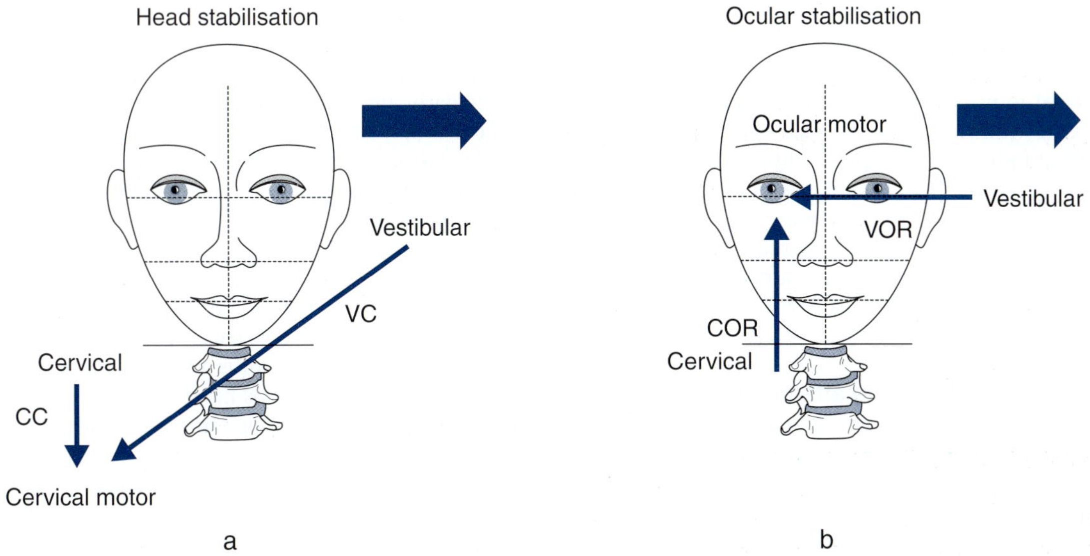

Figure 7.2 Reflex activity relating to the control of (a) head and (b) eye movement. COR = cervico-ocular reflex; VOR = vestibuloocular reflex; CCR = cervicocollic reflex; VCR = vestibulocollic reflex.

movement results in equal but opposite movement of the eyes. Through this connection, clear vision is maintained during head movement. The COR is evoked through stretching the neck muscles and acts on the extraocular muscles via their nuclei.[63]

Cervical afferents are also thought to influence the OKR through the convergence of information from the cervical and optokinetic systems on the vestibular neurons. In turn, eye movements can generate activation of the cervical muscles while the head is still. A close relationship between the deep cervical extensors/rotators and horizontal eye movement has also been observed,[64] and it is thought that this synergy is mediated by tecto-reticulo-spinal nuclei at the brain stem.[65]

The TNR mediates alterations in limb muscle activity when the body moves with respect to the head and acts to maintain a stable posture. It is integrated with the vestibulospinal reflex (VSR) to achieve postural stability.[66] Again, it is thought that neck muscle spindle afferents primarily generate the signals for this reflex.[67]

Effects of artificial disturbance of cervical afferentation on postural control

The association between artificial disturbances to cervical afferentation and disturbances to sensorimotor control has been demonstrated in several ways. Sectioning of the cervical dorsal root ganglions or injections of anaesthetic into deep neck structures has also been shown to cause nystagmus and severe ataxia.[68, 69] Less invasive techniques, such as neck muscle vibration, which is considered to primarily stimulate the muscle spindle afferents, has been shown to induce prolonged eye position changes, and visual and head illusory movements,[70, 71] produce increased body sway,[72] and to influence velocity and direction of gait and running.[73, 74] Similarly, experimentally induced pain, muscle fatigue and restriction of range of motion have also demonstrated altered sensorimotor control.[75, 76] The induced sensorimotor changes are similar to those seen in people following a whiplash injury, which provides further support for the neck as a primary cause of the disturbances.

Mechanisms responsible for altered sensorimotor control due to disturbed cervical afferentation

Conflict between the converging input from the different sensory systems or a sensory mismatch is the mechanism thought to be responsible for disturbances in sensorimotor control following interference to the cervical afferents, such as could occur after a whiplash injury.[14] Since information from the muscle spindles is of primary importance for cervical afferent information, and this input interacts with vestibular and visual information, a changed or disturbed sensitivity of the muscle spindles may result in the complaint of dizziness and visual disturbances, as well as altered cervical joint position and movement sense, knowledge of head position, eye–head coordination and/or balance following a whiplash injury.

There is also some evidence that the neck may directly influence the function of the VOR and VCR.[46] It is proposed that altered neck input could give rise to a mismatch of sensory input, as well as asymmetry of these reflexes.[12, 46]

Mechanisms of cervical afferent disturbance

There appears to be evidence that sensorimotor control disturbances may result from either a decrease or an increase in cervical afferent activity. The crucial factor appears to be that afferent input is altered and abnormal. Studies where anaesthetics are applied to the cervical region suggest that a decrease in afferent activity is responsible for the symptoms.[69] However, others suggest that 'over'-excitation of the cervical afferents may create problems.[77] Of specific relevance to whiplash has been the postulation that the injury may cause a perpetual cycle of incorrect afferent information.[78, 79] The sudden barrage of input from the cervical proprioceptors to the sensorimotor control system could create incorrect afferent information followed by compensatory muscle tension generated by the sensorimotor control system to restore postural stability. This, in turn, could lead to further altered neck afferent input, perpetuating the cycle. The situation may be complicated further by the effects of pain and inflammation resulting from damage to neck structures.

Causes of abnormal cervical afferent input following a whiplash injury

The combined influence of direct trauma and/or functional impairment of the receptors as well as the role of changed reflex activity and somatosensory reorganisation within the CNS should not be underestimated in the role of sensorimotor control disturbances following a whiplash injury (Fig 7.3).

Alterations in the neuromuscular control of muscles, through desensitising the mechanoreceptors, are likely to be particularly important causes of ongoing disturbances to sensorimotor control.[80] Neuromuscular control can become impaired in those with neck pain via several mechanisms, including inhibition of the deep stabilising musculature,[81] altered feed-forward preparatory muscle activity,[82] compensatory increased activity in the superficial muscles,[83] and altered neuromuscular efficiency and fatigability.[83] Similarly, morphological changes in cervical muscles, particularly the suboccipital muscles, in those with whiplash may also alter their proprioceptive capabilities.[84, 85] It is possible that such changes occur in the acute stages and persist despite the patient reporting recovery from pain.[86] Recent studies have demonstrated the direct deleterious effects of neck extensor muscle fatigue or pain on standing balance.[75, 87] Specifically, McPartland et al.[88] determined a significant correlation between poor balance control and fatty infiltration of the rectus capitis posterior minor muscle.

Altered reflex responses have also been suggested as possible causes of sensorimotor control disturbances following a whiplash injury. Decreased range of motion,[89] voluntary guarding or increased superficial muscle activity[83, 90] in participants with persistent WAD could possibly lead to an alteration in the gain of the CCR and perhaps secondary changes to VCR activity.[46] Further, evidence of altered COR activity and lack of compensatory changes with the VOR have also been noted in some people with persistent whiplash, and are thought to be factors contributing to altered sensorimotor control.[91]

Inflammatory mediators released following the injury may also activate chemosensitive nerve endings in joints and muscles, leading to altered muscle spindle activity.[92, 93] In addition, the effects of inflammation on nociceptors and mechanoreceptors locally, at the spinal cord and within the CNS can also influence the modulation of afferent input and, thus, both neuromuscular and sensorimotor control.[57, 94]

At the local level, an increase in nociceptor input occurs as a result of a peripheral release of chemical mediators following injury. This increase in nociceptive input may also cause a decrease in non-nociceptive input; that is, an alteration of afferent input to the sensorimotor control system. Such changes may also result in perpetuating pain, as non-nociceptive input normally has an inhibitory effect on pain modulation.[95]

Increased nociceptive input from the periphery can also lead to altered processing in the spinal cord and brain.[96] In chronic pain, mechanical receptors can continue to be pain-sensitive, possibly due to changes in the CNS and decreased central inhibition.[97] This generalised sensitivity to a variety of stimuli often occurs at both local and remote regions to the original injury and has been shown to be a particularly early feature in some subjects with whiplash, as well as one of the predictive features for chronicity.[98] In turn, this may lead to further prolonged disruption of afferent input from the cervical region.

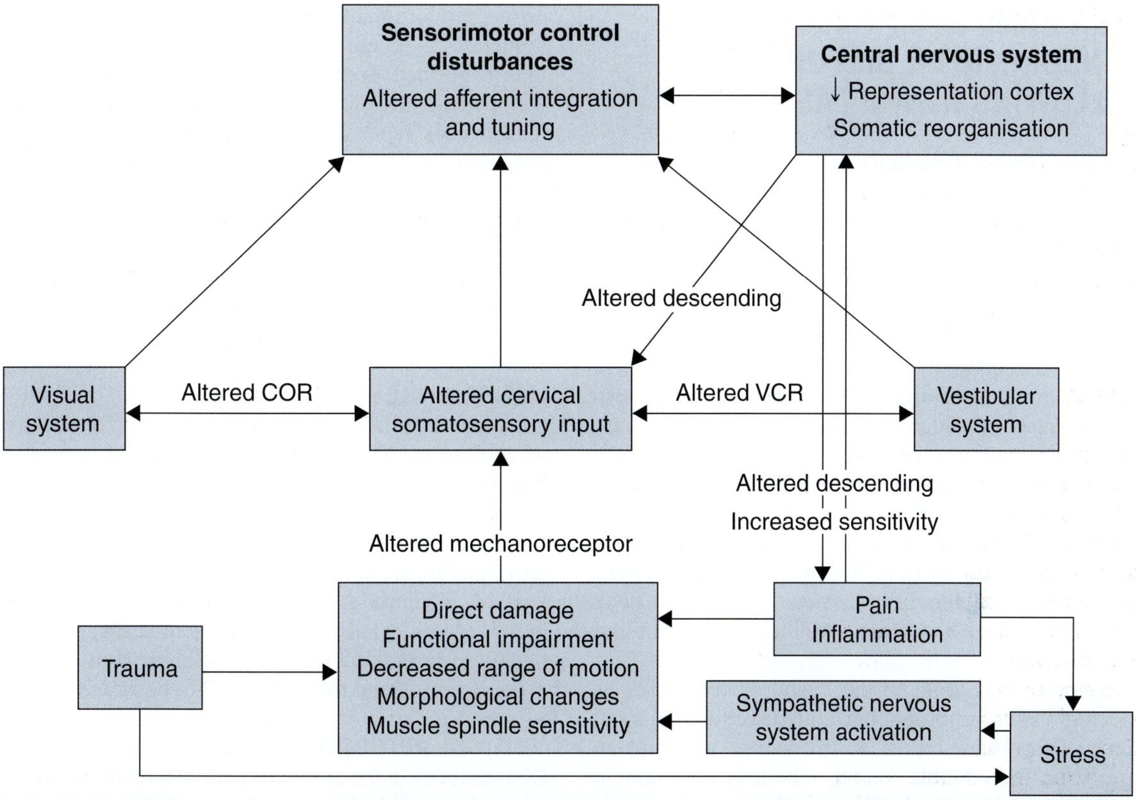

Figure 7.3 Causes of sensorimotor disturbance originating from the cervical region. COR = cervico-ocular reflex; VCR = vestibulocollic reflex.

Experimental pain has also been shown to influence muscle function.[94] Experimental neck pain in rats has demonstrated a direct and long-lasting influence on muscle spindle activity via excitation of chemosensitive afferents.[92, 93] This can also alter reflex muscle activity and adversely affect postural stability.[75] Pain has also been shown to alter spinal inhibitory effects, through the effect on the somatosensory cortex and other subcortical levels.[94] There is also evidence to suggest a possible role for pain in subcortical and cortical reorganisation at many levels of the somatosensory system in humans, and that both the removal of afferent inputs and the enhancement of nociceptive inputs could contribute to this neural reorganisation.[99]

Further, it is not uncommon for subjects with persistent whiplash to have elevated general and specific anxiety related to the accident.[100] Recently, it has been suggested that psychological stress may also influence cervical muscle spindle sensitivity via activation of the sympathetic nervous system and, thus, also contribute to altered cervical afferent input following a whiplash injury.[17]

In summary, several mechanisms could disturb cervical afferents in patients with neck pain following a whiplash injury. These include inflammation, direct damage, functional impairment and/or morphological changes to musculature, pain and psychological distress. These may alter proprioceptive capabilities, joint mechanics, CNS representation and muscle spindle sensitivity, and thus affect cervical afferent input to the sensorimotor control system. This, in turn, may also influence reflex connections to the visual and vestibular systems and subsequently cause secondary disturbances. Evidence to date would suggest altered cervical afferent input and its effect on the sensorimotor control system is the most likely primary cause of dizziness, unsteadiness, visual disturbances and altered balance, eye and head movement control that has been demonstrated in those following a whiplash injury, especially when there has been no associated mild head injury.

SIGNS AND SYMPTOMS OF SENSORIMOTOR DISTURBANCE FOLLOWING A WHIPLASH INJURY

Subjective complaints

Symptoms of dizziness and unsteadiness (cervical vertigo) are often present in patients with whiplash, especially in those with persistent pain and disability, and are present at a similar level of disability to those with chronic vestibular pathology.[1, 47] Such complaints have also been associated with reports of loss of balance and falls in some of these patients. Participants with whiplash generally report a pattern of dizziness considered characteristic of dizziness and/or unsteadiness of a cervical origin, which is different from patterns described by those with vestibular disturbances.[47] True vertigo, or spinning, is rarely described and generally the description is of a vague unsteadiness or lightheadedness.[1] Exacerbating features are generally related to increased neck pain or headache and/or neck-related movement and activity.[1, 47]

Symptoms relating to the visual system, such as blurred vision, photophobia and disordered fusion, have also been reported following a whiplash injury.[101] True double vision, which is common in patients with vertebrobasilar insufficiency, is rare in those with cervicogenic dizziness.[101]

Joint position sense

Cervical joint position sense (JPS) is considered to primarily reflect afferent input from the neck joint and muscle receptors and not to be particularly influenced by vestibular input, especially if neck movements are performed slowly when the vestibular system is below threshold.[102] Further, others have been able to demonstrate improvements in both the complaint of dizziness and cervical JPS following treatment directed at the cervical spine, such as manual therapy, acupuncture and specific neck muscle control exercises, suggesting that the effects were related more to changes in mechanoreceptor afferent input rather than changes in the vestibular system.[103, 104] However, there has been recent conflicting evidence of this in studies assessing cervical JPS in those with vestibular pathology.[47, 105]

The measure is based on the ability to relocate the natural head posture while vision is occluded.[106] Greater errors have been shown in subjects with both idiopathic neck pain and with persistent whiplash, although errors are thought to be greater in those with whiplash.[1, 2, 107] Sterling et al.[86] found JPS errors predominantly in those with whiplash with moderate-to-severe pain and disability early post injury. Further, Treleaven et al.[1] found that subjects with persistent whiplash complaining of dizziness had greater neck repositioning errors than those not complaining of dizziness, suggesting that subjects with complaints of dizziness and unsteadiness may have these symptoms as a result of a greater degree of abnormal afferent input from the cervical mechanoreceptors.

Position sense deficits have not been isolated to the neck, with deficits also seen in the shoulder and elbow in some patients with whiplash.[108, 109]

Cervical movement sense

Kristjansson et al.[107] reported on another dimension of neck proprioception where accuracy of reproduction of a neck-movement task was measured. This test showed that participants with whiplash had less accuracy in tracing a computer-generated movement pattern using the head when compared to control subjects. Further, Roren et al.[110] demonstrated no relationship between cervical JPS and movement sense, suggesting these tests are measuring different constructs of proprioception and that both need to be assessed.

Vertical perception

Disturbances in the ability of people with neck pain to correctly identify the vertical perception using the rod and frame test has been demonstrated and thought to be another test that reflects disturbed cervical proprioception.[111] It has been suggested that those with whiplash may also have greater deficits in this test, but this research is in its infancy and more work is required.

Standing balance

Several studies have demonstrated disturbed postural stability in patients with persistent whiplash,[3, 112, 113] especially in those complaining of dizziness.[18] Deficits were noted in most tests, including comfortable and tandem stances, but especially when vision was occluded. These deficits have also been demonstrated in those with recent whiplash but did not necessarily relate to pain and disability.[114, 115]

Furthermore, these static balance responses are likely to be primarily due to cervical afferent dysfunction rather than vestibular function, as they have been shown to differ between subjects with persistent WAD and those with unilateral vestibular pathology.[47] Others have also demonstrated improvements in sensorimotor control following treatment localised to the cervical spine.[116, 117] Fattori et al.[117] demonstrated that acupuncture to the cervical spine improved balance responses in subjects with whiplash, also supporting a cervical origin of the disturbances. Balance disturbances have also been related to dysfunction of the upper cervical extensor musculature,[87, 88] with a significant correlation found between poor balance control and fatty infiltration of the muscle in this small sample.[88]

Recently, dynamic and functional balance measures were assessed in those with persistent whiplash, and impairments in the step test, timed 10-metre walk with and without head turns, tandem walk and stair walking were demonstrated when compared to asymptomatic control subjects.[118] Delayed corrective responses to destabilising perturbations while sitting have also been seen in those with persistent whiplash.[119]

Eye movement control

Several alterations in oculomotor control have been demonstrated in those with whiplash, including disturbed eye follow, gaze stability, eye–head coordination and reflex activity. Abnormalities of eye follow during smooth pursuit eye movements may be present in disorders of the vestibular system, the CNS and as a result of abnormal afferent input from the cervical spine. A number of studies have identified abnormalities in patients with idiopathic cervical spine disorders, as well as in those with whiplash.[5, 79, 120] Tjell and Rosenhall[9] reported a method of testing—the smooth pursuit neck torsion (SPNT) test—which appears to be able to differentiate between smooth pursuit abnormalities of a vestibular or CNS cause from those of a cervical cause. To differentiate between these conditions, the researchers used a torsion manoeuvre of the neck, which would stimulate the cervical receptors but not the vestibular receptors. They demonstrated no change in smooth pursuit when measured in neutral and neck-torsioned positions in healthy asymptomatic participants or in participants with CNS or vestibular dysfunction, but there was a difference in participants with WAD. Subjects with whiplash not complaining of dizziness also demonstrated SPNT test abnormalities but to a lesser extent, suggesting that those complaining of dizziness have greater levels of abnormal cervical afferent input.[5, 79]

In another study using the SPNT test, this group of researchers suggested that cognitive disturbance, another common complaint post whiplash injury, might manifest from disturbed sensorimotor control due to abnormal cervical afferent input. Gimse et al.[40] demonstrated a close correlation between technical reading ability and information uptake, and disturbances in eye movement control of cervical origin (results of SPNT test) in participants with WAD. Similarly, driving skills and some cognitive disturbances were also shown to closely correlate with results of the SPNT test in the absence of other possible causes.[38, 121] Tjell et al.[79] hypothesised that the correlation between the SPNT results and reading, driving skills and cognition may be due to like areas of the brain being overloaded by the abnormal proprioceptive activity, which may lead to a decreased functional ability in areas controlling cognition.

However, there has not been universal agreement in the findings of research using the SPNT test in patients with whiplash, which may reflect methodological problems. For example, Prushansky et al.[122] demonstrated no change in eye movement performance with neck torsion in participants with whiplash using a fully automated analysis. In order to determine differences, it appears that trained observers are required to determine and extract the appropriate elements of the signal for analysis, so more research is required to refine and automate this measure.

There is also some evidence that eye movement dysfunction may be a feature of persistent problems following whiplash injury.[123] Hildingsson and Toolanen[123] followed 40 subjects from an average of 1.7 months (range 0.5–3 months) to 15 months (range 8–28 months) post whiplash injury. Smooth pursuit in neutral only (not torsion) and saccadic eye movement was measured. The subjects with eye movement dysfunction (20% of the cohort), measured on an initial assessment soon after the accident, had persistent disabling symptoms at the follow-up period (at least eight months post injury). In contrast, the 80% of subjects with normal eye movement function on initial assessment recovered fully or had only minor discomfort at follow-up.

While abnormalities in smooth pursuit have been linked with cervical afferent disturbances with the neck in torsion, it is possible that smooth pursuit abnormalities in neutral may reflect CNS lesions. Wieser et al.[124] contend that smooth pursuit abnormalities in neutral could be a clinical sign of brainstem involvement in subjects with migraine. There is some evidence that brainstem pathology might also exist in severe cases of persistent whiplash, but this is thought to be relatively uncommon.[10]

An increased gain of the COR has also been demonstrated in patients with whiplash.[125] In people with vestibular disorders and in older people, this is thought to be a compensatory response to a decrease in VOR gain.[91] Montfort et al.[91] have expanded on this work and recently found no compensatory decrease in the vestibulo-ocular gain in those with whiplash who have an increased cervico-ocular gain. They conclude that this phenomenon may be an important cause of disturbances to the visual system in those with whiplash.[91]

Recently, a pilot trial of case studies of individuals with whiplash reporting visual disturbances indicated deficits in gaze stability and head–eye coordination when compared to control subjects.[6] Specifically, decreased range of head movement while attempting gaze fixation, decreased head velocity during head–eye coordination, and compensatory head movements during isolated eye rotation were noted, which suggest disturbances in gaze stability and head–eye coordination in some of those with whiplash.[6] More work in this area is currently underway.

IMPLICATIONS FOR ASSESSMENT

Onset of impairments

The precise time of onset of symptoms of dizziness, unsteadiness and disturbances in measures of sensorimotor control needs to be further explored. Sterling et al.[86] demonstrated that changes in motor and sensory function occur soon after the whiplash injury, and that certain features were predictive of a poorer outcome. Dizziness was reported in 20% of the group complaining of moderate-to-severe pain and disability within one month of the injury. Cervical joint position error was also increased in these subjects.[86] Few subjects with milder complaints of neck pain and disability complained of dizziness or presented with deficits in cervical joint position error. Similarly, static balance deficits and some oculomotor deficits have been demonstrated in some people soon after the whiplash injury.[114, 115, 126]

Clinical assessment

Thus, early assessment of each of the tests of cervical joint position and movement sense, balance and oculomotor disturbances should be routine in all patients with whiplash. Such tests should not be confined to patients with symptoms of dizziness, as there is evidence for impairments in these measures in subjects who are not specifically complaining of any disturbances.[1, 5, 18, 127] Furthermore, the practice of using cervical joint position error tests to implicate other sensorimotor control deficits[2, 103] cannot be supported, as while it is feasible that abnormal cervical afferent input is the primary cause of the disturbances in subjects with persistent whiplash, the individual tests reflect different elements of sensorimotor control dysfunction. Some correlation between sensorimotor tests has been seen but prediction of abnormality between tests was limited.[110, 127]

Clinical assessment of cervical position and movement sense can be made by using a laser pointer mounted onto a lightweight headband.[106, 110] A difference between the starting and resting position of the laser beam on the wall of 4.5°, following an active movement with the eyes closed, is thought to suggest impairment in cervical position sense.[106, 110] Similarly, the laser method can be used to trace an intricate pattern, such as a figure of eight placed on the wall in front of the patient, to assess cervical movement sense. A subjective clinical judgment can be made based on the patient's ability to trace the pattern accurately and smoothly. A computerised method to measure head movement sense, 'the Fly', has also recently been developed.[107] It measures the patient's ability to correct cervical spine movements on a moment-to-moment basis, while moving the head and neck.

In the clinical assessment of static balance, a suite of tests, including altered visual, stance and surface conditions, is supported by the findings in the studies conducted and, thus, is the preferred protocol for testing.[1, 18, 128] Qualitative measures of balance, combined with the ability to maintain the test for 30 seconds, may also be useful in the clinical situation. Measures of dynamic and functional balance, such as the step test, stairs and timed 10-metre walk, may also be useful.[118]

Similarly, qualitative evaluation of smooth pursuit eye movement in neutral compared to torsioned positions,[5] gaze stability while moving the head and head–eye coordination should be used.[6, 129]

Differential diagnosis

The clinician should also consider the other possible causes of the disturbances discussed above, including vertebral artery insufficiency and peripheral or central vestibular pathology, and interview the patient and choose tests accordingly to determine the most likely cause.

Although there is some evidence that the neck may directly influence vestibular functioning,[12] primary vestibular pathology is possible and additional tests, such as the VOR and Hallpike–Dix manoeuvre,[130] may be necessary. Referral for a more thorough investigation of the vestibular apparatus or CNS may also be warranted.

IMPLICATIONS FOR MANAGEMENT

The management of WAD still challenges healthcare practitioners. No treatment to date has offered a panacea for whiplash. Improvements and new directions in management approaches are needed if the challenge of effective management of whiplash is to be met. Sensorimotor control can be impaired in people with whiplash, and this is likely to be due to abnormal cervical afferent input to the sensorimotor control system and different elements of dysfunction.

Thus, management of these disturbances may need to address not only the possible causes of abnormal cervical afferent input but also consider the effects that this may have in relation to the visual and vestibular systems and any secondary adaptive changes in the sensorimotor control system.

Addressing altered cervical afferent input

Several studies have demonstrated improvements in dizziness and/or sensorimotor control following treatment only localised to the cervical spine.[103, 116, 117] Acupuncture has been shown to improve neck joint position error, vertigo[103] and standing balance[117] in those with neck pain. Improvements in dizziness symptoms, cervical position sense and range of motion has also been demonstrated following neck manual therapy.[103, 131] Further, specific neuromuscular control training,[104] improved cervical position sense and cervical muscle endurance training improved balance in patients with whiplash.[132]

Addressing secondary adaptive changes in the sensorimotor control system

In contrast to the above, there is also evidence that specific treatment programs that emphasise gaze stability, eye–head coordination and/or head on trunk relocation practised in isolation without local cervical spine treatment have resulted in improvements not only in sensorimotor impairments but also improvements in range of motion, neck pain, drug intake and/or perceived disability.[50, 104, 133, 134]

Recently, a vestibular rehabilitation program improved balance and dizziness in patients with whiplash injury.[135] A novel method of training neck coordination may also be of benefit.[136] Again, it is unknown whether such an approach provided in isolation is able to address all the deficits or is the most efficient approach.

Combined local treatment and structured sensorimotor approach

Studies that have included eye–head coupling and coordination exercises as part of a multimodal approach have demonstrated improvements in neck pain and joint position error.[103, 137] There is also evidence that an exercise program combining manipulation, proprioceptive neuromuscular facilitation, acupressure on trigger points and range of motion exercises, intertwined with exercises to improve head relocation accuracy, was efficacious for neck pain.[138] Recently, a pilot trial of a combined approach demonstrated significant improvements in postural stability in those with chronic whiplash.[139]

Combined local and tailored sensorimotor approach

Such a combined approach of the above may be more suitable. However, the lack of direct correlation between sensorimotor measures[127] would imply that treatment directed to improve, for example, eye movement control, may not necessarily be the most effective to improve impairment in balance or joint position error. Thus, a tailored approach with exercises aimed to improve identified sensorimotor control deficits in cervical joint position and movement sense, oculomotor and/or static and dynamic balance, may be superior and is currently recommended clinically.[129, 140, 141] This type of intervention is similar to programs used in vestibular rehabilitation, which are tailored to the individual and have been found to be effective.[130] Suggested exercises have been described in detail elsewhere.[129, 140, 141]

CONCLUSION

There is considerable evidence to support the importance of cervical afferent dysfunction in the development of dizziness, unsteadiness, visual disturbances and altered balance, eye and head movement control following a whiplash injury, especially in those with persistent complaints, although other possible causes should be considered in the differential diagnosis. It is important that such symptoms and impairments are adequately assessed and managed and this should become an essential part of the routine management of whiplash injuries. Research to assist differential diagnosis and to understand the most important contributing factors associated with abnormal cervical afferent input and subsequent disturbances to the sensorimotor control system, as well as the most efficacious management of such complaints and impairments, will be important directions for the future.

References

1. Treleaven J, Jull G, Sterling M. Dizziness and unsteadiness following whiplash injury: characteristic features and relationship with cervical joint position error. *J Rehabil Med* 2003;35(1):36–43.
2. Heikkila H & Astrom PG. Cervicocephalic kinesthetic sensibility in patients with whiplash injury. *Scand J Rehabil Med* 1996;28(3):133–8.

3. Sjöström HJ, Allum J, Carpenter MG, et al. Trunk sway measures of postural stability during clinical balance tests in patients with chronic whiplash injury symptoms. *Spine* 2003;28(15):1725–34.
4. Kristjansson E, Dall'Alba P, Jull G. A study of five cervicocephalic relocation tests in three different subject groups. *Clin Rehabil* 2003;17(7):768–74.
5. Treleaven J, Jull G, Low Choy N. Smooth pursuit neck torsion test in whiplash associated disorders – relationship to self reports of neck pain and disability, dizziness and anxiety. *J Rehabil Med* 2005;37(4):219–23.
6. Grip H, Jull G, Treleaven J. Head eye co-ordination and gaze stability using simultaneous measurement of eye in head and head in space movements – potential for use in subjects with a whiplash injury. *J Clin Monit Comput* 2009;23:31–40.
7. Tjell C. Diagnostic considerations on whiplash associated disorders. Skovde: Department of Otorhinolaryngology, Central Hospital, Skovde, 1998.
8. Ferrari R. The chronic whiplash syndrome – a case of attributional pathosis? *Cephalalgia* 2002;22(7):560–2.
9. Tjell C & Rosenhall U. Smooth pursuit neck torsion test: a specific test for cervical dizziness. *Am J Otol* 1998;19(1):76–81.
10. Wenngren B, Pettersson K, Lowenhielm G, Hildingsson C. Eye motiliy and auditory brainstem response dysfunction after whiplash injury. *Acta Orthop Scand* 2002;122(3):276–83.
11. Panjabi MM, Cholewicki J, Nibu K, et al. Mechanism of whiplash injury. *Clin Biomech* 1998;13(4–5):239–49.
12. Fischer A, Verhagen WIM, Huygen PLM. Whiplash injury. A clinical review with emphasis on neuro-otological aspects. *Clin Otolaryngol Allied Sci* 1997;22(3):192–201.
13. Blokhorst M, Swinkels M, Lof O, et al. The influence of "state" related factors on focused attention following whiplash associated disorder. *J Clin Exp Neuropsychol* 2002;24(4):471–8.
14. Baloh R & Halmagyi G. Disorders of the vestibular system. New York: Oxford University Press, 1996.
15. Furman JM & Jacob RG. A clinical taxonomy of dizziness and anxiety in the otoneurological setting. *J Anxiety Disord* 2001;(1–2):9–26.
16. Bracher ES, Almeida CI, Almeida RR, et al. A combined approach for the treatment of cervical vertigo. *J Manipulative Physiol Ther* 2000;23(2): 96–100.
17. Passatore M & Roatta S. Influence of sympathetic nervous system on sensorimotor function: whiplash associated disorders (WAD) as a model. *Eur J Appl Physiol* 2006;98:423–49.
18. Treleaven J, Jull G, Low Choy N. Standing balance in persistent WAD – comparison between subjects with and without dizziness. *J Rehabil Med* 2005;37(4):224–9.
19. Cassidy JD. Early intervention in whiplash-associated disorders – a comparison of two treatment protocols. *Spine* 2000;25(14):1786–7.
20. Sapir DA & Gorup JM. Radiofrequency medial branch neurotomy in litigant and nonlitigant patients with cervical whiplash; a prospective study. *Spine* 2001;26(12):268–73.
21. Endo K, Suzuki H, Yamamoto K. Consciously postural sway and cervical vertigo after whiplash injury. *Spine* 2008;33(16):E539–E542.
22. Ferrari R & Russell AS. Development of persistent neurologic symptoms in patients with simple neck sprain. *Arthritis Care Res* 1999;12(1):70–6.
23. Kloen P, Patterson JD, Wintman BI, et al. Closed cervical spine trauma associated with bilateral vertebral artery injuries. *Arch Orthop Trauma Surg* 1999;119(7–8):478–81.
24. Biffl WL, Moore EE, Elliott JP, et al. The devastating potential of blunt vertebral arterial injuries. *Ann Surg* 2000;231(5):672–81.
25. Panjabi MM, Cholewicki J, Nibu K, et al. Biomechanics of whiplash injury. *Orthopade* 1998;27(12):813–19.
26. Chong CL & Ooi SB. Neck pain after minor neck trauma—is it always neck sprain? *Eur J Emerg Med* 2000;7(2):147–9.
27. Chung YS & Han DH. Vertebrobasilar dissection: a possible role of whiplash injury in its pathogenesis. *Neurol Res* 2002;24(2):129–38.
28. De Decker K, Van Havenbergh T, D'Archambeau O, Jorens PG. Basilar artery thrombosis in a trauma patient. Case report and review of the literature. *Resuscitation* 2003;59(1):147–54.
29. Seric V, Blazic-Cop N, Demarin V. Haemodynamic changes in patients with whiplash injury measured by transcranial Doppler sonography (TCD). *Coll Antropol* 2000;24(1):197–204.
30. Michaud TC. Uneventful upper cervical manipulation in the presence of a damaged vertebral artery. *J Manipulative Physiol Ther* 2002;25(7):472–83.
31. Taylor J & Taylor M. Cervical spinal injuries: an autopsy study of 109 blunt injuries. *J Musculoskeletal Pain* 1996;4(4):61–79.
32. Hurley M. The effects of joint damage on muscle function, proprioception and rehabilitation. *Man Ther* 1997;2(1):11–17.
33. Fitzgerald DC. Head trauma: hearing loss and dizziness [see comments]. *J Trauma* 1996;40(3):488–96.

34. Ommaya A & Hirsch A. Tolerances for cerebral concussion from head impact and whiplash in primates. *J Biomech* 1971;4:13–18.
35. Szabo T & Welcher J, eds. Human subject kinematics and electromyographic activity during low speed rear impact. Washington, DC: Society of Automotive Engineers, 1996.
36. Grimm RJ. Inner ear injuries in whiplash. *J Whiplash Related Disorders* 2002;1(1):65–75.
37. Radanov B. Controversy about brain damage following cranio-cervical acceleration-deceleration trauma. *J Musculoskeletal Pain* 2000;8(1–2):179–92.
38. Gimse R, Björgen IA, Tjell C, et al. Reduced cognitive functions in a group of whiplash patients with demonstrated disturbances in the posture control system. *J Clin Exp Neuropsychol* 1997;19(6):838–49.
39. Sturzenegger M, Radanov BP, Winter P, et al. MRI-based brain volumetry in chronic whiplash patients: no evidence for traumatic brain injury. *Acta Neurol Scand* 2008;117(1):49–54.
40. Gimse R, Tjell C, Björgen IA, Saunte C. Disturbed eye movements after whiplash due to injuries to the posture control system. *J Clin Exp Neuropsychol* 1996;18(2):178–86.
41. Wenngren BI, Pettersson K, Lowenhielm G, Hildingsson C. Eye motility and auditory brainstem response dysfunction after whiplash injury. *Acta Otolaryngol (Stockh)* 2002;122(3):276–83.
42. Chester JB. Whiplash, postural control, and the inner-ear. *Spine* 1991;16(7):716–20.
43. Tranter R, Graham JR. A review of the otological aspects of whiplash injury. *J Forensic Leg Med* 2009;16(2):53–5.
44. Vibert D & Hausler R. Acute peripheral vestibular deficits after whiplash injuries. *Ann Otol Rhinol Laryngol* 2003;112(3):246–51.
45. Fischer A, Huygen PLM, Folgering HT, et al. Vestibular hyperreactivity and hyperventilation after whiplash injury. *J Neurol Sci* 1995;132(1):35–43.
46. Solarino B, Coppola F, Di Vella G, et al. Vestibular evoked myogenic potentials (VEMPs) in whiplash injury: a prospective study. *Acta Otolaryngol* 2008;Nov 13:1–6.
47. Treleaven J, Low Choy N, Darnell R, et al. Comparison of sensorimotor disturbance between subjects with persistent whiplash-associated disorder and subjects with vestibular pathology associated with acoustic neuroma. *Arch Phys Med Rehabil* 2008;89(3):522–30.
48. Padula WV & Argyris S. Post trauma vision syndrome and visual midline shift syndrome. *Neurorehabilitation* 1996;6(3):165–71.
49. Brown S. Effect of whiplash injury on accommodation. *Clin Experiment Ophthalmol* 2003;31(5):424–9.
50. Storaci R, Manelli A, Schiavone N, et al. Whiplash injury and oculomotor dysfunctions: clinical-posturographic correlations. *Eur Spine J* 2006;15(12):1811–16.
51. Peterson BW. Current approaches and future directions to understanding control of head movement. *Prog Brain Res* 2004;143:369–81.
52. Corneil BD, Olivier E, Munoz DP. Neck muscle responses to stimulation of monkey superior colliculus. I. Topography and manipulation of stimulation parameters. *J Neurophysiol* 2002;88(4):1980–99.
53. Kulkarni V, Chandy M, Babu K. Quantitative study of muscle spindles in suboccipital muscles of human foetuses. *Neurol India* 2001;49:355–9.
54. Boyd Clark L, Briggs C, Galea M. Muscle spindle distribution, morphology, and density in the longis colli and multifidus muscles of the cervical spine. *Spine* 2002;27(7):694–701.
55. Liu J, Thornell L, Pedrosa-Domellof F. Muscle spindles in the deep muscles of the human neck: a morphological and immunocytochemical study. *J Histochem Cytochem* 2003;51(2):175–86.
56. McLain RF. Mechanoreceptor endings in human cervical facet joints. *Spine* 1994;19(5):495–501.
57. Ageborg E. Consequences of a ligament injury on neuromuscular function and relevance to rehabilitation – using the anterior cruciate ligament-injured knee as a model. *J Electromyogr Kinesiol* 2002;12:205–12.
58. Sjölander P, Johansson H, Djupsjöbacka M. Spinal and supraspinal effects of activity in ligament afferents. *J Electromyogr Kinesiol* 2002;12:167–76.
59. Gdowski GT & McCrea RA. Neck proprioceptive inputs to primate vestibular nucleus neurons. *Exp Brain Res* 2000;135(4):511–26.
60. Isa T & Sasaki S. Brainstem control of head movements during orienting; organization of the premotor circuits. *Prog Neurobiol* 2002;66(4):205–41.
61. Hinoki M. Vertigo due to whiplash injury: a neuro-otological approach. *Acta Otolaryngol (Stockh)* 1975;419:9–29.
62. Peterson B, Goldberg J, Bilotto G, Fuller JH. Cervicocollic reflex: its dynamic properties and interaction with vestibular reflexes. *J Neurophysiol* 1985;54(1):90–108.
63. Mergner T, Schweigart G, Botti F, Lehmann A. Eye movements evoked by proprioceptive stimulation along the body axis in humans. *Exp Brain Res* 1998;120(4):450–60.

64. Corneil BD, Olivier E, Munoz DP. Visual responses on neck muscles reveal selective gating that prevents express Saccades. *Neuron* 2004;42(5): 831–41.
65. Berthoz A & Grantyn A. Neuronal mechanisms underlying eye-head coordination. *Prog Brain Res* 1986;64:325–43.
66. Yamagata Y, Yates BJ, Wilson VJ. Participation of Ia reciprocal inhibitory neurons in the spinal circuitry of the tonic neck reflex. *Exp Brain Res* 1991;84(2):461–4.
67. Chan YS, Kasper J, Wilson VJ. Dynamics and directional sensitivity of neck muscle-spindle responses to head rotation. *J Neurophysiol* 1987;57(6):1716–29.
68. Ishikawa K, Matsuzaki Z, Yokomizo M, et al. Effect of unilateral section of cervical afferent nerve upon optokinetic response and vestibular nystagmus induced by sinusoidal rotation in guinea pigs. *Acta Otolaryngol Suppl* 1998;537:6–10.
69. DeJong PT, DeJong JM, Cohen B, Jongkees LB. Ataxia and nystagmus induced by injection of local anaesthetics in the neck. *Ann Neurol* 1977;1(3): 240–6.
70. Lennerstrand G, Han Y, Velay JL. Properties of eye movements induced by activation of neck muscle proprioceptors. *Graefes Arch Clin Exp Ophthalmol* 1996;234(11):703–9.
71. Karnath HO, Reich E, Rorden C, et al. The perception of body orientation after neck-proprioceptive stimulation – effects of time and of visual cueing. *Exp Brain Res* 2002;143(3):350–8.
72. Kavounoudias A, Gilhodes JC, Roll R, Roll JP. From balance regulation to body orientation: two goals for muscle proprioceptive information processing? *Exp Brain Res* 1999;124(1):80–8.
73. Bove M, Courtine G, Schieppati M. Neck muscle vibration and spatial orientation during stepping in place in humans. *J Neurophysiol* 2002;88(5): 2232–41.
74. Courtine G, Papaxanthis C, Laroche D, Pozzo T. Gait-dependent integration of neck muscle afferent input. *Neuroreport* 2003;14(18):2365–8.
75. Vuillerme N & Pinsault N. Experimental neck muscle pain impairs standing balance in humans. *Exp Brain Res* 2009;192(4):723–9.
76. Schmid M & Schieppati M. Neck muscle fatigue and spatial orientation during stepping in place in humans. *J Appl Physiol* 2005;99(1):141–53.
77. Hinoki M & Niki H. Neurotological studies on the role of the sympathetic nervous system in the formation of traumatic vertigo of cervical origin. *Acta Otolaryngol Suppl* 1975;330:185–96.
78. Davis C. Chronic pain/dysfunction in whiplash-associated disorders. *J Manipulative Physiol Ther* 2001;24(1):44–51.
79. Tjell C, Tenenbaum A, Sandström S. Smooth pursuit neck torsion test—a specific test for whiplash associated disorders? *J Whiplash Associated Disorders* 2003;1(2):9–24.
80. Swanik C, Lephart F, Giannantonio F, Fu F. Re-establishing proprioception and muscle control in the ACL injured athlete. *J Sport Rehabil* 1997;6:182–206.
81. Falla D, Jull G, Dall'Alba P, et al. An electromyographic analysis of the deep cervical flexor muscles in performance of craniocervical flexion. *Phys Ther* 2003;83(10):899–906.
82. Falla D, Jull G, Hodges PW. Feedforward activity of the cervical flexor muscles during voluntary arm movements is delayed in chronic neck pain. *Exp Brain Res* 2004;157(1):43–8.
83. Falla D. Unravelling the complexity of muscle impairment in chronic neck pain. *Man Ther* 2004; 9(3):125–33.
84. Elliott J, Jull G, Noteboom JT, et al. Fatty infiltration in the cervical extensor muscles in persistent whiplash-associated disorders – a magnetic resonance imaging analysis. *Spine* 2006;31(22):E847–E855.
85. Uhlig Y, Weber BR, Grob D, Muntner M. Fiber composition and fiber transformation in neck muscles of patients with dysfunction of the cervical spine. *J Orthop Res* 1995;13:240–9.
86. Sterling M, Jull G, Vicenzino B, et al. Development of motor system dysfunction following whiplash injury. *Pain* 2003;103(1–2): 65–73.
87. Schieppati M, Nardone A, Schmid M. Neck muscle fatigue affects postural control in man. *Neuroscience* 2003;121(2):277–85.
88. McPartland JM, Brodeur RR, Hallgren RC. Chronic neck pain, standing balance, and suboccipital muscle atrophy – a pilot study. *J Manipulative Physiol Ther* 1997;20(1):24–9.
89. Dall'alba P, Sterling M, Treleaven J, Jull G. Cervical range of motion discriminates between asymptomatic and whiplash subjects. *Spine* 2001;26(19):2090–4.
90. Jull G. Deep cervical flexor muscle dysfunction in whiplash. *J Musculoskeletal Pain* 2000;8: 143–54.
91. Montfoort I, Van der Geest JN, Slijper HP, et al. Adaptation of the cervico- and vestibulo-ocular reflex in whiplash injury patients. *J Neurotrauma* 2008;25(6):687–93.

92. Thunberg J, Hellstrom F, Solander P, et al. Influences on the fusimotor-muscle spindle system from chemosensitive nerve endings in the cervical facet joints in the cat: possible implications for whiplash induced disorders. *Pain* 2001;91: 15–22.
93. Wenngren B, Pedersen J, Sjolander P, et al. Bradykinin and muscle stretch alter contralateral cat neck muscle spindle output. *Neurosci Res* 1998;32:119–29.
94. Le Pera D, Graven-Nielsen T, Valeriani M, et al. Inhibition of motor system excitability at cortical and spinal level by tonic muscle pain. *Clin Neurophysiol* 2001;112(9):1633–41.
95. Davis KD, Kiss ZH, Tasker RR, Dostrovsky JO. Thalamic stimulation-evoked sensations in chronic pain patients and in nonpain (movement disorder) patients. *J Neurophysiol* 1996;75(3):1026–37.
96. Woolf CJ. Evidence for a central component of post-injury pain hypersensitivity. *Nature* 1983;306(5944):686–8.
97. Curatolo M, Petersen-Felix S, Arendt-Nielsen L, et al. Central hypersensitivity in chronic pain after whiplash injury. *Clin J Pain* 2001;17(4):306–15.
98. Sterling M, Jull G, Vicenzino B, Kenardy J. Sensory hypersensitivity occurs soon after whiplash injury and is associated with poor recovery. *Pain* 2003;104(3):509–17.
99. Tinazzi M, Fiaschi A, Rosso T, et al. Neuroplastic changes related to pain occur at multiple levels of the human somatosensory system: a somatosensory-evoked potentials study in patients with cervical radicular pain. *J Neurosci* 2000;20(24):9277–83.
100. Sterling M, Kenardy J, Jull G, Vicenzino B. The development of psychological changes following whiplash injury. *Pain* 2003;106(3):481–9.
101. Hülse M. *Klinik der Funktionsstörungen des Kopfgelengbereichs*. In: Hülse M, Neuhuber WL, Wolff HD, eds. *Der kranio-zervikale Übergang*. Berlin: Springer, 1998: pp 43–97.
102. Blouin J, Okada T, Wolsley C, Bronstein A. Encoding target-trunk relative position: cervical versus vestibular contribution. *Exp Brain Res* 1998;122(1):101–7.
103. Heikkila H, Johansson M, Wenngren BI. Effects of acupuncture, cervical manipulation and NSAID therapy on dizziness and impaired head repositioning of suspected cervical origin: a pilot study. *Man Ther* 2000;5(3):151–7.
104. Jull G, Falla D, Treleaven J, Hodges P, Vicenzino B. Retraining cervical joint position sense: the effect of two exercise regimes. *J Orthop Res* 2007;25(3): 404–12.
105. Pinsault N, Vuillerme N, Pavan P. Cervicocephalic relocation test to the neutral head position: assessment in bilateral labyrinthine-defective and chronic, nontraumatic neck pain patients. *Arch Phys Med Rehabil* 2008;89(12):2375–8.
106. Revel M, Andre-Deshays C, Minguet M. Cervicocephalic kinesthetic sensibility in patients with cervical pain. *Arch Phys Med Rehabil* 1991;72:288–91.
107. Kristjansson E, Hardardottir L, Asmundardottir M, Gudmundsson K. A new clinical test for cervicocephalic kinesthetic sensibility: "The fly". *Arch Phys Med Rehabil* 2004;85(3):490–5.
108. Sandlund J, Djupsjobacka M, Ryhed B, et al. Predictive and discriminative value of shoulder proprioception tests for patients with whiplash-associated disorders. *J Rehabil Med* 2006;38(1):44–9.
109. Knox JJ, Beilstein DJ, Charles SD, et al. Changes in head and neck position have a greater effect on elbow joint position sense in people with whiplash-associated disorders. *Clin J Pain* 2006;22(6):512–18.
110. Roren A, Mayoux-Benhamou MA, Fayad F, et al. Comparison of visual and ultrasound based techniques to measure head repositioning in healthy and neck-pain subjects. *Man Ther* 2009;14(3):270–7.
111. Bagust J. Assessment of verticality perception by a rod-and-frame test: Preliminary observations on the use of a computer monitor and video eye glasses. *Arch Phys Med Rehabil* 2005;86(5):1062–4.
112. Madeleine P, Prietzel H, Svarrer H, Arendt-Nielsen L. Quantitative posturography in altered sensory conditions: a way to assess balance instability in patients with chronic whiplash injury. *Arch Phys Med Rehabil* 2004;85(3):432–8.
113. Michaelson P, Michaelson M, Jaric S, et al. Vertical posture and head stability in patients with chronic neck pain. *J Rehabil Med* 2003;35(5):229–35.
114. Cobo EP, Garcia-Alsina J, Almazan CG, et al. Postural control disorders in initial phases of whiplash. *Med Clin (Barc)* 2009;132(16):616–20.
115. Dehner C, Heym B, Maier D, et al. Postural control deficit in acute QTF grade II whiplash injuries. *Gait Posture* 2008;28(1):113–19.
116. Karlberg M, Magnusson M, Malmstrom EM, et al. Postural and symptomatic improvement after physiotherapy in patients with dizziness of suspected cervical origin. *Arch Phys Med Rehab* 1996;77(9):874–82.
117. Fattori B, Borsari C, Vannucci G, et al. Acupuncture treatment for balance disorders following whiplash injury. *Acupunct Electrother Res* 1996;21(3–4): 207–17.

118. Stokell R, Yu A, Treleaven J. Dynamic and functional balance tasks in subjects with persistent whiplash. MPA APA Conference, Sydney, October 2009.
119. Cote JN, Patenaude I, St-Onge N, Fung J. Whiplash-associated disorders affect postural reactions to antero-posterior support surface translations during sitting. *Gait Posture* 2009;29(4):603–11.
120. Heikkila HV & Wenngren BI. Cervicocephalic kinesthetic sensibility, active range of cervical motion, and oculomotor function in patients with whiplash injury. *Arch Phys Med Rehabil* 1998;79(9):1089–94.
121. Gimse R, Bjorgen I, Straume A. Driving skills after whiplash. *Scand J Psychol* 1997;38(3):165–70.
122. Prushansky T, Dvir Z, Pevzner E, Gordon CR. Electro-oculographic measures in patients with chronic whiplash and healthy subjects: a comparative study. *J Neurol Neurosurg Psychiatry* 2004;75(11):1642–4.
123. Hildingsson C & Toolanen G. Outcome after soft-tissue injury of the cervical spine: a prospective study of 93 car-accident victims. *Acta Orthop Scand* 1990;61(4):357–9.
124. Wieser T, Wolff R, Hoffmann KP, et al. Persistent ocular motor disturbances in migraine without aura. *Neurol Sci* 2004;25(1):8–12.
125. Montfoort I, Kelders WPA, van der Geest JN, et al. Interaction between ocular stabilization reflexes in patients with whiplash injury. *Invest Ophthalmol Vis Sci* 2006;47(7):2881–4.
126. Hildingsson C, Wenngren BI, Toolanen G. Eye motility dysfunction after soft-tissue injury of the cervical-spine – a controlled, prospective-study of 38 patients. *Acta Orthop Scand* 1993;64(2):129–32.
127. Treleaven J, Jull G, Low Choy N. The relationship of cervical joint position error to balance and eye movement disturbances in persistent whiplash. *Man Ther* 2006;11(2):99–106.
128. Field S, Treleaven J, Jull G. Standing balance: a comparison between idiopathic and whiplash-induced neck pain. *Man Ther* 2008;13(3):183–91.
129. Treleaven J. Sensorimotor disturbances in neck disorders affecting postural stability, head and eye movement control. *Man Ther* 2008;13(1):2–11.
130. Herdman S. Vestibular rehabilitation. Philadelphia: Davis, 2000.
131. Reid S, Rivett D, Katekar M, Callister R. Sustained natural apophyseal glides (SNAGs) are an effective treatment for cervicogenic dizziness. *Man Ther* 2008;13:357–66.
132. Stapley PJ, Beretta MV, Dalla Toffola E, Schieppati M. Neck muscle fatigue and postural control in patients with whiplash injury. *Clin Neurophysiol* 2006;47(3):610–22.
133. Revel M, Minguet M, Gergory P, et al. Changes in cervicocephalic kinesthesia after a proprioceptive rehabilitation program in patients with neck pain: a randomized controlled study. *Arch Phys Med Rehabil* 1994;75:895–9.
134. Humphreys B & Irgens P. The effect of a rehabilitation exercise program on head repositioning accuracy and reported levels of pain in chronic neck pain subjects. *J Whiplash Related Disorders* 2002;1(1):99–112.
135. Hansson EE, Mansson NO, Ringsberg KAM, Hakansson A. Dizziness among patients with whiplash-associated disorder: a randomized controlled trial. *J Rehabil Med* 2006;38(6):387–90.
136. Roijezon U, Bjorklund M, Bergenheim M, Djupsjobacka M. A novel method for neck coordination exercise – a pilot study on persons with chronic non-specific neck pain. *J Neuroeng Rehabil* 2008;5:36.
137. Provinciali L, Baroni M, Illuminati L, Ceravolo MG. Multimodal treatment to prevent the late whiplash syndrome. *Scand J Rehabil Med* 1996;28(2): 105–11.
138. Palmgren PJ, Sandstrom PJ, Lundqvist FJ, Heikkila H. Improvement after chiropractic care in cervicocephalic kinesthetic sensibility and subjective pain intensity in patients with nontraumatic chronic neck pain. *J Manipulative Physiol Ther* 2006;29(2):100–6.
139. Oddsdottir G. Cervical induced balance disturbances after motor vehicle collisions: the efficacy of two successive physical treatment approaches. Reykjavik: University of Iceland, 2006.
140. Jull G, Sterling M, Falla D, et al. Whiplash, headache and neck pain. London: Elsevier, 2008.
141. Treleaven J. Sensorimotor disturbances in neck disorders affecting postural stability, head and eye movement control – part 2: case studies. *Man Ther* 2008;13(3):266–75.

CHAPTER 8
Psychological aspects of whiplash associated disorders

Jan Buitenhuis, Peter de Jong, Jan Jaspers, Justin Kenardy

This chapter provides an overview of current scientific knowledge regarding psychological determinants of whiplash associated disorders (WAD) and the possible relationship with aetiology, symptom severity and course.

A distinct characteristic of whiplash injury, or WAD, when compared to other chronic pain conditions, is the relationship to an accident. As a consequence, there is usually a sudden onset of symptoms. Furthermore, in many cases the accident is caused by someone else, which can lead to negative feelings towards the responsible party. The latter situation can also lead to a liability claim, which could further influence the course of symptoms.[1]

Dealing with an accident requires certain emotional and stress management skills. The onset of acute or post-traumatic stress symptoms can influence the experience of symptoms and, thus, their course. Neck pain can be named or labelled in several ways. This process can lead to or be the result of anxiety, dysfunctional beliefs and negative expectations regarding the experienced symptoms.

In research on low back pain, it is well established that psychological factors are related to chronic pain and disability.[2] Given that chronic whiplash is also chronic musculoskeletal pain related to the spine without clear identification of a somatic cause, it seems reasonable to hypothesise that psychological parameters may play a role in the aetiology and course of persisting whiplash symptoms. Although a recent review of predictive factors for developing chronic whiplash complaints revealed only limited evidence for psychosocial variables, such as personality traits and psychosocial work factors, there is evidence that psychological distress, including affective disturbances, anxiety and depression, are associated with persistent whiplash symptoms.[3–5] It is becoming apparent that psychological factors, such as initial and persisting post-traumatic stress, may be involved in the aetiology and maintenance of chronic whiplash symptoms.[6] Identification of these and other psychological factors is, therefore, of paramount importance in the facilitation of prevention and/or treatment.

ACCIDENT-RELATED PSYCHOLOGICAL FACTORS

Acute and post-traumatic stress disorder

An important factor to consider is that neck complaints in whiplash follow an accident. An accident can be a frightening and sometimes even a terrifying experience. It is, therefore, not surprising that such an experience often gives rise to post-traumatic anxiety symptoms. Experiencing a traumatic event can also lead to the onset of a so-called acute stress disorder (ASD). The essential features of ASD are the development of anxiety, dissociative and other symptoms that occurs within one month after exposure to an extreme traumatic stressor.[7] Following the American Psychiatric Association's DSM IV classification, the specific diagnosis requires several criteria, including derealisation, depersonalisation or dissociative amnesia where an important aspect of the trauma cannot be recalled; recurrent images, thoughts, dreams, illusions or flashback episodes; marked avoidance of stimuli that arouse recollections of the trauma; and marked symptoms of anxiety or increased arousal. These symptoms cause clinically significant distress or impairment in social, occupational or other important areas of functioning.[7] Also, when the formal diagnostic criteria are not met, there can obviously still be acute stress symptoms. Although research on early stress symptoms (< one month) in whiplash is rather scarce, the available evidence suggests that there is a moderate-to-severe acute stress response in about 13% of whiplash cases.[8] Thus far it is largely unclear if acute stress symptoms are associated with whiplash symptom severity or have any predictive value regarding recovery.

Stress symptoms that persist for more than one month may eventually evolve into post-traumatic stress disorder (PTSD). PTSD is an anxiety disorder that requires a response of fear at the time of trauma together with three symptom clusters: re-experiencing, avoidance and hyperarousal symptoms. PTSD is a relatively common condition following traffic accidents.[9–12] As many as 23% of traffic accident victims develop PTSD, which is known to have high psychiatric and medical comorbidity.[13–16] Post-traumatic stress symptoms may give rise to increased anxiety and vigilance levels, thereby fuelling catastrophic, dysfunctional interpretations of acute neck pain. PTSD shares several symptoms with whiplash, including sleep disorder, irritability and problems with attention and concentration. Therefore, it is also conceivable that post-traumatic stress symptoms may be erroneously attributed to whiplash.

There is evidence to indicate that post-traumatic stress symptoms (i.e. re-experiencing and avoidance symptoms) are related to whiplash.[6, 17] More specifically, the re-experiencing and avoidance subscales of the Impact of Event Scale (IES) were found to be associated with relatively persistent whiplash complaints at six months follow-up.[18] Unfortunately, many studies use the IES, thereby only testing two of the three PTSD symptom scales; the hyperarousal symptom cluster scale is not included in the IES. Nonetheless, other research has shown hyperarousal symptoms to be highly relevant in the relationship between PTSD and whiplash.[19]

Since anxiety is an important feature of PTSD and is known to influence the perception and experience of pain, post-traumatic stress symptoms may also alter the perception and experience of acute neck pain.[20, 21] It has been shown that PTSD is more prevalent among car-accident victims who have post-whiplash syndrome compared to car-accident victims experiencing other symptoms. Moreover, the presence of PTSD is associated with more severe post-whiplash symptoms.[6, 17, 19] Additionally, the hyperarousal symptoms cluster has been found to have predictive validity for the persistence and severity of post-whiplash symptoms six and 12 months after the accident.[19] This predictive validity cannot be readily attributed to either the severity of the accident or the severity of the sustained injury, as these aspects have been found to be largely independent of the development of PTSD.[22] This seems to correspond with earlier research that suggests that victims with post-whiplash syndrome generally considered the accident more frightening than did other car-accident victims, suggesting the presence of higher fear levels, which in turn may elicit or indicate post-traumatic stress.[23]

Because perceived threat is of paramount importance in the aetiology of PTSD, it can be hypothesised that the presence of whiplash complaints is threatening and induces anxiety complaints. This would make the accident even more frightening and could subsequently lead to more post-traumatic stress symptoms. The presence of PTSD was found to be associated with more severe whiplash complaints and poor functional recovery.[6, 19] Results from research on the specific relevance of the three symptom clusters is still ambiguous. One study found that avoidance behaviour may have a stronger influence on recovery.[6] In another study, which controlled for all three symptoms clusters, only the hyperarousal cluster was found to have predictive validity.[19] Hyperarousal symptoms also include hypervigilance, which is known to be correlated with higher reported pain intensity and catastrophic thinking.[24] Therefore, it could be that hypervigilance results in symptom amplification, fuelling perceived symptom severity, thereby contributing to a process that leads to chronic complaints.

In the sympathetic arousal hypothesis, hypervigilance is labelled as sensory hypersensitivity. There is consistent evidence of sensory disturbances indicative of central nervous system hyperexcitability as a characteristic of whiplash. Studies have shown lowered pain thresholds and pain tolerance to various stimuli. Specific sensory features, such as cold hyperalgesia and intolerance, seem predictive of poor functional recovery.[25, 26] Early sympathetic disturbance was found to be associated with persistent post-traumatic stress symptoms, leading to speculation of a biological vulnerability that may trigger persistent post-traumatic stress.[27] All in all, studies from several directions point to a mechanism characterised by hyperarousal, hypervigilance or nociceptive sensitisation related to the prognosis of whiplash symptoms.

It is important to note that within PTSD, hyperarousal symptoms closely resemble symptoms that are often attributed to post-whiplash syndrome, such as difficulty concentrating or nervousness. It is, therefore, conceivable that these symptoms often associated with whiplash are actually related to post-traumatic stress. It is also possible that the predictive value of hyperarousal symptoms is merely due to these symptoms resembling symptoms associated with or often attributed to post-whiplash syndrome. The intensity of these symptoms is known to be related to a poor prognosis.

Anger and blame

Whiplash is, by definition, preceded by an accident. In many cases an accident may have an external cause, involving another person or persons. Feelings of anger towards those perceived to be responsible are often expressed in clinical practice. Furthermore, it has been argued that chronic whiplash symptoms seldom present in drivers who have caused the collision. Therefore, attributed blame may be associated with the prognosis.[28] It has been demonstrated that perceived responsibility for a traffic accident was associated with lower PTSD levels six months after the accident.[29] Research in other chronic pain conditions has shown that anger is associated with heightened pain expression.[30] In whiplash, anger was found to be associated with physical and psychological complaints six months after a motor vehicle crash (MVC).[31] In summary, research suggests that anger is an emotion that can influence the experienced pain and is associated with persistent symptoms. This is especially so in the context of legal liability.

COPING

Coping can be defined as the way in which an individual behaviourally, cognitively and emotionally adapts to manage external or internal stressors.[32] The accident itself, as well as the pain afterwards, can be considered an external stressor and, therefore, requires coping efforts. Research in the context of chronic low back pain showed that individuals' coping style is an important moderator of the course of pain symptoms and the outcome of treatment.[33, 34] Because in whiplash the onset of complaints is often related to a stressful accident, this may place an even higher demand on existing coping skills. Accidents can lead to physical complaints or to temporary or long-term disability, all demanding satisfactory coping.

The experience of neck pain may be more frightening than low back pain, which, while more common, is usually believed to be benign in nature. Depending on the cultural context, acute neck pain can be associated with persistent complaints and disability, making the complaints even more frightening. Dysfunctional coping styles could lead to worsened pain experience or catastrophic interpretations of symptoms, thereby contributing to a bad prognosis. An active coping style is usually considered preferable, and improving active coping strategies is often advised as a main treatment goal.[35] Dysfunctional coping styles could lead to a heightened pain experience or catastrophic interpretations of symptoms, thereby contributing to a bad prognosis.

The use of passive coping styles is associated with prolonged symptoms.[36, 37] Previous research has shown that patients who believe they can control their pain, who avoid catastrophising about their condition and who believe they are not severely disabled appear to function better than those who do not. Such beliefs may mediate some of the relationships between pain severity and adjustment.[38] This finding suggests that there is a possible relationship with expectations and, hence, causal attribution. However, other research has found no evidence that coping styles influenced the outcome. This may be due to differences in the questionnaires used and, hence, in the definitions and participants.[39]

CATASTROPHISING AND KINESIOPHOBIA

The fear-avoidance model was developed in relation to low back pain to provide an integrated model of the risk factors known to be associated with pain.[40, 41] When acute pain is not perceived as threatening, patients usually continue daily activities, thereby promoting functional recovery. However, when pain is catastrophically misinterpreted, a vicious circle may be initiated in which catastrophising leads to pain-related fear, which leads to avoidance behaviour, including the avoidance of movement and physical activity, resulting in disuse and continuing pain. In support of the fear-avoidance model, studies on chronic pain conditions suggest that excessive pain catastrophising and fear of movement/(re) injury (*kinesiophobia*) are important in the aetiology of chronic symptoms.[42] Pain catastrophising has consistently been associated with disability in patients experiencing pain.[43, 44] In avoidance behaviour, activities that are thought to increase or cause pain are avoided. Various studies demonstrate that patients with chronic low back pain avoid behavioural performance tasks.[40] In cases of low back pain, fear-avoidance beliefs are identified as risk factors for chronic low back pain, suggesting that these factors play a critical role.

Patients with chronic low back pain who retrospectively reported a sudden traumatic pain onset exhibited more kinesiophobia than patients who reported that the pain had started gradually.[45] In the case of whiplash, the onset of pain is often described as sudden, possibly setting the stage for the development of kinesiophobia, which in turn may contribute to a chronic course. Patients who are fearful of pain may focus on possible threats, thereby not only disrupting attentional processes, and thus leaving less attention available for other tasks but, also, experiencing intensified pain.[46, 47]

Pain catastrophising refers to an exaggerated negative interpretation of actual or anticipated pain.[48] Earlier research has found that the habitual tendency to make catastrophic interpretations of pain is associated with a heightened pain experience in various patient groups.[49] Furthermore, catastrophising has been associated with heightened disability in chronic pain, independent of the level of actual physical impairment.[50–52]

Because of the apparent role of kinesiophobia in the transition from acute to chronic low back pain, it may play a role in recovery from acute neck pain as well.[53] However, current research demonstrates ambiguous results. Some studies found kinesiophobia to be related to the development of chronic whiplash symptoms or disability.[54, 55] However, other studies showed no predictive value for kinesiophobia.[26, 56]

One possible explanation for the possible limited role of kinesiophobia in whiplash could be that anxiety-related factors play a more prominent role than in low back pain. Because neck pain starts or is attributed to an often stressful MVC, this distinguishes it from most cases of low back pain and could give rise to more or different forms of anxiety. The sudden, traumatic onset could give rise to stronger somatic beliefs and related fears regarding recovery. Furthermore, it may be that neck pain in itself is experienced as more frightening than low back pain. All in all, the available research suggests that anxiety is associated with recovery from whiplash but that fear of pain or (re)injury specifically seems unrelated to the prognosis of post-traumatic neck pain.

Earlier work in the context of chronic disorders characterised by unexplained physical complaints, such as chronic low back pain, has provided evidence to suggest that pain catastrophising and attributional bias are of great importance in the development of chronic complaints.[57] It has been found that the habitual tendency to make catastrophic interpretations of pain is associated with a heightened pain experience in various patient groups.[49] Furthermore, catastrophising has been associated with greater disability in chronic pain, independent of the level of actual physical impairment.[50, 52, 58] It has been shown that, consistent with research into chronic pain, pain catastrophising is related to concurrent neck disability.[50, 52] Catastrophising may lead to increased physical complaints, thereby indirectly contributing to a delayed recovery. Both catastrophising and fear of movement have been found to be predictors of disability and depression.[55] However, other research suggests that pain catastrophising is associated with neck disability but has no independent predictive value regarding recovery.[59] In summary, the fear-avoidance model and its components show some promise in helping to understand cases of whiplash-related neck pain.

ATTRIBUTIONS, BELIEFS AND EXPECTATIONS

In the above-mentioned fear-avoidance model, the pathway from pain experience to fear, anxiety and avoidance, leading ultimately to disuse and disability, is moderated by catastrophising and threatening illness beliefs.[40] Causal illness beliefs can be defined as the patient's ideas about the origin or cause of the symptoms or illness experienced.

The causal beliefs of the patient seem very relevant in relation to the persistence of complaints, especially when no organic cause has been identified. When patients are diagnosed with an illness, they generally develop an organised pattern of beliefs about their condition. These illness perceptions or cognitive representations directly influence behavioural and emotional responses.[60]

In chronic fatigue syndrome, for example, it has been found that somatic illness beliefs are associated with increased symptoms and functional impairment, poorer subjective and objective outcomes, and a poor prognosis.[61, 62] In somatoform disorders, organic causal attributions are associated with a need for medical diagnostic examinations, increased expression of complaints and body scanning.[63] In addition, inadequate illness beliefs were found to be associated with heart-focused anxiety.[64] In a similar vein, dysfunctional causal beliefs may also apply to neck complaints after MVCs.

Health professionals and patients may hold many different beliefs regarding the cause and course of whiplash symptoms. Causal beliefs lead to expectations regarding the course of complaints. Negative expectations may give rise to avoidance behaviour, leading to the avoidance of movement and physical activity, and ultimately leading to disuse and a heightened state of fear. For example, when the cause of acute post-traumatic neck complaints is attributed to a severe neural or irreparable cause, dysfunctional beliefs and expectations could arise. Therefore, given the possible importance of causal attribution, dysfunctional beliefs may play an important role in the prognosis of whiplash.

In the large body of research on whiplash, its cultural dependence is often a subject of discussion.[65] There seems to be a considerable cultural variation regarding whiplash. For example, whiplash only seems to occur in a restricted number of countries and runs an apparently different course in various countries. This suggests that the cultural context is a major factor to be considered.[66–69] However, the actual nature of that cultural context has never been subject to research. Causal illness beliefs are obviously shaped by cultural factors. Beliefs and expectations regarding whiplash were found to vary profoundly across countries, thereby providing a cultural parameter relevant to the prognosis of muscular neck pain.[67, 70–72]

The medical interpretation and explanation of myogenic neck pain after an MVC, provided by general practitioners or emergency room staff, as well as commonly held knowledge and culture-defined ideas, may give rise to dysfunctional illness beliefs regarding the cause of the neck complaints, which in turn may elicit negative expectations contributing to a chronic course.[65] In addition, it may be that pain catastrophising leads to more dysfunctional causal beliefs. The tendency to attribute neck complaints to irreparable or severe causes, in turn, may elicit catastrophic interpretations of potentially benign muscular symptoms. Catastrophising and dysfunctional causal beliefs could, thus, lead to a negative spiral, augmenting symptom severity and discharging into irrational expectations regarding the course of the symptoms and disability, thereby fuelling a chronic course.[40, 73]

In the context of post-whiplash symptoms, dysfunctional causal beliefs can be defined as the attribution of the cause of acute muscle-related neck complaints to severe, neural or irreparable causes. At the chronic stage of post-whiplash syndrome, somatic or organic beliefs, in general, could be considered dysfunctional, since no somatic cause can be identified. Causal beliefs are assumed to fuel anxiety regarding the origin and expected course of whiplash symptoms.

To test the role of causal illness beliefs in the persistence of post-whiplash syndrome, the Causal Beliefs Questionnaire-Whiplash (CBQ-W) was developed.[59] Research indicated that attributing early neck complaints to whiplash or psychological factors has a predictive value over and above the intensity of initial complaints. This finding not only supports theories regarding the potential influence of culturally embedded causal beliefs, but could also have important implications for management and treatment. It suggests that modifying symptom expectations regarding whiplash and altering the causal attribution applied to initial muscle-related neck complaints are two possible therapeutic strategies. The findings are also in line with the 'nocebo hypothesis', in which it is proposed that expectations of sickness and the affective state associated with such expectations can cause sickness in the patient.[74]

Causal beliefs–anxiety model

The possible involvement of causal beliefs can be integrated in the 'causal beliefs–anxiety model' (Fig 8.1). In this model, causal beliefs play an important role because they are proposed to be the main factor leading from neck pain to the conviction that the pain is caused by 'whiplash'. Accordingly, these beliefs are assumed to function as the gatekeeper, guarding the entrance to the chronic pain circle. This illness belief is moderated by culturally embedded beliefs. Once the belief is established, catastrophising fuels the process, leading to anxiety. Increased anxiety levels have been shown to give rise to increased attention and focus on the perceived symptoms, which is further enhanced by hypervigilance.[46] Increased anxiety levels lead to kinesiophobia and cognitive symptoms due to attention interference, as well as increased muscle tension, which leads to increased or continued neck pain. Eventually, the process of focusing on perceived pain and anxiety results in central sensitisation, in which case nociceptive neurons of pain-modulating systems in the central nervous system are thought to become sensitised.[75] Central sensitisation provides a theoretical explanation for unexplained chronic pain.

CONCLUSION

Whiplash is a heterogeneous condition featuring a broad range of physical and psychological symptoms. Although whiplash could be considered a chronic pain condition originating in the musculoskeletal system, it seems to have unique psychological factors contributing to the aetiology and development of chronic symptoms. Accident-related psychological distress, as well as specific illness beliefs, are factors that show promise in explaining symptom severity and the ultimate course of symptoms.

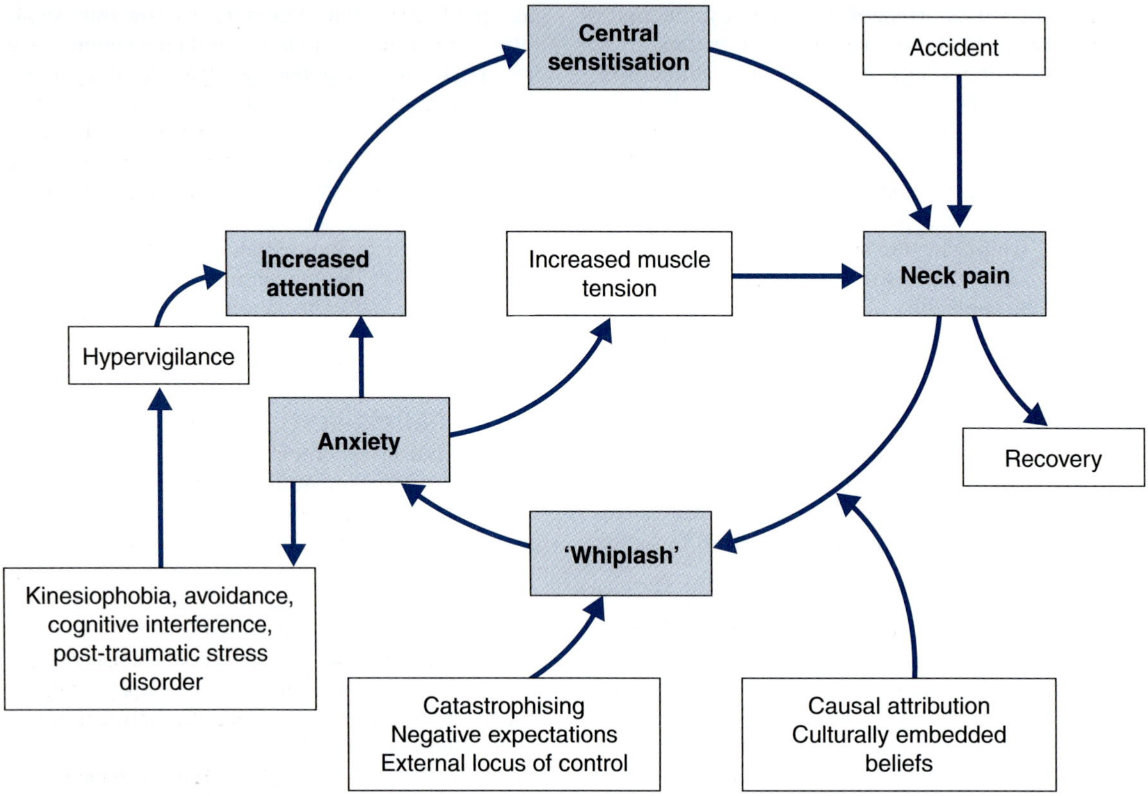

Figure 8.1 The causal beliefs–anxiety model.

References

1. Joslin CC, Khan SN, Bannister GC. Long-term disability after neck injury. a comparative study. *J Bone Joint Surg Br* 2004;86(7):1032–4.
2. Linton SJ. Do psychological factors increase the risk for back pain in the general population in both a cross-sectional and prospective analysis? *Eur J Pain* 2005;9(4):355–61.
3. Williamson E, Williams M, Gates S, Lamb SE. A systematic literature review of psychological factors and the development of late whiplash syndrome. *Pain* 2008;135(1–2):20–30.
4. Scholten-Peeters GG, Verhagen AP, Bekkering GE, et al. Prognostic factors of whiplash-associated disorders: a systematic review of prospective cohort studies. *Pain* 2003;104(1–2):303–22.
5. Peebles JE, McWilliams LA, MacLennan R. A comparison of symptom checklist 90—revised profiles from patients with chronic pain from whiplash and patients with other musculoskeletal injuries. *Spine* 2001;26(7):766–70.
6. Sterling M, Kenardy J, Jull G, Vicenzino B. The development of psychological changes following whiplash injury. *Pain* 2003;106(3):481–9.
7. American Psychiatric Association. *Diagnostic and statistical manual of mental disorders*. 4th edn. Washington, DC: APA, 1993.
8. Kongsted A, Bendix T, Qerama E, et al. Acute stress response and recovery after whiplash injuries. A one-year prospective study. *Eur J Pain* 2008;12(4):455–63.
9. Brom D, Kleber RJ, Hofman MC. Victims of traffic accidents: incidence and prevention of post-traumatic stress disorder. *J Clin Psychol* 1993;49(2):131–40.
10. Mayou RA. Psychiatric consequences of motor vehicle accidents. *Psychiatr Clin North Am* 2002;25(1):27–41, vi.
11. Mayou RA, Black J, Bryant B. Unconsciousness, amnesia and psychiatric symptoms following road traffic accident injury. *Br J Psychiatry* 2000;177:540–5.
12. Mayou R, Bryant B, Duthie R. Psychiatric consequences of road traffic accidents. *Br Med J* 1993;307(6905):647–51.
13. Blanchard EB, Buckley TC, Hickling EJ, Taylor AE. Posttraumatic stress disorder and comorbid major depression: is the correlation an illusion? *J Anxiety Disord* 1998;12(1):21–37.
14. Blanchard EB, Hickling EJ, Freidenberg BM, et al. Two studies of psychiatric morbidity among motor vehicle accident survivors 1 year after the crash. *Behav Res Ther* 2004;42(5):569–83.

15. Blaszczynski A, Gordon K, Silove D, et al. Psychiatric morbidity following motor vehicle accidents: a review of methodological issues. *Compr Psychiatry* 1998;39(3):111–21.
16. Mayou R, Bryant B, Ehlers A. Prediction of psychological outcomes one year after a motor vehicle accident. *Am J Psychiatry* 2001;158(8):1231–8.
17. Drottning M, Staff PH, Levin L, Malt UF. Acute emotional response to common whiplash predicts subsequent pain complaints. *Nord J Psychiatry* 1995;49:293–9.
18. Sundin EC, Horowitz MJ. Horowitz's Impact of Event Scale evaluation of 20 years of use. *Psychosom Med* 2003;65(5):870–6.
19. Buitenhuis J, de Jong PJ, Jaspers JP, Groothoff JW. Relationship between posttraumatic stress disorder symptoms and the course of whiplash complaints. *J Psychosom Res* 2006;61(5):681–9.
20. Chibnall JT & Duckro PN. Post-traumatic stress disorder in chronic post-traumatic headache patients. *Headache* 1994;34(6):357–61.
21. Sterling M & Kenardy J. The relationship between sensory and sympathetic nervous system changes and posttraumatic stress reaction following whiplash injury—a prospective study. *J Psychosom Res* 2006;60(4):387–93.
22. Ehlers A, Mayou RA, Bryant B. Psychological predictors of chronic posttraumatic stress disorder after motor vehicle accidents. *J Abnorm Psychol* 1998;107(3):508–19.
23. Mayou R & Bryant B. Psychiatry of whiplash neck injury. *Br J Psychiatry* 2002;180:441–8.
24. Crombez G, Eccleston C, Van den Broeck A, et al. Hypervigilance to pain in fibromyalgia: the mediating role of pain intensity and catastrophic thinking about pain. *Clin J Pain* 2004;20(2):98–102.
25. Kasch H, Qerama E, Bach FW, Jensen TS. Reduced cold pressor pain tolerance in non-recovered whiplash patients: a 1-year prospective study. *Eur J Pain* 2005;9(5):561–9.
26. Sterling M, Jull G, Vicenzino B, et al. Physical and psychological factors predict outcome following whiplash injury. *Pain* 2005;114(1–2):141–8.
27. Sterling M & Kenardy J. Physical and psychological aspects of whiplash: important considerations for primary care assessment. *Man Ther* 2008;13(2): 93–102.
28. Ferrari R & Russell AS. Why blame is a factor in recovery from whiplash injury. *Med Hypotheses* 2001;56(3):372–5.
29. Schnyder U, Wittmann L, Friedrich-Perez J, et al. Posttraumatic stress disorder following accidental injury: rule or exception in Switzerland? *Psychother Psychosom.* 2008;77(2):111–18.
30. van Middendorp H, Lumley MA, Moerbeek M, et al. Effects of anger and anger regulation styles on pain in daily life of women with fibromyalgia: a diary study. *Eur J Pain* 2010;14(2):176–82.
31. Vangronsveld K. By accident. Pain catastrophizing and fear of movement in patients with neck pain after a motor vehicle accident. Maastricht, Netherlands: University of Maastricht, 2007.
32. Folkman S, Lazarus RS, Dunkel-Schetter C, et al. Dynamics of a stressful encounter: cognitive appraisal, coping, and encounter outcomes. *J Pers Soc Psychol* 1986;50(5):992–1003.
33. Wessels T, van Tulder M, Sigl T, et al. What predicts outcome in non-operative treatments of chronic low back pain? A systematic review. *Eur Spine J* 2006;15(11):1633–44.
34. van der Hulst M, Vollenbroek-Hutten MM, IJzerman MJ. A systematic review of sociodemographic, physical, and psychological predictors of multidisciplinary rehabilitation–or, back school treatment outcome in patients with chronic low back pain. *Spine* 2005;30(7):813–25.
35. Scholten-Peeters GG, Bekkering GE, Verhagen AP, et al. Clinical practice guideline for the physiotherapy of patients with whiplash-associated disorders. *Spine* 2002;27(4):412–22.
36. Carroll LJ, Cassidy JD, Côté P. The role of pain coping strategies in prognosis after whiplash injury: passive coping predicts slowed recovery. *Pain* 2006;124(1–2):18–26.
37. Buitenhuis J, Spanjer J, Fidler V. Recovery from acute whiplash: the role of coping styles. *Spine* 2003;28(9):896–901.
38. Jensen MP, Turner JA, Romano JM, Karoly P. Coping with chronic pain: a critical review of the literature. *Pain* 1991;47(3):249–83.
39. Kivioja J, Jensen I, Lindgren U. Early coping strategies do not influence the prognosis after whiplash injuries. *Injury* 2005;36(8):935–40.
40. Vlaeyen JW & Linton SJ. Fear-avoidance and its consequences in chronic musculoskeletal pain: a state of the art. *Pain* 2000;85(3):317–32.
41. Leeuw M, Goossens ME, Linton SJ, et al. The fear-avoidance model of musculoskeletal pain: current state of scientific evidence. *J Behav Med* 2007;30(1):77–94.
42. Picavet HS, Vlaeyen JW, Schouten JS. Pain catastrophizing and kinesiophobia: predictors of chronic low back pain. *Am J Epidemiol* 2002;156(11):1028–34.
43. Peters ML, Vlaeyen JW, Weber WE. The joint contribution of physical pathology, pain-related fear and catastrophizing to chronic back pain disability. *Pain* 2005;113(1–2):45–50.

44. Sullivan MJ, Lynch ME, Clark AJ. Dimensions of catastrophic thinking associated with pain experience and disability in patients with neuropathic pain conditions. *Pain* 2005;113(3):310–15.
45. Crombez G, Vlaeyen JW, Heuts PH, Lysens R. Pain-related fear is more disabling than pain itself: evidence on the role of pain-related fear in chronic back pain disability. *Pain* 1999;80(1–2):329–39.
46. van Damme S, Crombez G, Eccleston C. Retarded disengagement from pain cues: the effects of pain catastrophizing and pain expectancy. *Pain* 2002;100(1–2):111–18.
47. Arntz A, Dreesen L, de Jong PJ. The influence of anxiety on pain: attentional and attributional mediators. *Pain* 1994;56:307–14.
48. Sullivan MJ & Pivik J. The Pain Catastrophizing Scale: development and validation. *Psychol Assess* 1995;7(4):524–32.
49. Sullivan MJ, Thorn B, Haythornthwaite JA, et al. Theoretical perspectives on the relation between catastrophizing and pain. *Clin J Pain* 2001;17(1):52–64.
50. Sullivan MJ, Stanish W, Waite H, et al. Catastrophizing, pain, and disability in patients with soft-tissue injuries. *Pain* 1998;77(3):253–60.
51. Sullivan MJ, Stanish W, Sullivan ME, Tripp D. Differential predictors of pain and disability in patients with whiplash injuries. *Pain Res Manag* 2002;7(2):68–74.
52. Severeijns R, Vlaeyen JW, van den Hout MA, Weber WE. Pain catastrophizing predicts pain intensity, disability, and psychological distress independent of the level of physical impairment. *Clin J Pain* 2001;17(2):165–72.
53. Vangronsveld K, Peters M, Goossens M, et al. Applying the fear-avoidance model to the chronic whiplash syndrome. *Pain* 2007;131(3):258–61.
54. Nederhand MJ, IJzerman MJ, Hermens HJ, et al. Predictive value of fear avoidance in developing chronic neck pain disability: consequences for clinical decision making. *Arch Phys Med Rehabil* 2004;85(3):496–501.
55. Nieto R, Miro J, Huguet A. The fear-avoidance model in whiplash injuries. *Eur J Pain* 2009;13(5):518–23.
56. Buitenhuis J, Jaspers JP, Fidler V. Can kinesiophobia predict the duration of neck symptoms in acute whiplash? *Clin J Pain* 2006;22(3):272–7.
57. Vlaeyen JW, Kole-Snijders AM, Boeren RG, van Eek H. Fear of movement/(re)injury in chronic low back pain and its relation to behavioral performance. *Pain* 1995;62(3):363–72.
58. Sullivan MJ, Stanish W, Sullivan ME, Tripp D. Differential predictors of pain and disability in patients with whiplash injuries. *Pain Res Manag* 2002;7(2):68–74.
59. Buitenhuis J, de Jong PJ, Jaspers JP, Groothoff JW. Catastrophizing and causal beliefs in whiplash. *Spine* 2008;33(22):2427–33.
60. Petrie KJ & Weinman J. Why illness perceptions matter. *Clin Med* 2007;6(6):536–9.
61. Vercoulen JH, Swanink CM, Fennis JF, et al. Prognosis in chronic fatigue syndrome: a prospective study on the natural course. *J Neurol Neurosurg Psychiatry* 1996;60(5):489–94.
62. Butler JA, Chalder T, Wessely S. Causal attributions for somatic sensations in patients with chronic fatigue syndrome and their partners. *Psychol Med* 2001;31(1):97–105.
63. Rief W, Nanke A, Emmerich J, et al. Causal illness attributions in somatoform disorders: associations with comorbidity and illness behavior. *J Psychosom Res* 2004;57(4):367–71.
64. Eifert GH, Hodson SE, Tracey DR, et al. Heart-focused anxiety, illness beliefs, and behavioral impairment: comparing healthy heart-anxious patients with cardiac and surgical inpatients. *J Behav Med* 1996;19(4):385–99.
65. Ferrari R. Whiplash cultures. *Can Med Assoc J* 1999;161(4):368.
66. Giebel GD, Bonk AD, Edelmann M, Huser R. Whiplash injury. *J Rheumatol* 1999;26(5):1207–8.
67. Partheni M, Constantoyannis C, Ferrari R, et al. A prospective cohort study of the outcome of acute whiplash injury in Greece. *Clin Exp Rheumatol* 2000;18(1):67–70.
68. Obelieniene D, Schrader H, Bovim G, et al. Pain after whiplash: a prospective controlled inception cohort study. *J Neurol Neurosurg Psychiatry* 1999;66(3):279–83.
69. Schrader H, Obelieniene D, Bovim G, et al. Natural evolution of late whiplash syndrome outside the medicolegal context. *Lancet* 1996;347(9010):1207–11.
70. Ferrari R & Lang C. A cross-cultural comparison between Canada and Germany of symptom expectation for whiplash injury. *J Spinal Disord Tech* 2005;18(1):92–7.
71. Ferrari R, Constantoyannis C, Papadakis N. Laypersons' expectation of the sequelae of whiplash injury: a cross-cultural comparative study between Canada and Greece. *Med Sci Monit* 2003;9(3):CR120–CR124.
72. Ferrari R, Obelieniene D, Russell A, et al. Laypersons' expectation of the sequelae of whiplash injury. A cross-cultural comparative study between Canada and Lithuania. *Med Sci Monit* 2002;8(11):CR728–CR734.
73. Leeuw M, Goossens ME, Linton SJ, et al. The fear-avoidance model of musculoskeletal pain: current state of scientific evidence. *J Behav Med* 2007;30(1):77–94.
74. Hahn RA. The nocebo phenomenon: concept, evidence, and implications for public health. *Prev Med* 1997;26:607–11.
75. Nijs J, Van OJ, De HW. Rehabilitation of chronic whiplash: treatment of cervical dysfunctions or chronic pain syndrome? *Clin Rheumatol* 2009;28(3):243–51.

CHAPTER 9
Potential role of stress systems in the pathogenesis of whiplash associated disorders

Samuel McLean

Consistent with the term 'whiplash associated disorders' (WAD), biological mechanisms influencing neck pain and coincident somatic symptoms after a motor vehicle crash (MVC) have traditionally been conceptualised as related to cervical sprain/strain during the MVC event. However, in addition to subjecting soft tissues to biomechanical strain, an MVC event is also an acute stressor that activates physiological stress response systems. It is increasingly appreciated that these systems modulate *neurosensory* processing and are capable of increasing pain sensitivity (causing hyperalgesia) and of causing normally non-painful sensations to become painful (causing allodynia). This chapter reviews the evidence that physiological systems involved in the stress response may contribute to the development of the hyperalgesia and allodynia seen in people with WAD after an MVC.

Several concepts are important when considering the potential role of stress systems in the development of WAD:

1. The term 'stress systems' refers to the physiological processes that modulate neurosensory processing when an organism experiences a stressful event, such as a potentially life-threatening MVC. These systems are extremely useful in optimising the response of an organism to immediate environmental circumstances. However, it appears that the activation of these potent modulatory systems may cause and/or contribute to hyperalgesia and allodynia, which are long-lasting and deleterious.
2. The available evidence suggests that stress system activation may, by itself, be capable of causing long-lasting changes in pain processing, even in the absence of tissue trauma. For example, in an animal model of stress exposure, exposing Sprague-Dawley rats to 10–20 minutes of forced swimming (inescapable, non-painful, moderate swim stress) for three days produced hyperalgesia to both thermal and chemical stimuli.[1] In vulnerable individuals, stress system activation in response to a potentially life-threatening MVC may, by itself, be sufficient to cause WAD symptoms.
3. The evidence also suggests that the influence of stress response system components on central nervous system (CNS) processes may be time-dependent. For example, since the middle of the last century, it has been appreciated that adrenergic nervous system activation can produce immediate analgesia.[2, 3] Indeed, it is part of common lay understanding that such analgesia is a component of the 'fight or flight' response. In contrast, only during the past two decades have animal and human studies revealed that adrenergic nervous system activation may also cause marked hyperalgesia and allodynia.[4–10] These opposing effects of stress systems on neurosensory processing are consistent with recent work demonstrating the opposing, time-dependent effects of stress response elements on other CNS processes. For example, in order to form long-lasting memories ('flashbulb memories') of traumatic events, the same set of stress response effectors produces, first, a brief period of marked memory formation and then a period of marked memory inhibition.[11, 12]

In the sections that follow, the available evidence is reviewed regarding the potential influence of specific stress system components on neurosensory processing after stress exposure. It is hoped that, in aggregate, these data will support the plausibility of a contribution of stress systems to the alterations in neurosensory processing which characterise WAD. In the final sections, the potential clinical implications of these findings, as well as the current research needs and future directions, are discussed.

SYMPATHETIC NERVOUS SYSTEM

Non-genetic studies

Acute stressors activate the sympathetic nervous system and adrenomedullary hormonal system, resulting in the release of adrenaline and noradrenaline.[13, 14]

These catecholamines produce immediate adaptive benefits, such as increased vigilance and energy mobilisation.[13, 14] In addition, catecholamines have also long been known to be capable of producing immediate analgesia.[2, 3] However, sympathetic activation can also have adverse consequences. For example, sympathetic activation in the setting of a surgical stressor has been shown to increase both immediate and long-term cardiovascular sequelae.[15, 16] As described below, it is also being increasingly recognised that sympathetic activation may contribute to the development of hyperalgesia and allodynia after stressful events, such as an MVC.[17]

Catechol-o-methyltransferase (COMT) is the primary enzyme that degrades catecholamines. In animal studies, increasing catecholamine levels via the inhibition of this enzyme has been shown to produce allodynia and hyperalgesia.[4] The increase in pain sensitivity produced by elevated catecholamines was found to be comparable in magnitude to that produced by the intraplantar injection of carrageenan (an inflammatory agent).[4] Similarly, in humans the chronic administration of β–adrenergic receptor agonists has been shown to produce a painful arthritis-like syndrome.[18]

In addition to these direct effects on pain sensitivity, catecholamines have been shown to enhance pain due to tissue inflammation. In animal models of rheumatoid arthritis, the sustained bioavailability of adrenaline (either released from the adrenal medulla or administered exogenously) substantially augments inflammatory mediator-induced hyperalgesia.[5, 6] Similarly, increasing catecholamine levels has been shown to increase carrageenan-induced pain.[4]

Just as increased catecholamines have been shown to increase pain, a reduction in catecholamine effects has been shown to reduce pain and/or prevent enhanced pain sensitivity. Denervation of sympathetic noradrenergic fibres and the depletion of peripheral adrenaline have been found to attenuate arthritic responses.[7, 8] Nackley-Neely et al.[4] showed that the allodynia and hyperalgesia induced by increasing catecholamine levels could be prevented by the administration of selective β_2 and β_3 antagonists. In humans, sympathetic blockade or the administration of the β-adrenergic receptor antagonist propranolol has been observed to reduce the severity of arthritis and joint responses to injury, and to provide pain relief for patients with chronic musculoskeletal pain syndromes.[19–22]

Genetic studies

Another way to assess the association between elevated catecholamine levels and vulnerability to develop immediate and persistent pain is to examine the association between genetic polymorphisms that determine adrenergic system function and patient outcomes. If adrenergic systems influence pain processing, then genetic variations influencing adrenergic system function may be associated with individual variation in pain sensitivity and vulnerability to develop persistent pain.

Catecholamine levels in the synaptic cleft are influenced by the activity of enzymes that degrade catecholamines. Such enzymes include COMT, which is located on the postsynaptic membrane, and monoamine oxidases A and B (MAO-A and MAO-B), which are located on the outer membrane of mitochondria in the presynaptic cell. Catecholamine concentrations are also influenced by the activity of transporters, such as the noradrenaline (norepinephrine) transporter (NET), which transports noradrenaline from the synaptic cleft to presynaptic storage vesicles for later use. If adrenergic pathways activated by the stress response influence pain processing, then genetic variations in COMT, MAO-A/B and NET may be associated with individual variation in pain sensitivity and vulnerability to develop persistent pain. The available evidence suggests that this is, indeed, the case, as outlined below.

- *COMT*: Previous work has identified three common variations, or haplotypes, of the *COMT* gene that code for different levels of enzymatic activity and are associated with differences in pain sensitivity.[10] The *LPS haplotype* codes for the highest enzyme activity and is associated with the highest pain tolerance. The *APS haplotype* codes for comparably less enzyme activity and is associated with average pain tolerance. The *HPS haplotype* codes for the least enzyme activity and is associated with the lowest pain tolerance.[10] In a recent prospective cohort study, the presence of even a single LPS haplotype was found to diminish, by as much as 2.3 times, the risk of developing a common musculoskeletal pain condition, myogenous temporomandibular joint disorder (TMD).[10] Preliminary evidence also suggests that genetic variations in *COMT* function influence vulnerability to acute and chronic WAD symptoms after an MVC.[23]
- *MAO and NET*: Polymorphisms of the gene encoding MAO-B, *MAO-B*, have been associated with pain intensity after tonsillectomy and third molar extraction.[24, 25] NET inhibition has been shown to alleviate mechanical allodynia[26] and to augment endogenous analgesia.[27] The analgesic affect of NET inhibition is believed to occur, at least in part, via bulbospinal noradrenergic projections that activate α_{2A}-adrenoreceptors in the spinal cord

dorsal horn.[26, 28] The analgesia produced by several common analgesics is believed to be due, in part, to NET inhibition.[27, 29]

Adrenergic receptors activate (transduce) the cellular response to catecholamines. If adrenergic pathways involved in the stress response influence pain sensitivity and vulnerability to develop persistent pain, then pain processing would also be expected to be influenced by the function of adrenergic receptors. The available evidence suggests that this is, indeed, the case, as outlined below.

- *α_1-adrenoceptors*: α_1-adrenoceptor activity has been shown to sensitise nociceptive neurotransmission at numerous CNS sites[30] and to upregulate known pain and inflammatory mediators, such as STAT and cytokines.[31] Consistent with these findings, α_1-adrenoceptor agonists, such as phenylephrine, generally have a pro-nociceptive effect.[32–38] α_1-adrenoceptors are subclassified as α_{1A}, α_{1B} and α_{1D}. α_{1A} and α_{1D} receptors have been shown to contribute to inflammatory pain[32] and heat pain[39] sensitivity, respectively. In addition, the three α_1-adrenoceptor subtypes have been shown to be differentially expressed in response to painful nerve damage, suggesting that it is likely that nociceptive stimulation regulates the expression of these genes.[40] In a recent prospective study, genetic variations in α_{1A} receptors were found to be associated with up to a nine-fold increase in vulnerability to develop a common musculoskeletal pain condition, myogenous TMD.[41] Further assessments of the influence of genetic variations in α_{1A} receptors on acute pain and vulnerability to persistent pain after an MVC are needed.
- *α_2-adrenoceptors*: α_2-adrenoceptor agonists, such as clonidine, are widely used as analgesics.[42] α_2-adrenoceptors are subclassified as α_{2A}, α_{2B} and α_{2C}. α_{2A} receptors have received the most study, and have been shown to help mediate adrenergic antinociception.[43, 44] Little work has been done on examining the influence of specific α_2 genes on pain sensitivity, with the exception of a single study that found that variations in α_{2A} and α_{2C} receptors were associated with somatic symptom scores in patients with irritable bowel disease.[45]
- *β_2 and β_3 adrenoceptors*: The β_2-adrenoceptor has received relatively more study, and has been associated with variation in nociceptive function.[9, 46] Cardiovascular function, particularly arterial blood pressure, appears to be regulated by β_2-adrenoceptors,[46] and cardiovascular and pain regulatory systems are closely associated with one another.[47, 48] A recent prospective study of the development of a common musculoskeletal pain disorder found that variation in the gene encoding the β_2-adrenoceptor is associated with vulnerability to develop persistent pain.[9] In addition, a recent report identified an association between clinical conditions characterised by musculoskeletal pain and somatic symptoms and the minor allele for the gene encoding the β_3-adrenoceptor.[49] More work assessing the association between genetic variations influencing β_2 and β_3 adrenoceptor function and acute and persistent WAD symptoms after an MVC is needed.

NEUROPEPTIDE Y

Neuropeptide Y is a small, 36-amino acid peptide that is present both in the brain and in the neurons of the peripheral autonomic nervous system.[50] Neuropeptide Y has been shown to be present in areas of the brain critical to pain modulation, including the periaqueductal grey and nucleus raphe magnus, and is thought to play an important role in pain processing.[51] Administration of neuropeptide Y in these areas results in a reduction in both acute[52] and ongoing[53] inflammatory pain. In the periphery, it is found in particularly large quantities in the sympathetic nervous system, where it is co-stored and co-released with noradrenaline in response to stress.[50] Neuropeptide Y expression has been shown to be markedly altered by tissue injury.[54–57] Evidence suggests that increased levels of neuropeptide Y after stress exposure may be associated with a reduced vulnerability to post-traumatic stress disorder (PTSD) symptoms.[58, 59] This finding is of particular interest because evidence from several studies indicates that PTSD symptoms in the early aftermath of an MVC predict persistent WAD symptoms.[17] To date, no studies have examined the potential influence of variations in the biology of neuropeptide Y pathways on the development of WAD.

HPA axis/glucocorticoids

Acute stressors trigger the release of corticotrophin-releasing factor, which initiates the activation of the hypothalamic–pituitary–adrenocortical (HPA) axis and the release of cortisol.[14] Variation in the function of the HPA axis has been shown to predict the development of pain and somatic symptoms in large population-based studies,[60] in patients undergoing surgery,[61] and in experimental studies of patients exposed to standardised stressors.[62] Individual variation in cortisol levels after an MVC may influence the balance of peripheral pro-inflammatory cytokines, which may contribute to pain symptoms via peripheral or central mechanisms.[63]

Another important source of individual variation in pain vulnerability after an MVC may be variation in the function of glucocorticoid receptors. There is increasing appreciation that the physiology of glucocorticoid receptors is highly complex.[64] Glucocorticoid receptors are located throughout the CNS, including both the brain and spinal cord dorsal horn. The activation of central glucocorticoid receptors has been shown to reduce systemic mechanical pain thresholds.[65] Glucocorticoid receptors in the spinal cord dorsal horn respond to peripheral nociceptive stimulation,[66, 67] and are capable of inducing antinociception.[68–70] In addition, there appear to be substantial functional interactions between central glucocorticoid and opioid analgesic systems.[71] Several genetic variations in glucocorticoid receptors and associated regulatory elements have been associated with an altered HPA axis stress response.[72, 73] More work is needed examining the associations between genetic polymorphisms related to the function of the HPA axis and the development of acute and chronic WAD symptoms after an MVC.

SEROTONIN

Serotonin is primarily located in nine clusters of cells in the brainstem, termed the raphe nuclei, which extend projections to almost all areas of the brain and throughout the spinal cord.[74, 75] Some raphe nuclei are stimulated by corticotrophin-releasing factor, and the activation of serotonin pathways is part of the acute stress response.[76] Serotonergic projections to the spinal cord are believed to play an important role in the inhibition and/or facilitation of nociceptive inputs (reviewed in Millan[75]) and, thus, play an important role in enhancing/prolonging or extinguishing acute pain. This role is achieved, at least in part, via influencing the antinociceptive effects of opioids at the spinal cord level.[77, 78] Serotonin reuptake inhibition is believed to be an important component of the analgesic efficacy of commonly used analgesic medications. A genetic variation in the serotonin transporter that results in relatively low levels of serotonin availability has been found to be associated with several chronic pain conditions, including fibromyalgia,[79] irritable bowel syndrome[80] and tension headache.[81]

CLINICAL IMPLICATIONS

The above evidence demonstrates that primary components of the stress response, including the adrenergic nervous system, HPA axis, neuropeptide Y and serotonin pathways, have consistently been shown to influence neurosensory processing. After an MVC, the influence of such stress system components may interact with the acute physical and emotional effects of the MVC, and the outcomes of these interactions, together with post-collision behaviours and cognitions, may be important components in determining symptom persistence versus recovery. If this is the case, then treatments that dampen the effect of these systems may provide another 'arrow in our quiver' of multimodal therapeutic interventions to help individuals who are at risk of chronic symptom development.

In the animal model of stress-induced sensory changes mentioned in the introduction, it has been shown that the changes in sensory threshold and muscle hyperalgesia induced by stress exposure can be attenuated or prevented by pretreatment with medications that influence stress system biology.[1, 82] For example, animal pretreatment with medications that augment central serotonin (e.g. fluoxetine) has been shown to attenuate sensory threshold changes and to reduce muscle hyperalgesia caused by stress exposure.[1, 82] Whether the use of medications that modify the influence of the stress response *after* stress exposure in humans can improve WAD outcomes is unknown. However, it is possible that, in selected patients, such interventions may be useful adjuncts to current treatments and improve WAD outcomes.

CURRENT RESEARCH NEEDS AND FUTURE RESEARCH DIRECTIONS

This chapter presents a great deal of evidence supporting the potential influence of stress systems on neurosensory processing and the development of hyperalgesia and allodynia. However, none of this data was obtained from patient cohorts experiencing MVC. Current research efforts in this area should include studies that assess the ability of measures of stress system function to predict persistent WAD symptom outcomes after an MVC. This would provide more evidence that stress system function influences WAD outcomes. Such measures of stress system function might include assessments of HPA axis function (e.g. cortisol levels) and/or autonomic nervous system function (e.g. heart rate variability assessment) collected around the time of the MVC. Other studies that would provide useful information regarding the importance of stress systems in the pathophysiology of WAD are ones that assess whether genetic variations determining the function of important components of these systems are associated with the risk of the development of WAD symptoms. These studies should simultaneously examine a range of outcomes after an MVC, including both regional and widespread pain and psychological sequelae, so that the potential influence of stress system function across a range of important patient outcomes can be assessed. Similarly, the potential interaction between stress system measures and other patient characteristics (e.g. psychological and cognitive–behavioural characteristics) in shaping patient outcomes should also be examined.

If such observational studies indicate that stress systems may play an important role in the pathophysiology of WAD, either alone or via interactions with other factors, then studies providing interventions for selected high-risk individuals which target one or more stress system components may be worthwhile. The identification of those high-risk individuals who are most likely to benefit from the intervention is likely to be crucial in this regard. This is because patients with WAD, like patients with other common musculoskeletal pain conditions, are likely to be heterogenous. Thus, the contribution of a particular aetiological factor or biological pathway to patient outcomes may vary a great deal from patient to patient.

References

1. Quintero L, Moreno M, Avila C, et al. Long-lasting delayed hyperalgesia after subchronic swim stress. *Pharmacol Biochem Behav* 2000;67:449–58.
2. Ivy AC, Gorrzl FR, Burmill DY. The analgesic effect of intracarotid and intravenous infection of epinephrine in dogs and of subcutaneous injection in man. *Quart Bull Northw Univ Med Sch* 1944;18: 298–306.
3. Leimdorfer A & Metzner WR. Analgesia and anesthesia induced by epinephrine. *Am J Physiol* 1949;157:116–21.
4. Nackley-Neely AG, Tan KS, Fecho K, et al. Catechol-O-methyltransferase inhibition increases pain sensitivity through activation of both β_2 and β_3 adrenergic receptors. *Pain* 2007;128(3):199–208.
5. Khasar SG, Green PG, Miao FJ, Levine JD. Vagal modulation of nociception is mediated by adrenomedullary epinephrine in the rat. *Eur J Neurosci* 2003;17:909–15.
6. Khasar SG, McCarter G, Levine JD. Epinephrine produces a beta-adrenergic receptor-mediated mechanical hyperalgesia and in vitro sensitization of rat nociceptors. *J Neurophysiol* 1999;81: 1104–12.
7. Levine JD, Dardick SJ, Roizen MF, et al. Contribution of sensory afferents and sympathetic efferents to joint injury in experimental arthritis. *J Neurosci* 1986;6:3423–9.
8. Coderre TJ, Basbaum AI, Dallman MF, et al. Epinephrine exacerbates arthritis by an action at presynaptic B2-adrenoceptors. *Neuroscience* 1990;34:521–3.
9. Diatchenko L, Anderson AD, Slade GD, et al. Three major haplotypes of the β_2 adrenergic receptor define psychological profile, blood pressure, and the risk for development of a common musculoskeletal pain disorder. *Am J Med Genet B Neuropsychiatr Genet* 2006;141B(5):449–62.
10. Diatchenko L, Slade GD, Nackley AG, et al. Genetic basis for individual variations in pain perception and the development of a chronic pain condition. *Hum Mol Genet* 2005;14:135–43.
11. Diamond DM, Campbell AM, Park CR, et al. The temporal dynamics model of emotional memory processing: a synthesis on the neurobiological basis of stress-induced amnesia, flashbulb and traumatic memories, and the Yerkes-Dodson law. *Neural Plast* 2007;2007:60803.
12. Joels M, Pu Z, Wiegert O, et al. Learning under stress: how does it work? *Trends Cogn Sci* 2006;10:152–8.
13. Goldstein DS. Catecholamines and stress. *Endocr Regul* 2003;37:69–80.
14. Chrousos GP. Stressors, stress, and neuroendocrine integration of the adaptive response. The 1997 Hans Selye Memorial Lecture. *Ann N Y Acad Sci* 1998;851:311–35.
15. Mangano DT, Layug EL, Wallace A, Tateo I. Effect of atenolol on mortality and cardiovascular morbidity after noncardiac surgery. Multicenter Study of Perioperative Ischemia Research Group. *N Engl J Med* 1996;335:1713–20.
16. Grassi G. Sympathetic overdrive and cardiovascular risk in the metabolic syndrome. *Hypertens Res* 2006;29:839–47.
17. McLean SA, Clauw DJ, Abelson JL, Liberzon I. The development of persistent pain and psychological morbidity after motor vehicle collision: integrating the potential role of stress response systems into a biopsychosocial model. *Psychosom Med* 2005;67: 783–90.
18. Vyden J, Groseth-Dittrich M, Callis G, et al. The effect of propranolol on peripheral hemodynamics in rheumatoid arthritis. *Arthritis Rheum* 1971;14:420.
19. Baerwald CG, Laufenberg M, Specht T, et al. Impaired sympathetic influence on the immune response in patients with rheumatoid arthritis due to lymphocyte subset-specific modulation of beta 2-adrenergic receptors. *Br J Rheumatol* 1997;36:1262–9.
20. Kaplan R, Robinson CA, Scavulli JF, Vaughan JH. Propranolol and the treatment of rheumatoid arthritis. *Arthritis Rheum* 1980;23:253–5.

21. Levine JD, Fye K, Heller P, et al. Clinical response to regional intravenous guanethidine in patients with rheumatoid arthritis. *J Rheumatol* 1986;13:1040–3.
22. Tchivileva IE, Lim PF, Kasravi P, et al. Propranolol in temporomandibular joint disorder treatment. American Pain Society Meeting, San Diego, CA, 2009.
23. McLean SA, Diatchenko L, Reed C, et al. Catechol-O-Methyltransferase (COMT) met/met genotype influences cortisol response and pain symptoms after minor motor vehicle collision (MVC). American Pain Society Meeting, Tampa Bay, FL, 2008.
24. Sery O, Hrazdilova O, Didden W, et al. The association of monoamine oxidase B functional polymorphism with postoperative pain intensity. *Neuro Endocrinol Lett* 2006;27:333–7.
25. Kim H, Lee H, Rowan J, et al. Genetic polymorphisms in monoamine neurotransmitter systems show only weak association with acute post-surgical pain in humans. *Mol Pain* 2006;2:24.
26. Nielsen CK, Lewis RJ, Alewood D, et al. Anti-allodynic efficacy of the chi-conopeptide, Xen2174, in rats with neuropathic pain. *Pain* 2005;118:112–24.
27. Bohn LM, Xu F, Gainetdinov RR, Caron MG. Potentiated opioid analgesia in norepinephrine transporter knock-out mice. *J Neurosci* 2000;20: 9040–5.
28. Tyce GM & Yaksh TL. Monoamine release from cat spinal cord by somatic stimuli: an intrinsic modulatory system. *J Physiol* 1981;314:513–29.
29. Sagata K, Minami K, Yanagihara N, et al. Tramadol inhibits norepinephrine transporter function at desipramine-binding sites in cultured bovine adrenal medullary cells. *Anesth Analg* 2002;94:901–6.
30. Pertovaara A. Noradrenergic pain modulation. *Prog Neurobiol* 2006;80:53–83.
31. Gonzalez-Cabrera PJ, Gaivin RJ, Yun J, et al. Genetic profiling of alpha 1-adrenergic receptor subtypes by oligonucleotide microarrays: coupling to interleukin-6 secretion but differences in STAT3 phosphorylation and gp-130. *Mol Pharmacol* 2003;63:1104–16.
32. Hong Y & Abbott FV. Contribution of peripheral alpha 1A-adrenoceptors to pain induced by formalin or by alpha-methyl-5-hydroxytryptamine plus noradrenaline. *Eur J Pharmacol* 1996;301:41–8.
33. Mailis-Gagnon A & Bennett GJ. Abnormal contralateral pain responses from an intradermal injection of phenylephrine in a subset of patients with complex regional pain syndrome (CRPS). *Pain* 2004;111:378–84.
34. Ali Z, Ringkamp M, Hartke TV, et al. Uninjured C-fiber nociceptors develop spontaneous activity and alpha-adrenergic sensitivity following L6 spinal nerve ligation in monkey. *J Neurophysiol* 1999;81:455–66.
35. Pluteanu F, Ristoiu V, Flonta ML, Reid G. Alpha(1)-adrenoceptor-mediated depolarization and beta-mediated hyperpolarization in cultured rat dorsal root ganglion neurones. *Neurosci Lett* 2002;329: 277–80.
36. Sagen J & Proudfit HK. Evidence for pain modulation by pre- and postsynaptic noradrenergic receptors in the medulla oblongata. *Brain Res* 1985;331: 285–93.
37. Hedo G & Lopez-Garcia JA. Alpha-1A adrenoceptors modulate potentiation of spinal nociceptive pathways in the rat spinal cord in vitro. *Neuropharmacology* 2001;41:862–9.
38. Kingery WS, Guo TZ, Davies MF, et al. The alpha(2A) adrenoceptor and the sympathetic postganglionic neuron contribute to the development of neuropathic heat hyperalgesia in mice. *Pain* 2000;85:345–58.
39. Harasawa I, Honda K, Tanoue A, et al. Responses to noxious stimuli in mice lacking alpha(1d)-adrenergic receptors. *Neuroreport* 2003;14:1857–60.
40. Xie J, Ho Lee Y, Wang C, et al. Differential expression of alpha1-adrenoceptor subtype mRNAs in the dorsal root ganglion after spinal nerve ligation. *Brain Res Mol Brain Res* 2001;93:164–72.
41. Smith S, Slade G, Belfer I, et al. ADRA1A polymorphisms associated with multiple psychological and nociceptive phenotypes predict vulnerability to an idiopathic pain condition. American Pain Society Meeting, Washington, DC, 2007.
42. Crassous PA, Denis C, Paris H, Senard JM. Interest of alpha2-adrenergic agonists and antagonists in clinical practice: background, facts and perspectives. *Curr Top Med Chem* 2007;7:187–94.
43. Millan MJ, Bervoets K, Rivet JM, et al. Multiple alpha-2 adrenergic receptor subtypes. II. Evidence for a role of rat R alpha-2A adrenergic receptors in the control of nociception, motor behavior and hippocampal synthesis of noradrenaline. *J Pharmacol Exp Ther* 1994;270: 958–72.
44. Graham BA, Hammond DL, Proudfit HK. Differences in the antinociceptive effects of alpha-2 adrenoceptor agonists in two substrains of Sprague-Dawley rats. *J Pharmacol Exp Ther* 1997;283:511–19.
45. Kim HJ, Camilleri M, Carlson PJ, et al. Association of distinct alpha(2) adrenoceptor and serotonin transporter polymorphisms with constipation and somatic symptoms in functional gastrointestinal disorders. *Gut* 2004;53:829–37.
46. Small KM, McGraw DW, Liggett SB. Pharmacology and physiology of human adrenergic receptor polymorphisms. *Ann Rev Pharmacol Toxicol* 2003;43:381–411.

47. Bruehl S & Chung OY. Interactions between the cardiovascular and pain regulatory systems: an updated review of mechanisms and possible alterations in chronic pain. *Neurosci Biobehav Rev* 2004;28: 395–414.
48. Hagen K, Zwart JA, Holmen J, et al. Does hypertension protect against chronic musculoskeletal complaints? The Nord-Trondelag Health Study. *Arch Intern Med* 2005;165:916–22.
49. Clauw DJ, Belfer I, Max MB, et al. Increased frequency of the minor allele for beta-3 adrenergic receptors in individuals with fibromyalgia and related syndromes. Boston, MA; American College of Rheumatology, 2007.
50. Silva AP, Cavadas C, Grouzmann E. Neuropeptide Y and its receptors as potential therapeutic drug targets. *Clin Chim Acta* 2002;326:3–25.
51. Zhang Y, Lundeberg T, Yu L. Involvement of neuropeptide Y and Y1 receptor in antinociception in nucleus raphe magnus of rats. *Regul Pept* 2000;95:109–13.
52. Taiwo OB & Taylor BK. Antihyperalgesic effects of intrathecal neuropeptide Y during inflammation are mediated by Y1 receptors. *Pain* 2002;96: 353–63.
53. Mahinda TB & Taylor BK. Intrathecal neuropeptide Y inhibits behavioral and cardiovascular responses to noxious inflammatory stimuli in awake rats. *Physiol Behav* 2004;80:703–11.
54. Zhang X, Shi T, Holmberg K, et al. Expression and regulation of the neuropeptide Y Y2 receptor in sensory and autonomic ganglia. *Proc Natl Acad Sci U S A* 1997;94:729–34.
55. Zhang X, Bean AJ, Wiesenfeld-Hallin Z, Hokfelt T. Ultrastructural studies on peptides in the dorsal horn of the rat spinal cord—IV. Effects of peripheral axotomy with special reference to neuropeptide Y and vasoactive intestinal polypeptide/peptide histidine isoleucine. *Neuroscience* 1995;64:917–41.
56. Hokfelt T, Zhang X, Wiesenfeld-Hallin Z. Messenger plasticity in primary sensory neurons following axotomy and its functional implications. *Trends Neurosci* 1994;17:22–30.
57. Ji RR, Zhang X, Wiesenfeld-Hallin Z, Hokfelt T. Expression of neuropeptide Y and neuropeptide Y (Y1) receptor mRNA in rat spinal cord and dorsal root ganglia following peripheral tissue inflammation. *J Neurosci* 1994;14:6423–34.
58. Morgan CA, 3rd, Rasmusson AM, Wang S, et al. Neuropeptide-Y, cortisol, and subjective distress in humans exposed to acute stress: replication and extension of previous report. *Biol Psychiatry* 2002;52:136–42.
59. Morgan CA, 3rd, Wang S, Southwick SM, et al. Plasma neuropeptide-Y concentrations in humans exposed to military survival training. *Biol Psychiatry* 2000;47:902–9.
60. McBeth J, Chiu YH, Silman AJ, et al. Hypothalamic-pituitary-adrenal stress axis function and the relationship with chronic widespread pain and its antecedents. *Arthritis Res Ther* 2005;7:R992–R1000.
61. Geiss A, Rohleder N, Kirschbaum C, et al. Predicting the failure of disc surgery by a hypofunctional HPA axis: evidence from a prospective study on patients undergoing disc surgery. *Pain* 2005;114:104–17.
62. Glass JM, Lyden AK, Petzke F, et al. The effect of brief exercise cessation on pain, fatigue, and mood symptom development in healthy, fit individuals. *J Psychosom Res* 2004;57:391–8.
63. Watkins LR, Maier SF, Goehler LE. Immune activation: the role of pro-inflammatory cytokines in inflammation, illness responses and pathological pain states. *Pain* 1995;63:289–302.
64. Biddie SC & Hager GL. Glucocorticoid receptor dynamics and gene regulation. *Stress* 2009;12: 193–205.
65. Myers B, Greenwood-Van Meerveld B. Divergent effects of amygdala glucocorticoid and mineralocorticoid receptors in the regulation of visceral and somatic pain. *Am J Physiol Gastrointest Liver Physiol* 2010;298(2):G295–303.
66. De Nicola AF, Moses DF, Gonzalez S, Orti E. Adrenocorticoid action in the spinal cord: some unique molecular properties of glucocorticoid receptors. *Cell Mol Neurobiol* 1989;9:179–92.
67. Cintra A, Molander C, Fuxe K. Colocalization of Fos- and glucocorticoid receptor-immunoreactivities is present only in a very restricted population of dorsal horn neurons of the rat spinal cord after nociceptive stimulation. *Brain Res* 1993;632:334–8.
68. Capasso A, Di Giannuario A, Loizzo A, et al. Central interaction of dexamethasone and RU-38486 on morphine antinociception in mice. *Life Sci* 1992;51:PL 139–43.
69. Pieretti S, Capasso A, Di Giannuario A, et al. The interaction of peripherally and centrally administered dexamethasone and RU 38486 on morphine analgesia in mice. *Gen Pharmacol* 1991;22:929–33.
70. Lim G, Wang S, Zeng Q, et al. Evidence for a long-term influence on morphine tolerance after previous morphine exposure: role of neuronal glucocorticoid receptors. *Pain* 2005;114(1–2):81–92.
71. Capasso A & Loizzo A. Functional interference of dexamethasone on some morphine effects: hypothesis for the steroid-opioid interaction. *Recent Pat CNS Drug Discov* 2008;3:138–50.

72. van Rossum EF & Lamberts SW. Polymorphisms in the glucocorticoid receptor gene and their associations with metabolic parameters and body composition. *Recent Prog Horm Res* 2004;59:333–57.
73. Wust S, Van Rossum EF, Federenko IS, et al. Common polymorphisms in the glucocorticoid receptor gene are associated with adrenocortical responses to psychosocial stress. *J Clin Endocrinol Metab* 2004;89:565–73.
74. Filip M & Bader M. Overview on 5-HT receptors and their role in physiology and pathology of the central nervous system. *Pharmacol Rep* 2009;61:761–77.
75. Millan MJ. Descending control of pain. *Prog Neurobiol* 2002;66:355–474.
76. Chaouloff F. Serotonin, stress and corticoids. *J Psychopharmacol* 2000;14:139–51.
77. Hain HS, Belknap JK, Mogil JS. Pharmacogenetic evidence for the involvement of 5-hydroxytryptamine (Serotonin)-1B receptors in the mediation of morphine antinociceptive sensitivity. *J Pharmacol Exp Ther* 1999;291:444–9.
78. Song B, Chen W, Marvizon JC. Inhibition of opioid release in the rat spinal cord by serotonin 5-HT(1A) receptors. *Brain Res* 2007;1158:57–62.
79. Buskila D & Neumann L. Genetics of fibromyalgia. *Curr Pain Headache Rep* 2005;9:313–15.
80. Yeo A, Boyd P, Lumsden S, et al. Association between a functional polymorphism in the serotonin transporter gene and diarrhoea predominant irritable bowel syndrome in women. *Gut* 2004;53:1452–8.
81. Park JW, Kim JS, Lee HK, et al. Serotonin transporter polymorphism and harm avoidance personality in chronic tension-type headache. *Headache* 2004;44:1005–9.
82. Suarez-Roca H, Quintero L, Arcaya JL, et al. Stress-induced muscle and cutaneous hyperalgesia: differential effect of milnacipran. *Physiol Behav* 2006;88:82–7.

CHAPTER 10
Prognostic indicators of non-recovery following whiplash injury

Michele Sterling

The capacity to predict outcome following whiplash injury is important for several reasons. Predictive factors may be modifiable or non-modifiable, and treatments directed at the former factors may improve outcomes for those identified as at risk of poor recovery. This, in turn, may assist in the curtailment of both personal and financial costs associated with the condition. The identification of those who show good potential for recovery is also important so that both injured people and clinicians can have greater confidence in a good outcome. An understanding of prognostic indicators for both outcomes will allow the appropriate allocation of resources by policy-makers.

Fifteen years ago, the Quebec Task Force identified predictive studies as an area requiring urgent investigation in whiplash research.[1] Since that time the number of cohort studies has substantially increased and now several systematic reviews of prognosis are available.[2–6] However, these have not been undertaken without difficulty owing to shortcomings in some of the primary cohort studies, including inconsistencies between studies in time from injury until baseline data collection, time to follow-up and use of various and sometimes unvalidated outcome measures.[5] There is also variation between the systematic reviews, with some performing meta-analysis,[5] others indicating that due to heterogeneity data pooling could not be undertaken,[3, 4] and others comprising task force findings that were not peer reviewed.[7] Nevertheless, the findings of the various reviews have generally been in agreement that the factors of higher initial pain and/or disability are the most consistent predictors of poor functional recovery.[2–6]

It is not the aim of this chapter to conduct another systematic review of currently available cohort studies. Rather, it is to present an overview of systematic review findings, discuss emerging factors that show potential for prognostic capacity of both recovery and non-recovery, and outline the clinical implications for the recognition of prognostic indicators.

PROGNOSTIC FACTORS FOR NON-RECOVERY

Presenting signs and symptoms

Clearly, the most consistent predictor of poor functional recovery is the intensity of neck pain at the initial or baseline assessment point.[2–6] Walton et al.[5] synthesised the data from eight cohorts and established a cut-off point of 55 out of 100 or 5 out of 10 on a visual analogue pain scale. These authors report that a pain intensity of greater than 55 out of 100 demonstrated a nearly sixfold (OR, 5.77; 95% CI: 2.89–11.52) increase in the risk of persistent pain or disability at follow-up. This factor was slightly more robust at predicting an outcome of disability when compared to pain outcomes.[5] Initially, moderate-to-high levels of pain-related disability have also shown predictive capacity.[8]

Some reviews pointed to other symptoms, such as the presence of headache,[5] or neurological symptoms, such as arm pain or paraesthesia, as also showing predictive capacity.[2] The Quebec Task Force classification (see Chapter 1 for description), a predominantly symptom-based system, was evaluated in two reviews, with the authors concluding that increasing grades of whiplash associated disorders (WAD) predicted increasingly higher pain intensities and disability two years later.[5, 7] Walton et al.[5] reported that the size of effect was significant when WAD grades II and III were compared against grades I and 0, and this effect was consistent at various follow-up time points.

Other symptoms, such as dizziness, reported sleep disturbances and cognitive difficulties, have not emerged from the systematic reviews as showing any predictive capacity.[2–6]

Crash-related factors

Numerous crash-related factors have been investigated for their predictive capacity. Some of these include the vehicle being stationary when hit, a frontal collision, a rear-end collision, side or other collision, being unprepared for the collision, no seat belt use and no head restraint. However, few of these factors have demonstrated significant predictive power. The exceptions to this are not wearing a seat belt, which was reported to nearly double the risk of developing persistent pain or disability.[5] This is an interesting finding as, in certain jurisdictions where compulsory seat belt use is legislated, the voluntary admission of not wearing a seat belt would not be expected to be common, particularly in jurisdictions operating under a fault-based system. Thus, it is possible that the risk of developing a chronic condition associated with not wearing a seat belt may be even higher than that reported by Walton and colleagues.[5] Scholten-Peeters et al.[4] reported some limited prognostic value for accidents that occur on a highway, but also reported that there was strong evidence that rear-end collisions *have no* predictive value for poor functional recovery.

Thus, the weight of evidence indicates that crash-related factors are of limited value in attempting to predict poor recovery following whiplash injury.

Sociodemographic factors

The predictive capacity of sociodemographic factors has been studied extensively in musculoskeletal pain conditions, and whiplash is no exception. Older age (>50 years), while showing predictive value in some original studies,[8, 9] when subjected to systematic review seems to not be a strong prognostic factor,[5] with some reporting that there is strong evidence for no predictive value of this factor.[4] Similar conclusions have been made for female gender,[4, 5] with only one review reporting predictive value of either of these factors.[2] Since this review by Côté et al. was the first to be conducted for WAD, later systematic reviews will have included a greater number of primary studies, which would suggest that at this point in time these factors should not be considered as having predictive capacity.

Lower education level, defined as no post secondary education, has been identified in five cohorts and appears to be a risk factor for poor recovery,[5] although it is possible that this factor may be mediated by the type of occupation held by those with this risk factor.[7] The clinical usefulness of this prognostic indicator is questionable as its modification cannot be achieved in the context of the clinical management of WAD.

Potentially modifiable risk factors, such as obesity, have not shown a significant effect on outcomes in three different cohorts.[5]

Health status prior to whiplash injury

It would seem feasible that poorer health status prior to the motor vehicle crash (MVC) may have a detrimental influence on recovery, and this issue has been explored in relation to the onset of more widespread pain conditions.[10] Most studies of whiplash have focused on the existence of previous neck pain or headache and the determination of these prior conditions was usually by patient self-report, which may be associated with recall bias.[5] While individual studies have reported conflicting findings, the general consensus of most systematic reviews is that these factors do not have predictive value.[4, 5, 7] The review that performed meta-analysis found only a small, yet significant, risk of developing persistent whiplash pain if the individual reported prior neck pain but no significant effect for prior headache.[5]

Few studies have investigated the predictive capacity of pre-existing neck 'pathology' or structural changes, and Carroll et al.[7] noted that they could find no scientifically admissible studies addressing this factor. One recent study not included in the systematic reviews found that pre-existing degeneration, identified using magnetic resonance imaging (MRI), is not associated with prognosis.[11]

Physical factors

The physical manifestations of the whiplash condition have been extensively studied and it is clear that a variety of impairments may be present, including: motor/movement dysfunction;[12, 13] postural control disturbances, including balance loss, head repositioning errors and disturbed eye movement control;[14–16] and sensory disturbances.[17, 18] These characteristics have been discussed in earlier chapters.

Despite the frequent presence of these factors, few have demonstrated consistent predictive value. Decreased cervical range of movement is the physical factor most commonly investigated for its predictive capacity. An earlier review found only limited evidence for the prognostic capacity of this factor,[4] and this is supported by more recent reviews where the general consensus is that this factor is not a strong predictor of poor recovery.[3, 5] However, a recent cohort study conducted in a clinical environment, which measured cervical range of movement with a simple clinical device, showed that the relative risk for a one-year disability increased by 4.6 times with reduced initial movement.[19]

Features such as altered muscle activation patterns and greater head repositioning errors have been shown in one cohort to not be predictive of poor functional recovery at six months post accident.[8]

Similarly, disturbed eye movement control measured with the smooth pursuit test demonstrated no predictive capacity for pain or disability at 12 months post injury in a large (n = 262) cohort study,[20] despite showing some promise as a predictor in an earlier, much smaller, study.[21]

The exception to the lack of predictive capacity of physical measures is some measures of sensory disturbance. Increased sensitivity to cold stimulation measured via both lowered cold pain thresholds and decreased cold pain tolerance has been shown to be a significant predictor of non-recovery.[8, 22] Relevant systematic reviews indicated that further research was required before this measure could be considered to have consistent predictive value.[3, 5] In a later study it has been shown that cold hyperalgesia (cold pain threshold of >13°C) increases the risk of developing a chronic moderate-to-severe pain and disability pathway by 13-fold.[23] Additionally, classifying injured people at three to four weeks post accident based on the presence of cold hyperalgesia and higher levels of pain identified over 80% of those who had persistent moderate-to-severe symptoms at six months post injury.[24] This factor will, no doubt, appear in future systematic reviews. The mechanisms underlying the presence of cold hyperalgesia are far from clear but may be a reflection of augmented central processing mechanisms.[25]

Other sensory measures, such as mechanical hyperalgesia (lowered pressure pain thresholds), have not demonstrated significant predictive value.[8, 26]

Psychological factors

The earlier systematic reviews found only limited evidence for factors such as nervousness and previous psychological problems,[2, 4] which likely reflects the fact that at the time of these reviews few cohort studies had included psychological factors. This situation has improved and now numerous psychological factors have been studied for their predictive capacity. A systematic review by Williamson et al.[6] is unique in that psychological factors alone were reviewed for their predictive capacity. These authors concluded that there was some evidence to support lower self-efficacy and symptoms of post-traumatic stress as being associated with the development of chronic whiplash, although no meta-analysis was performed. They also reported that evidence for factors such as depression, fear-avoidance behaviours, coping strategies and pain catastrophising was inconclusive, mainly due to conflicting findings within studies or low-quality primary studies.[27] In contrast, Walton et al.[5] concluded that pain catastrophising is a significant risk factor based on the data of three cohorts; these authors also concluded that depression appeared to play no role in outcome following whiplash injury.

Studies published since those included in the systematic reviews have provided additional information. Buitenhuis et al.[28] found that pain catastrophising is predominantly related to concurrent disability rather than a predictor of outcome. This research group also further explored the role of post-traumatic stress symptoms and found that the hyperarousal symptom cluster predicted symptom persistence at six and 12 month follow-up.[29] Hyperarousal symptoms include feelings of irritability, being easily startled and physical signs, such as sweating and a pounding heart. Kongsted et al.[30] also found a weak but significant relationship between acute post-traumatic stress symptoms and recovery.

In summary, it would appear that there is a link between pain-related psychological factors and outcome following whiplash injury. Additionally, the psychological response to the car crash itself seems also to be associated with long-lasting physical symptoms, and this factor should be taken into account in the management of whiplash-injured people.[30, 31]

Expectations of recovery

A recent series of studies has explored the concept of the injured individual's expectations of recovery and/or return to work in compensable cohorts in Canada and Sweden.[32, 33] Participants were those who had made a claim for whiplash injury within 30 to 42 days post the MVC. Those who consented to be involved were followed by structured interview[32] or via postal questionnaire,[33] which comprised a single question of whether or not the participant expected to get better. These studies report a strong relationship between participants not expecting to recover and ongoing pain and disability, even after controlling for variables such as symptom severity, sociodemographic and crash-related variables.[32, 33] A later study from the Canadian group in a similar compensable cohort has shown that expecting to return to work was associated with a quicker recovery.[34]

The results of these studies are tempting to use in order to provide a straightforward explanation for the problem of chronicity following whiplash injury in that simply improving an injured person's expectations will lead to better outcomes. However, the studies were conducted in compensable environments where all participants had filed a claim. It is feasible that accurate answers were not provided by participants in case they perceived this may jeopardise their claim. Additionally, two of the studies[33, 34] used an unvalidated self-report measure of recovery, which is at odds with current calls for the use of validated tools in the measurement of whiplash outcomes.[3, 4] The study by Ozegovic et al.[34] also reported a 42% quicker recovery in those with expectations of return to work but this is not quantified, thus making it difficult to determine whether or not the difference in time to recovery is clinically relevant. Thus, replication of these results in other jurisdictions and in non-compensable environments is required.

Compensation-related factors

Controversy surrounds the relationship between compensation-related factors and outcome following whiplash injury. While some systematic reviews have reported that compensation-related factors are predictive of poor recovery,[2, 7] others have concluded that they have no prognostic value for poor or delayed recovery,[4, 5] and yet others determine that such factors cannot be included as predictor variables due to the varying time frames post injury in which individuals may submit a claim.[3] Spearing and Connelly[35] outline in detail the difficulties of issues surrounding compensation and litigation (see also Chapter 14) and how few cohort studies have considered these problems. Additionally, recent evidence suggests that there may be a differential association between compensation claim submission and severity levels. In whiplash, it has been shown that lodgement of a compensation claim, while associated with increased pain and disability in those with mild-to-moderate symptoms and recovery, had no significant effect on those who developed a more severe pain and disability profile.[36] A recent study provides some support for these findings, where it was shown that access to compensation was not associated with poorer recovery in people with motor vehicle injuries.[37] Thus, the relationship between compensation and health outcomes is complex and requires further research to elucidate these relationships.

Genetic factors

While no studies have yet investigated genetic factors and whiplash outcomes, interest in recent times has focused on the possibility that some individuals may be genetically predisposed to developing chronic pain conditions.[38] This could be one explanation as to why people with similar pathologies or injuries can show very different clinical presentations and outcomes.[38] Genetic variation in the function of the hypothalamic–pituitary–adrenal (HPA) axis has been shown to be associated with musculoskeletal pain.[39] However, genetic risk factors for pain sensitivity have been found to have no association with the development of chronic widespread pain.[40] In Chapter 9, McLean reports on some interesting preliminary data with respect to whiplash, and this will be an important research area to watch for further developments

PREDICTION OF OUTCOMES OTHER THAN PAIN AND DISABILITY

Most predictive studies have used pain and disability measures in some form as their outcome for recovery. This approach is reasonable considering the cardinal symptom of whiplash is neck pain and associated disability. However, whiplash is also characterised by the presence of psychological distress, and the recognition of underlying risk factors may assist healthcare providers to predict the course of psychological reactions and to provide effective interventions.

Only one systematic review reported on the prediction of psychological outcomes. The authors concluded that mental health problems present before the injury were predictive of later depressive symptomatology at one year follow-up.[7] In a later study, older age, greater initial neck pain, post-crash dizziness, vision and hearing problems, numbness/tingling in arms/hands, anxiety, prior mental health problems, and poorer general health predicted persistent depressive symptoms at 12 months post injury.[41] Other studies have used post-traumatic stress as the psychological outcome and have demonstrated a link between initial pain and disability levels and later persistent post-traumatic stress symptoms at six months post injury.[23, 42] Interestingly, there also seems to be a relationship between sensory hypersensitivity and post-traumatic stress.[23, 42] Together, these findings suggest a close relationship between the development of pain/disability, sensory disturbance and stress responses. This may have implications for the management of whiplash, where targeting one 'system', for example, post-traumatic stress via psychological interventions, may influence other manifestations of the condition, and further investigation of these possibilities is underway.

CLINICAL IMPLICATIONS

Knowledge and understanding of the factors associated with poor recovery following whiplash injury has increased in recent times; however, caution is required in the interpretation of these factors. Most of the systematic reviews of prognosis following whiplash injury have made comment on the moderate or lower quality of many of the primary studies from which data was extracted.[3–5] Furthermore, only one systematic review performed meta-analysis,[5] with others citing the heterogeneity of the studies in terms of outcome measures, prognostic factors and methods used.[3, 4, 6] This area of research is also devoid of studies that aim to validate previously identified prognostic indicators in a new and independent cohort. This is a necessary requirement before prognostic models are recommended for use in clinical practice, as various factors can lead to a model performing poorly when applied to other patients.[43] Thus, it would appear that further research is required before we can predict with confidence those individuals who will fail to recover.

As discussed in this chapter, the most consistent predictor of poor recovery is initial levels of pain and/or disability and, contrary to most other factors, this predictor has been validated in several high-quality studies.[5] For clinicians, Walton et al.[5] have proposed a cut-off of 55 out of 100 on a visual analogue pain scale based on data from eight cohorts. However, it should be noted that initially high pain levels do not automatically condemn the patient to a life of chronic pain. Inspection of data from some primary studies shows that initial pain intensity alone explained only 15.7% of the variance in pain and disability at 12 months post injury,[44] and successfully classified only 37% of participants who developed moderate-to-severe symptoms at six months post injury.[8] In this latter study, the classification rate improved to 69% when additional factors of cold pain threshold and post-traumatic stress symptom scores were added to the model.[8] For clinical purposes, it may be more useful to monitor a change in pain levels, and those who fail to show improvement in pain levels in the early weeks post injury may be the patients who clinicians should be concerned about. Current clinical guidelines for whiplash make this recommendation.[45]

It would seem that a combination of factors will likely offer the best predictive capacity. However, various studies include different combinations of variables, making interpretation of the most optimal predictive set difficult. Furthermore, interactions between predictor variables are likely to exist and many studies are not large enough (or have too many predictor variables) to investigate interactions in any meaningful way. For example, people classified as WAD grade III will likely report higher pain levels than those with a lower WAD grade; thus, WAD grade may be a predictor only due to its association with pain levels.

One aim of having a knowledge of predictors of outcome for any condition is that this may, in turn, provide indication for the most appropriate types of interventions, which could, in turn, modify the prognostic indicators and improve outcomes. For whiplash, this is an area that is lacking at present. Some factors that have evidence of predictive capacity offer no guidance with respect to modification (e.g. no post secondary education, prior neck pain, older age). Even the presence of high initial pain levels offers no information on the underlying reasons for high pain levels, which may be targeted for intervention. Intuitively, it would seem that medication may be able to modify pain levels but few trials of medication use have been conducted for WAD and, at this point, the most appropriate medication for use is unknown. For other predictive factors (e.g. cold hyperalgesia), interventions that can achieve modification are unknown.

CONCLUSION

While predictive studies have certainly improved our understanding of injured people at risk of poor recovery, there is still some way to go before we have clear modifiable risk factors that can be targeted with early interventions.

References

1. Spitzer WO, Skovron ML, Salmi LR, et al. Scientific Monograph of Quebec Task Force on Whiplash Associated Disorders: redefining "Whiplash" and its management. *Spine* 1995;20(8 Suppl):1S–73S.
2. Côté P, Cassidy D, Carroll L, et al. A systematic review of the prognosis of acute whiplash and a new conceptual framework to synthesize the literature. *Spine* 2001;26(19):E445–58.
3. Kamper S, Rebbeck T, Maher C, et al. Course and prognostic factors of whiplash: a systematic review and meta-analysis. *Pain* 2008;138(3):617–29.
4. Scholten-Peeters G, Verhagen A, Bekkering G, et al. Prognostic factors of whiplash associated disorders: a systematic review of prospective cohort studies. *Pain* 2003;104(1–2):303–22.
5. Walton D, Pretty J, MacDermid J, Teasell R. Risk factors for persistent problems following whiplash injury: results of a systematic review and meta-analysis. *J Orthop Sports Phys Ther* 2009;39(5): 334–50.
6. Williamson E, Williams M, Gates S, Lamb S. A systematic review of psychological factors and the development of late whiplash syndrome. *Pain* 2008;135:20–30.
7. Carroll L, Holm L, Hogg-Johnson S, et al. Course and prognostic factors for neck pain in whiplash-associated disorders (WAD). Results of the Bone and Joint Decade 2000–2010 Task Force on Neck Pain and Its Associated Disorders. *Spine* 2008;33(42): 583–92.

8. Sterling M, Jull G, Vicenzino B, et al. Physical and psychological factors predict outcome following whiplash injury. *Pain* 2005;114:141–8.
9. Hartling L, Pickett W, Brison R. Derivation of a clinical decision rule for whiplash associated disorders among individuals involved in rear-end collisions. *Accid Anal Prev* 2002;34:531–9.
10. Wynne-Jones G, Jones G, Wiles N, et al. Predicting new onset of widespread pain following a motor vehicle collision. *J Rheumatol* 2006;33:968–74.
11. Kongsted A, Sorensen J, Andersen H, et al. Are early MRI findings correlated with long-lasting symptoms following whiplash injury? A prospective trial with 1-year follow-up. *Eur Spine J* 2008;17(8):996–1005.
12. Nederhand M, Hermens H, IJzerman M, et al. Cervical muscle dysfunction in chronic whiplash associated disorder grade 2. The relevance of trauma. *Spine* 2002;27(10):1056–61.
13. Sterling M, Jull G, Vicenzino B, et al. Development of motor system dysfunction following whiplash injury. *Pain* 2003;103:65–73.
14. Treleaven J, Jull G, Low Choy N. Standing balance in persistent whiplash: a comparison between subjects with and without dizziness. *J Rehabil Med* 2005;37:224–9.
15. Treleaven J, Jull G, Low Choy N. The relationship of cervical joint position error to balance and eye movement disturbances in persistent whiplash. *Man Ther* 2006;11(2):99–106.
16. Treleaven J, Jull G, Low Choy N. Smooth pursuit neck torsion test in whiplash associated disorders: relationship to self-reports of neck pain and disability, dizziness and anxiety. *J Rehabil Med* 2005;37:219–23.
17. Koelbaek-Johansen M, Graven-Nielsen T, Schou-Olesen A, Arendt-Nielsen L. Muscular hyperalgesia and referred pain in chronic whiplash syndrome. *Pain* 1999;83:229–34.
18. Sterling M, Jull G, Vicenzino B, Kenardy J. Sensory hypersensitivity occurs soon after whiplash injury and is associated with poor recovery. *Pain* 2003;104: 509–17.
19. Kasch H, Qerama E, Kongsted A, et al. Clinical assessment of prognostic factors for long-term pain and handicap after whiplash injury: a 1-year prospective study. *Eur J Neurol* 2008;15(11):1222–30.
20. Kongsted A, Leboeuf-Yde C, Korsholm L, Bendix T. Are altered smooth pursuit eye movements related to chronic pain and disability following whiplash injuries? A prospective trial with one-year follow-up. *Clin Rehabil* 2008;22:469–79.
21. Hildingsson C, Wenngren B, Toolanen G. Eye motility dysfunction after soft-tissue injury of the cervical spine. *Acta Orthop Scand* 1993;64(2):129–32.
22. Kasch H, Qerama E, Bach F, Jensen T. Reduced cold pressor pain tolerance in non-recovered whiplash patients: a 1 year prospective study. *Eur J Pain* 2005;9(5):561–9.
23. Sterling M, Hendrikz J, Kenardy J. Developmental trajectories of pain and disability and posttraumatic stress symptoms following whiplash injury. In: Williamson O (ed.). Australian Spine Society Annual Meeting, Brisbane, 2009.
24. Chien A, Eliav E, Sterling M. The development of sensory hypoaesthesia following whiplash injury. *Clin J Pain* 2010;26:722–8.
25. Sterling M, Jull G, Vicenzino B, Kenardy J. Sensory hypersensitivity occurs soon after whiplash injury and is associated with poor recovery. *Pain* 2003;104: 509–17.
26. Kasch H, Stengaard-Pedersen K, Arendt-Nielsen L, Staehelin Jensen T. Pain thresholds and tenderness in neck and head following acute whiplash injury: a prospective study. *Cephalalgia* 2001;21:189–97.
27. Williams M, Williamson E, Gates S, et al. A systematic literature review of physical prognostic factors for the development of late whiplash syndrome. *Spine* 2007;32(25):E764–80.
28. Buitenhuis J, de Jong P, Jaspers J, Groothoff W. Catastrophizing and causal beliefs in whiplash. *Spine* 2008;33(22):2427–33.
29. Buitenhuis J, DeJong J, Jaspers J, Groothoff J. Relationship between posttraumatic stress disorder symptoms and the course of whiplash complaints. *J Psychosom Res* 2006;61(3):681–9.
30. Kongsted A, Bendix T, Qerama E, et al. Acute stress reponse and recovery after whiplash injuries. A one year propsective study. *Eur J Pain* 2008;12: 455–63.
31. Sterling M & Kenardy J. Physical and psychological aspects of whiplash: important considerations for primary care assessment. *Man Ther* 2008;13(2): 93–102.
32. Carroll L, Holm L, Ferrari R, et al. Recovery in whiplash-associated disorders: do you get what you expect? *J Rheumatol* 2009;36:1063–70.
33. Holm L, Carroll L, Cassidy D, et al. Expectations for recovery important in the prognosis of whiplash injuries. *Plos Med* 2008;5(5):e105.
34. Ozegovic D, Carroll L, Cassidy D. Does expecting mean achieving? The association between expecting to work and recovery in whiplash associated disorders: a population-based prospective cohort study. *Eur Spine J* 2009;18:893–9.
35. Spearing N & Connelly L. Is compensation "bad for health"? A systematic meta-review. *Injury* 2010;41(7): 683–92.

36. Sterling M, Hendrikz J, Kenardy J. Developmental trajectories of pain/disability and PTSD symptoms following whiplash injury. *Pain* 2010;150:22–8.
37. O'Donnell M, Creamer M, McFarlane A, et al. Does access to compensation have an impact on recovery outcomes after injury? *Med J Aust* 2010;192(6):328–33.
38. Hocking L, Smith B, Jones G, et al. Genetic variation in the beta2-adrenergic receptor but not catecholamine-O-methyltransferase predisposes to chronic pain: Results from the 1958 British Birth Cohort Study. *Pain* 2010;149(1):143–51.
39. Holliday K, Nicholl B, Macfarlane G, et al. Genetic variation in HPA stress axis influences susceptibility to musculoskeletal pain: results from the EPIFUND study. *Ann Rheum Dis* 2010;69:556–60.
40. Holliday K, Nicholl B, Macfarlane G, et al. Do genetic predictors of pain sensitivity associate with persistent widespread pain? *Molecular Pain* 2009;5:56.
41. Phillips L, Carroll L, Cassidy D, Côté P. Whiplash-associated disorders: who gets depressed? Who stays depressed? *Eur Spine J* 2010;19(6):945–56.
42. Sterling M & Kenardy J. The relationship between sensory and sympathetic nervous system changes and acute posttraumatic stress following whiplash injury – a prospective study. *J Psychosom Res* 2006;60:387–93.
43. Altman D, Vergouwe Y, Royston P, Moons K. Prognosis and prognostic research: validating a prognostic model. *Br Med J* 2009;338:b605.
44. Hendricks E, Scholten-Peeters G, van der Windt D, et al. Prognostic factors for poor recovery in acute whiplash patients. *Pain* 2005;114:408–16.
45. TRACsa. A clinical pathway for best practice management of acute and chronic whiplash-associated disorders. Adelaide: South Australian Centre for Trauma and Injury Recovery, 2008.

CHAPTER 11
Primary care management of acute whiplash injury

Michele Sterling and Justin Kenardy

Primary care practitioners are often the first healthcare contact for individuals who have sustained a whiplash injury. While somewhat dependent upon jurisdictions, injured individuals may see community general practitioners, community allied health practitioners, including physiotherapists, chiropractors and osteopaths among others, or visit an accident and emergency department of a hospital.

The personal and economic costs associated with whiplash associated disorders (WAD) are a significant health burden, due in most part to the numbers of individuals who develop a chronic pain condition—estimated to be approximately 50%.[1] Systematic review data indicate that most recovery following whiplash injury occurs in the first two to three months, with a general plateau in symptoms occurring after this time.[2] More recently, trajectory modelling analyses have been used to identify distinct recovery pathways following injury. Three recovery pathways have been identified:

1. *Mild*: mild or negligible pain/disability for the entire 12 months (45%)
2. *Moderate*: initial moderate pain/disability that decreased to mild-to-moderate levels by three months (39%)
3. *Chronic–severe*: severe pain/disability persisting at moderate-to-severe levels for 12 months (16%).[3]

Of note was the finding that, in all trajectories, the most rapid recovery occurred within the first three months post injury (see Fig 2.1). Thus, the early two-to-three month period after injury seems a crucial time frame to potentially avert the course to chronic pain development following whiplash injury. The primary care provider most commonly sees the patient at this point of time and, thus, plays a vital role in the quest to reduce chronicity associated with the whiplash condition.

Although there is considerable uncertainty about the best management approaches for acute whiplash, most guidelines recommend early return to activity, exercise and education/advice based on the evidence available at the time of their development.[4–6] It has been argued that this approach may be sufficient for those with a less severe condition but for patients with a more complex condition characterised by higher pain and disability levels and more profound physical and psychological changes, additional management strategies will be necessary.[7]

Of course, WAD grade IV[8] (fracture or dislocation) must be recognised, and guidelines recommend the use of the Canadian C-spine rule to decide if an X-ray is required.[5] In this chapter, only WAD grades I to III are considered.[8] (For a description of WAD grades see Chapter 2, Table 2.1.)

This chapter outlines the current evidence for the management of acute whiplash, particularly in the primary care setting. The implications for management in accordance with the current knowledge of the heterogeneity of the whiplash condition, in terms of both physical and psychological features, as well as future treatment directions, are discussed.

CURRENT EVIDENCE FOR THE MANAGEMENT OF ACUTE WAD

A recent Cochrane review of conservative management for WAD included 21 studies, evaluating a broad variety of conservative treatment approaches for acute and subacute whiplash.[9] Interventions were divided into passive interventions (e.g. rest, immobilisation, ultrasound) and active interventions (e.g. exercises, act as usual approach), and were compared with no treatment, a placebo or each other. Only eight studies were deemed to be of a high quality. The authors reported that data pooling was not possible due to clinical and statistical heterogeneity and that, while individual studies demonstrated the effectiveness of one treatment over another, the comparisons were varied and the results inconsistent. Their conclusions were that the evidence neither supports nor refutes the effectiveness of either passive or active treatments to relieve the symptoms of WAD, grades I or II.[9]

A frequent criticism of Cochrane reviews and other systematic reviews is that, in spite of their methodological rigor, they fail to provide clear clinical answers, or lack appropriate translation of the evidence into the realities of clinical practice. It is common to read in reviews that 'the methodological quality of the evidence is limited, there are too few studies of merit, and there are no clear evidence-based answers'.[10] To overcome this problem, Gross et al.[10] attempted to translate findings from systematic reviews of neck pain management to clinical practice by the publication of a supplementary 'Tool Kit' with simplified summaries and practical application tips specifically aimed at clinicians. For acute whiplash, they reported strong evidence for active interventions, such as exercise, and that advice to rest and the wearing of neck collars should not be recommended.[10] These findings are consistent with recent clinical guidelines for whiplash management, which promote education and assurance to the patient, the maintenance of activity levels, general and specific exercises, simple analgesics and the promotion of coping strategies for acute WAD.[4–6, 11]

On closer inspection of data from randomised controlled trials included in the above-mentioned reviews, despite a particular intervention showing efficacy, a significant proportion of injured people still develop chronic pain and disability.[12–15] For example, in the study by Proviniciali et al.,[12] approximately 18% of participants were worse or only reported minimal improvement following a multimodal treatment intervention. In the study by Rosenfeld et al.,[15] 48% of participants receiving an active exercise intervention still reported greater than low pain levels following treatment. Additionally, there is evidence available to indicate that the introduction of evidence-based clinical guidelines for the management of WAD (based on the promotion of activity as discussed above) did not either improve health outcomes for injured people or decrease costs.[16] Thus, the current advocated approach is clearly not a panacea for whiplash.

The emerging multifactorial nature of WAD suggests that while the current guidelines may benefit some whiplash patients, they are likely to be inadequate for the management of those with a more complex condition, including both marked physical impairment and psychological distress. This has been recognised in more recent clinical guidelines, which have attempted to include recommendations for the identification of factors such as sensory disturbance and psychological distress, although they fall short of recommending what treatment should be provided to those with this clinical presentation.[4] The now greater understanding of the physical and psychological characteristics of the condition offers the opportunity to guide the development of improved management approaches in the acute/subacute stage of injury.

THE PROVISION OF ADVICE AND EDUCATION

Clinical guidelines for whiplash recommend the provision of education and advice for individuals who have sustained a whiplash injury.[4–6] A recent qualitative study in Western Australia that explored the experiences of patients with acute whiplash in relation to the management of injuries, as well as general practitioners, indicated that injured people sought reassurance and understanding of the implications of their condition.[17] However, a number of the general practitioners interviewed were unaware of their patients' concerns, feelings and fears about the injury.[17] Few qualitative studies of whiplash are available, so this one is important in that it suggests that this disconnection between patient and practitioner may challenge quality patient-centred care and detrimentally influence outcomes.[17] The findings of this study are supported by a survey of emergency departments in the United Kingdom, where it was found that inconsistent advice was often provided to patients with acute WAD and that advice about return to activity and appropriate use of collars was rarely provided.[18] Of interest was the common encouragement to pursue a personal injury claim, even extending to the sponsorship of advice leaflets by personal injury solicitors.[18] This may potentially facilitate delayed recovery in view of recent findings that poor expectations of recovery are associated with persistent pain and disability.[19]

These two studies were conducted in very specific geographical areas, so it is not known whether the results are transferable to other jurisdictions. Nevertheless, it is concerning that whiplash-injured people may not be receiving appropriate and helpful information. In saying this, a recent Cochrane review concluded that there was moderate evidence of no effect on outcomes for various forms of advice alone, focusing on resumption of activity in acute WAD, although this conclusion was based on the results of just two studies.[20] One study used a mailed-out video,[21] and the other an educational pamphlet provided in the emergency department.[22] Other forms of education, such as internet delivery or education about the pain neurophysiology, have not been investigated in patients with WAD, although these approaches show benefit for other conditions, such as low back pain.[23, 24]

In summary, although patients understandably want advice on the prognosis and implications of their injury,[17] it is not clear that advice per se will improve outcomes, and the most effective form and nature of the advice/education remains to be established.

IS PAIN CONTROL IMPORTANT?

The most consistent predictor of poor functional recovery following whiplash injury is initial levels of pain and disability.[1, 2, 25] Reported pain levels do not have to be high, as moderate or greater levels of pain and disability (pain: visual analogue pain scale >5 out of 10; disability: neck disability index >30%) demonstrate prognostic capacity.[25, 26] It would seem logical that a primary aim of early whiplash management would be to decrease levels of pain. Consistent with this are current recommendations for pain management that advocate adequate pain relief following acute injury.[27, 28] Despite this, very few trials of pain relief using medication in the early stages of whiplash have been conducted. One study showed that infusion of methylprednisone, provided in a hospital accident and emergency setting, for patients with acute whiplash resulted in fewer sick days over six months and less disabling pain than in those in the placebo group.[29] While interesting, this seems a rather drastic management approach that would not be feasible in community primary care settings. In a recent randomised controlled trial, little benefit (pain relief) was found from the use of muscle relaxants (cyclobenzaprine), either alone or combined with non-steroidal anti-inflammatory drugs (NSAIDs), for patients with acute neck strain in emergency departments.[30]

Some clinical guidelines recommend that analgesics can be used for acute whiplash but not routinely, and only when there is documented improvement in patient outcomes;[5] few include pain relief as an aim of treatment.[6] Such recommendations are predominantly consensus-based due to the lack of high-quality trials.[4, 5] This seems at odds to recommendations for acute pain after other injuries or surgery, where pain relief is seen as mandatory.[28] There seems to be a disparity between recommendations for other painful conditions and whiplash with respect to pain management. Presumably, this discrepancy has arisen due to the lack of randomised controlled trials specifically investigating pain control for patients with acute WAD. Thus, it is clear that further investigations of early pain-relief strategies for patients with acute whiplash are required.

Of course, pain relief can be achieved or enhanced via means other than medication, including advice and education,[28] or via some physical interventions, including exercise.[31] Therefore, by whatever means, decreasing pain should be an aim of management, particularly for those individuals reporting moderate or greater levels of pain.

PHYSICAL CHARACTERISTICS OF ACUTE WAD AND IMPLICATIONS FOR MANAGEMENT

It is clear that motor and postural control impairments, including movement loss, altered cervical and shoulder girdle muscle recruitment patterns, kinaesthetic deficits and disturbed eye movement control, have been identified in individuals with an acute whiplash injury;[32, 33] these have been discussed in detail in Chapter 7. The presence of such findings suggests that rehabilitation strategies directed at ameliorating these impairments may enhance recovery. However, as outlined above, while interventions based on trying to increase activity and restore movement have been shown to be somewhat beneficial in reducing pain and disability, significant numbers of patients still make the transition to chronicity.[12, 15] A trial of specific neck exercises and manual therapy for patients with chronic whiplash demonstrated only a modest effect on pain and disability, with preliminary data suggesting that this intervention was ineffective for those with associated sensory hypersensitivity.[34] Although it should be noted that this latter study involved patients with chronic WAD, such a trial for patients with acute WAD, where participants are subgrouped according to their sensory presentation, is yet to be reported. Additionally, motor or movement impairments have been shown not to be predictive of poor recovery.[26, 32] Together, these findings suggest that motor deficits, although present, may not play a key role in the development or maintenance of chronic symptoms following whiplash injury. This is not to say that treatment directed at ameliorating motor dysfunction should not be provided to whiplash-injured people, but, rather, that the identification of such impairments may not equip the primary care provider with useful information on either prognosis or treatment responsiveness.

Identification of sensory hypersensitivity

The early presence of sensory hypersensitivity (widespread decreased pain threshold to several stimuli) has been shown to be a feature of individuals with acute whiplash and higher levels of pain and disability,[33] and is associated with poor functional recovery.[35, 36] These changes are indicative of augmented central pain-processing mechanisms; these phenomena are discussed in depth in Chapter 5.

These sensory disturbances have implications for the management of acute WAD. As sensory hypersensitivity is not present in all those with an acute injury,[36] it is important for clinicians to be able to identify such processes in individual patients. Unfortunately, at this stage, there is no 'gold standard' per se for the assessment of central hyperexcitability. Clues as to its presence can be gained from both the patient interview and physical examination. Patient reports of mechanical and thermal allodynia, high irritability of the pain and sleep disturbances may be indicative of augmented central pain-processing mechanisms (Table 11.1).[7]

Neuropathic pain questionnaires, while not yet frequently used in the assessment of common musculoskeletal pain conditions, may provide an indication of central hyperexcitability. Thirty per cent of an acute whiplash cohort reported features indicative of neuropathic pain (S-LANSS ≥ 12).[37] This group showed higher levels of pain and disability, cold hyperalgesia and heightened bilateral responses with the brachial plexus provocation test (BPPT).[37]

The physical examination also provides additional clues. The presence of allodynia with manual light touch of the patient is indicative of disturbed central pain-processing mechanisms.[38] Pressure pain thresholds can be measured with commercially available pressure algometers, with control and whiplash data available for comparison (Fig 11.1).[39, 40] Clinical measurement of cold pain thresholds is more difficult. The use of thermorollers, which can be set at predetermined temperatures, has been suggested,[41] but at this stage no clinical test is available with which to quantify cold pain threshold. The BPPT has been proposed as a measure of central hyperexcitability,[42, 43] as hypersensitive responses to this test have been demonstrated in people with acute and chronic whiplash.[36, 44] A bilateral loss of range of movement (elbow extension) has been shown to be associated with decreased pressure and cold pain thresholds in whiplash.[42] In view of these findings and the familiarity of many musculoskeletal practitioners with the test, it is suggested that it may be a useful clinical tool in the assessment of hypersensitivity in neck pain. Table 11.2 summarises physical tests that may be useful in the evaluation of central hyperexcitability.

Table 11.1 Findings from patient interviews that may be suggestive of central hyperexcitability

Symptom	Example of patient report
Mechanical allodynia/ hyperalgesia	Pain with touch Pain from clothes or bedclothes
Thermal allodynia/ hyperalgesia	Pain with cold (e.g. ice, cold weather)
Irritable condition	Pain that is easily aggravated but difficult to settle infers the presence of sensitisation
Sleep disturbances	Difficulty sleeping due to pain

Central hyperexcitability—implications for management

Once central hyperexcitability has been identified, it may be necessary to modify the nature of the rehabilitation interventions usually provided to people with whiplash. While the resumption of activity is almost universally recommended, this should be undertaken with care in patients with signs of central hyperexcitability. The application of non-judicious, physical mechanically stimulating treatments may serve to maintain and prolong this hyperexcitability and have a deleterious effect on the patient's long-term outcome. It is not suggested that these patients avoid activity, as the maintenance of activity levels opposed to rest and the use of a collar has been shown to be important in the management of acute whiplash.[14] However, activity and exercise may need to be introduced more slowly, and the intensity and frequency gradually increased. Zusman[45] proposes that movement (activity, exercises) should be relatively pain-free to avoid long-lasting changes in neuronal synaptic memory. Certainly, studies investigating fibromyalgia, a condition also proposed to have disturbed central pain-processing mechanisms, have shown that sensory hypersensitivity increases following some forms of exercise, including isometric and submaximal aerobic exercise.[46]

In addition to modifying treatment approaches in this patient group, the question of whether or not the early modulation of central hyperexcitability

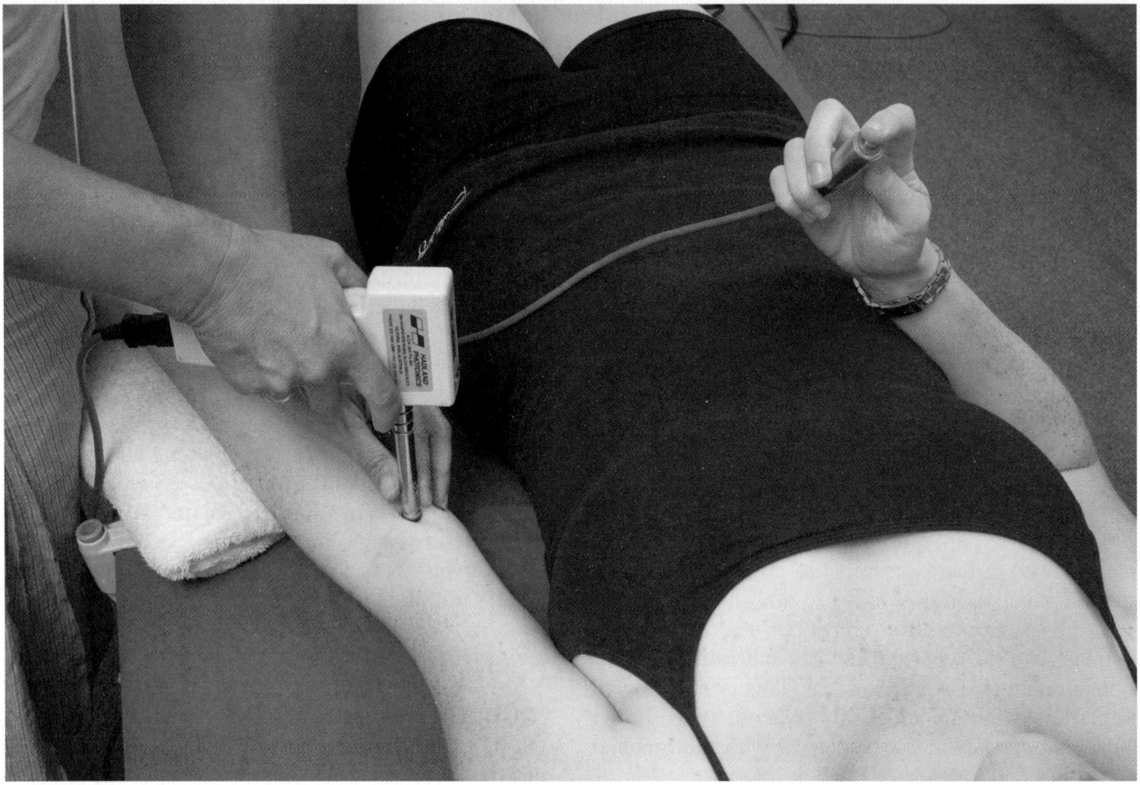

Figure 11.1 Measurement of pressure pain thresholds (PPT) over the median nerve trunk with an electronic pressure algometer. (Somedic AB, Sweden)

would lead to improved outcomes for these patients is frequently asked.[47] Possible treatment modalities for central hyperexcitability found in musculoskeletal pain conditions are largely unexplored. Pharmacological management approaches have been suggested[48] but the effectiveness of this form of treatment is yet to be investigated in patients with WAD. Furthermore, the side-effects of some drug therapy approaches are daunting.[46] In an ongoing randomised controlled trial for acute whiplash that included drug prescription (ranging from simple analgesics to opioids) conducted in our laboratory, many participants failed to adhere to their prescribed medication, citing side-effects such as drowsiness and nausea as the main reason for non-compliance. Thus, a predominantly medication-based approach to management, particularly in the acute stage, may not be feasible.

An important unanswered question is whether non-pharmacological interventions have the capacity to modulate central hyperexcitability in WAD. Spinal manual therapy exerts an immediate hypoalgesic effect on mechanical hyperalgesia[49] but it appears that it does not have similar hypoalgesic effects on either heat or cold hyperalgesia in patients with whiplash.[50] However, a spinal manual therapy technique (lateral glide) has been shown to modulate spinal cord hyperexcitability, at least in the short term, and further investigation of possible sustained effects is warranted.[50] It is not advocated that this form of treatment will ever be used as a sole therapy approach for the management of whiplash. Rather, if some modulation of central hyperexcitability can be achieved, then it is possible that additional treatments, such as exercise and functional restoration, may be more beneficial. At the present time, there is evidence to suggest that manual therapy has a better overall effect on neck pain when used in conjunction with exercise.[5, 51] The modulatory capacity of other modalities on central hyperexcitability is not yet known. Theoretically, physical interventions such as transcutaneous electrical nerve stimulation (TENS) and acupuncture may also be useful in modulating sensory hypersensitivity, and these have not been specifically investigated in WAD.

Table 11.2 Findings from physical examination that may be indicative of central hyperexcitability

Clinical tests	Interpretation
Manual examination of the neck	Presence of allodynia (pain with light touch) infers central hyperexcitability
Manual examination of structures away from the neck (e.g. upper limb nerve trunks)	Presence of allodynia/hyperalgesia infers central hyperexcitability
Pressure pain thresholds	Decreased pain thresholds at sites away from the neck may indicate central hyperexcitability
Cold sensitivity measured with thermorollers	Pain with thermorollers at 20°C—cold hyperalgesia
Brachial plexus provocation test (BPPT)	Bilaterally reduced elbow extension infers central hyperexcitability of motor responses

The primary care provider should not overlook the potential of cognitive behavioural strategies in addressing central hyperexcitability. Psychological factors, including post-traumatic stress symptoms,[26] pain catastrophising,[52] high levels of distress[53] and expectations for recovery,[20] have all demonstrated predictive capacity for poor recovery in various studies. While the central nervous system changes seen in people with whiplash are likely to reflect biological processes,[54] psychological factors can influence these processes. Relationships have been demonstrated between various psychological factors and sensory hypersensitivity in WAD.[54, 55] Furthermore, pain catastrophisation and post-traumatic stress have been shown to be associated with increased levels of inflammatory biomarkers.[56, 57] Thus, it would seem plausible that early cognitive behavioural-based interventions that aim to decrease early psychological distress may be helpful in attenuating central hyperexcitability and improve the course of recovery for those at risk.[58] However, to date, no studies have investigated this proposal.

PSYCHOLOGICAL CHARACTERISTICS OF ACUTE WAD AND IMPLICATIONS FOR MANAGEMENT

The psychological presentation in patients with whiplash can be equally as diverse as the physical presentation, with some individuals showing marked distress and others seeming resilient to the injury.[3, 59] Psychological factors, such as high levels of pain catastrophising,[60] fear of movement,[61] lower pain self-efficacy[62] and distress,[53] have been shown to be associated with more pain and disability in cases of acute WAD. Depressive symptoms are common in acute whiplash injury[63] and may be associated with prior mental health problems and poorer general health,[63] as well as post-injury adjustment.[64] The role of coping styles or strategies in patients with whiplash is unclear. Some data indicate that a palliative reaction (e.g. seeking palliative relief of symptoms, such as distraction, smoking or drinking) was associated with longer symptom duration.[65, 66] In contrast, Kivioja et al.[64] found no evidence that different coping styles in the early stage of injury influenced the outcome at one year post accident. The different cohort inception times of these studies may account for the differences in findings, indicating that coping strategies may vary depending on the stage of the condition, and this requires further investigation.

Whiplash injury differs from most other musculoskeletal pain syndromes in that it is generally precipitated by a traumatic event, typically a motor vehicle crash (MVC). The effect of the psychological stress surrounding the crash itself, as opposed to or in addition to distress about neck pain complaints, may have a significant influence on outcome. Post-traumatic stress disorder (PTSD) is a common sequelae of severe injuries following an MVC.[67] Yet, it is only recently that evidence has emerged that it may also play a role in less severe road accident injuries, including whiplash. A recent prospective cohort study of 155 participants identified three distinct trajectories for post-traumatic stress measured using the Post-Traumatic Stress Disorder Diagnostic Scale (PDS). These trajectories (see Fig. 2.2) are outlined below:

1. *Resilient*: mild symptoms throughout the 12 month study period (40%)
2. *Recovering*: initially moderate symptoms, declining to mild levels by three months (43%)
3. *Chronic moderate-to-severe*: persistent moderate-to-severe symptoms throughout 12 months (17%).[3]

Thus, 60% of this cohort showed an initial moderate post-traumatic stress reaction three weeks post injury.

Not all whiplash-injured people show elevated levels of distress,[3, 59] making it important for the primary care provider to be able to identify those patients who are distressed. In a busy primary care practice, it is not feasible to administer numerous questionnaires to patients to cover all possible psychological domains. It may be more efficient for clinicians to choose the most relevant screening questionnaire based on the individual patient's presentation. Such an approach is recommended in current clinical guidelines, which also provide recommendations for several relevant questionnaires.[4, 5] For example, the patient who indicates that they are troubled by nightmares about the MVC, which is possibly indicative of post-traumatic stress symptoms, could be further evaluated using a concise and easily scored questionnaire, such as the Impact of Events Scale–Revised (IES–R)[68] or the Trauma Screening Questionnaire (TSQ),[69] which are both readily available on the internet. Questionnaires that may be suitable for use in the assessment of individuals with acute whiplash are provided in Table 11.3.

Once the presence of psychological factors that may impede recovery has been identified, the primary care provider must then decide upon a course of action. Options may include an early referral to a psychologist or continued monitoring or management by the primary care provider, and decisions of which option to take may need to be based on the nature and/or severity of the psychological distress. Data available from the literature on acute/subacute low back pain indicates that early targeting of pain-related psychological factors (e.g. fear of movement and pain-coping strategies) with a cognitive behavioural approach delivered by physiotherapists may improve outcomes.[77, 78] However, no studies have investigated this approach for patients with acutc WAD. Nevertheless, the inclusion of management directed at behavioural and psychological responses to pain delivered in a primary care setting would seem to be a reasonable approach. In the case of more serious psychological factors, such as depression and post-traumatic stress, the injured person will likely require referral for more specialised psychological evaluation and management from a clinical psychologist or, perhaps, a general practitioner with skills and expertise in psychological care.

Assessment for the presence of acute post-traumatic stress symptoms may be unfamiliar to primary care providers but recent investigations indicate that clinicians will also need to consider this factor in their management of individuals with acute whiplash injury.[3, 79] A moderate or high level of symptoms assessed via the IES–R is not grounds for a diagnosis of PTSD to be made. This can only be achieved via comprehensive assessment, including clinical interview by a qualified mental health professional.[80] The general consensus indicates that a patient with an early post-traumatic stress reaction should be reassured and allowed some time for natural recovery to occur. It should be noted that psychological debriefing with a focus on recounting the traumatic event should not be offered on a routine basis as it can exacerbate stress symptoms.[81] If recovery is not apparent within three to four weeks, guidelines suggest that referral for specialist psychological or psychiatric care should be instigated.[4] For primary care providers this may mean that symptoms indicative of post-traumatic

Table 11.3 Psychological questionnaires that may be useful in the assessment of patients with acute whiplash

Psychological substrate	Questionnaire
Fear of movement	Tampa Scale of Kinesiophobia (TSK)[70] Pictorial Fear of Activity Scale-Cervical (PFACTS)[71]
Pain catastrophising	Pain catastrophising scale (PCS)[72]
Pain coping strategies	The Coping Strategies Questionnaire (CSQ)[73]
Self-efficacy	The Pain Self-Efficacy Questionnaire[74]
Post-traumatic stress symptoms	Impact of Events Scale–Revised (IES–R)[67] Trauma Screening Questionnaire (TSQ)[68]
Depression/distress symptoms	Patient Health Questionnaire–9 (PHQ–9)[75] The Kessler Psychological Distress Scale (K10)[76]

stress should be just monitored in the early post-injury period. Additionally, sound advice and assurance from primary care providers in this important early post-injury phase may assist in decreasing stress symptoms,[82] but this is yet to be tested in an experimental context for whiplash.

Pharmacological interventions provided immediately after a traumatic event have shown the capacity to prevent the development of subsequent PTSD. In a recent study of military personnel in Iraq, the administration of morphine during early post-trauma care was significantly associated with a lower risk of PTSD after injury.[83] There is also emerging evidence that pharmacotherapy aimed at attenuating the initial stress response of sympathetic arousal with drugs such as beta blockers (propranolol) may also prevent the development of PTSD.[84] However, at this stage the routine use of these types of pharmacological interventions preventively is not recommended. As outlined earlier in this chapter, investigations of pharmacotherapy of any kind for acute whiplash are scant, but data from other traumatic injuries provide a basis for the justification of similar trials to be conducted for cases of acute whiplash injury.

In some cases it may be advisable to defer physical rehabilitation until improvements in psychological status are gained. There is data available to indicate that trauma-focused cognitive behavioural therapy may potentially have an effect not only on PTSD symptoms but also on pain and disability. The results of a recent empirical examination explored directional relationships between PTSD and chronic pain in 323 survivors of accidents.[85] The results indicated a mutual maintenance of pain intensity and post-traumatic stress symptoms at five days post injury but by six months post injury (chronic stage), PTSD symptoms impacted significantly on pain but not vice versa. While this study did not specifically focus on whiplash injury, it provides indication that addressing PTSD symptoms may allow for a decrease in levels of pain, thus facilitating the potential effects of more pain/disability-focused approaches to management, such as exercise. Such an approach that combines both physical rehabilitation and psychological management may achieve better results, but this is yet to be evaluated.

Thus, in the early acute/subacute stage post whiplash injury, primary care providers play an important role in identifying psychological factors that may impede recovery. Their role also extends to the provision of initial psychological support and advice. The primary care provider should also identify patients who are not showing psychological recovery, and these individuals should be referred for more specific psychological management. The management of the psychological sequelae of chronic whiplash injury is discussed in Chapter 13.

EARLY MULTIDISCIPLINARY MANAGEMENT

The more complex presentation of the whiplash-injured person with higher levels of pain and disability, central hyperexcitability, movement disturbances and psychological distress suggests that an early multidisciplinary management approach will be required. Few studies have investigated the efficacy of such an approach, although recent data indicate that this may not be straightforward. A recent series of studies in one jurisdiction in Canada have reported that the delivery of early intensive interventions (defined as the frequency of treatments) provided in the acute injury stage was associated with poorer health outcomes and prolonged disability.[86, 87] These studies reported that greater frequency of treatment from general practitioners and/or chiropractors and/or medical specialists was associated with slower recovery.[86, 87] In another study, the authors reported intensive fitness training and multidisciplinary outpatient rehabilitation were also associated with slower recovery,[88] although these interventions were provided up to three months post injury and not in the early post-injury stage. These studies are not randomised controlled trials and all have involved retrospective inspection of insurance data. There has also been criticism of their methodologies, including the use of 'time to claim closure' as an outcome measure.[89, 90] Another aspect worth consideration is the heterogeneity of acute whiplash, which was not considered in these studies.[36] As argued, the pain of patients with features of central hyperexcitability may be exacerbated by exercise and other physical interventions.[43, 91] This may be one reason for the slower recovery when more frequent and/or intense physical-type interventions are provided.

A recent quasi-experimental study from Norway has found similar results, where the provision of early multidisciplinary assessment and advice showed an increased risk of chronic pain development three years post injury (relative risks ranged from 1.7 [95% CI: 1.0–2.6] to 2.6 [95% CI: 1.5–4.0]).[92] The intervention used in this study consisted of comprehensive testing by a general practitioner and physiotherapist for 2.5 hours, with some patients also being assessed by a neurologist or rehabilitation physician.[92] The authors suggest that the intensive assessment may have increased patient concerns of serious injury and this may have contributed further to poor recovery.[92] The nature of the interventions provided after patient assessment are not clearly detailed in this study and, while the authors acknowledge the presence of various psychological factors in whiplash-injured people, no psychological intervention was provided apart from 'advice-giving', the nature of which was also not described.[92] This latter point is important as, despite there being little dispute as to the presence of various psychological factors in patients with WAD, which are present from the early injury stage,[92, 93] there is yet to be a trial that specifically investigates specific and targeted psychological interventions in the acute/subacute stage.

While the results of these studies need to be confirmed in randomised controlled trials, they are nevertheless concerning for the management of patients with acute whiplash and the aim to decrease the transition to chronicity. However, numerous treatment models are yet to be investigated. Some options may include: the inclusion of controlled early medication use either alone or in conjunction with other interventions; the inclusion of specific psychological interventions; and the development of integrated care models where practitioners engage with the patients, their family and other practitioners to provide more patient-centred care. Another option may be the upskilling of certain practitioners on other areas of management, such that these practitioners provide most of the care or at least coordinate different care options in close liaison with the injured person. This role is often left to the general practitioner, where time constraints on this provider group may not make this the best option for individuals with whiplash injury.

SUMMARY

The most optimal management of acute WAD remains to be elucidated. While the facilitation of activity and exercise in conjunction with advice and assurance will likely be the mainstays of a management approach, it is apparent that, for some whiplash-injured people, this approach will require modification. In those individuals with moderate or greater pain and disability levels, central hyperexcitability and elevated levels of distress, care will need to be taken to avoid provocation of their condition, perhaps via a more gradual and graded progression of activity. This may be one reason for the reported slower recovery seen in patients in some studies with the provision of 'intensive' early physical-based interventions. These complex patients may not need more frequent treatment but, perhaps, more specific treatment that takes into account individual clinical presentations. This may include strategies to decrease pain (including medication but not restricted to medication) and a more specific approach to psychological distress if resolution is not apparent within several weeks. Such approaches will require careful 'coordinated' care that involves and includes the patient in treatment decisions, rather than a more 'ad hoc' multidisciplinary approach. New models of care for patients with whiplash in the primary care setting may need to be developed. It is clear that primary care providers play a vital role in the management of patients with acute whiplash injury and, more importantly, in the quest to prevent the transition to chronicity which so often occurs.

References

1. Carroll L, Holm L, Hogg-Johnson S, et al. Course and prognostic factors for neck pain in whiplash-associated disorders (WAD). Results of the Bone and Joint Decade 2000–2010 Task Force on Neck Pain and Its Associated Disorders. *Spine* 2008;33(42):583–92.
2. Kamper S, Rebbeck T, Maher C, et al. Course and prognostic factors of whiplash: a systematic review and meta-analysis. *Pain* 2008;138(3):617–29.
3. Sterling M, Hendrikz J, Kenardy J. Developmental trajectories of pain/disability and PTSD symptoms following whiplash injury. *Pain* 2010;in press.
4. NSW Motor Accident Authority. Guidelines for the management of whiplash associated disorders. Sydney: MAA, 2007.
5. South Australian Centre for Trauma and Injury Recovery. A clinical pathway for best practice management of acute and chronic whiplash-associated disorders. Adelaide: TRACsa, 2008.
6. Moore A, Jackson A, Jordan J, et al. Clinical guidelines for the physiotherapy management of whiplash associated disorder. London: The Chartered Society of Physiotherapy, 2005.
7. Sterling M & Kenardy J. Physical and psychological aspects of whiplash: important considerations for primary care assessment. *Man Ther* 2008;13(2):93–102.
8. Spitzer W, Skovron M, Salmi L, et al. Scientific Monograph of Quebec Task Force on Whiplash Associated Disorders: redefining "Whiplash" and its management. *Spine* 1995;20(8 Suppl):S1–S73.
9. Verhagen A, Scholten-Peeters G, van Wijngaarden S, et al. Conservative treatments for whiplash. *Cochrane Database Syst Rev* 2007(2):CD003338.
10. Gross A, Haines T, Goldsmith C, et al. Knowledge to action: a challenge for neck pain treatment. *J Orthop Sports Phys Ther* 2009;39(5):351–63.

11. Scholten-Peeters G, Bekkering G, Verhagen A, et al. Clinical practice guideline for the physiotherapy of patients with whiplash associated disorders. *Spine* 2002;27(4):412–22.
12. Provinciali L, Baroni M, Illuminati L, Ceravolo M. Multimodal treatment to prevent the late whiplash syndrome. *Scand J Rehabil Med* 1996;28(2):105–11.
13. Rosenfeld M, Gunnarsson R, Borenstein P. Early intervention in whiplash-associated disorders. A comparison of two protocols. *Spine* 2000;25:1782–7.
14. Rosenfeld M, Seferiadis A, Carllson J, Gunnarsson R. Active intervention in patients with whiplash associated disorders improves long-term prognosis: a randomised controlled clinical trial. *Spine* 2003;28(22):2491–8.
15. Rosenfeld M, Seferiadis A, Gunnarsson R. Active involvement and intervention in patients exposed to whiplash trauma in automobile crashes reduces costs. *Spine* 2006;31(16):1799–804.
16. Rebbeck T, Maher C, Refshauge K. Evaluating two implementation strategies for whiplash guidelines in physiotherapy: a cluster randomised trial. *Aust J Physiother* 2006;52(3):165–74.
17. Russell G & Nicol P. 'I've broken my neck or something!' The general practice experience of whiplash. *Fam Pract* 2009;26:115–20.
18. Lamb S, Williams M, Withers E, et al. A national survey of clinical practice for the management of whiplash-associated disorders in UK emergency departments. *Emerg Med J* 2009;26:644–7.
19. Holm L, Carroll L, Cassidy D, et al. Expectations for recovery important in the prognosis of whiplash injuries. *Plos Med* 2008;5(5):e105.
20. Haines T, Gross A, Burnie S, et al. Patient education for neck pain with or without radiculopathy. *Cochrane Database Syst Rev* 2009;CD005106.
21. Brison R, Hartling L, Dostaler S, et al. A randomised controlled trial of an educational intervention to prevent the chronic pain of whiplash associated disorders following rear-end motor vehicle collisions. *Spine* 2005;30(16):1799–807.
22. Ferrari R, Rowe B, Majumdar SR, et al. Simple educational intervention to improve the recovery from acute whiplash: results of a randomized, controlled trial. *Acad Emerg Med* 2005;12:699–706.
23. Buhrman M, Faltenhag S, Strom L, Andersson G. Controlled trial of Internet-based treatment with telephone support for chronic back pain. *Pain* 2004;111:368–77.
24. Moseley G, Nicholas M, Hodges P. A randomised controlled trial of intensive neurophysiology education in chronic low back pain. *Clin J Pain* 2004;20(5):324–30.
25. Walton D, Pretty J, MacDermid J, Teasell R. Risk factors for persistent problems following whiplash injury: results of a systematic review and meta-analysis. *J Orthop Sports Phys Ther* 2009;39(5):334–50.
26. Sterling M, Jull G, Vicenzino B, et al. Physical and psychological factors predict outcome following whiplash injury. *Pain* 2005;114:141–8.
27. Australian Acute Musculoskeletal Guidelines Group. Evidence-based management of acute musculoskeletal pain. Brisbane: Australian Academic Press, 2004.
28. Macintyre P, Scott D, Schug S, et al. Acute pain management: scientific evidence. Melbourne: ANZVA & FPM, 2010.
29. Pettersson K & Toolanen G. High-dose methylprednisolone prevents extensive sick leave after whiplash injury. *Spine* 1998;23(9):984–9.
30. Khwaja S, Minnerop M, Singer A. Comparison of ibuprofen, cyclobenzaprine or both in patients with acute cervical strain: a randomized controlled trial. *Can J Emerg Med* 2010;12(1):39–44.
31. O'leary S, Falla D, Hodges P, et al. Specific therapeutic exercise of the neck induces immediate local hyperalgesia. *J Pain* 2007;8(11):832–9.
32. Kongsted A, Jørgensen LV, Leboeuf-Yde C, et al. Are altered smooth pursuit eye movements related to chronic pain and disability following whiplash injuries? A prospective trial with one-year follow-up. *Clin Rehabil* 2008;22:469–79.
33. Sterling M, Jull G, Vicenzino B, Kenardy J. Characterisation of acute whiplash associated disorders. *Spine* 2004;29(2):182–8.
34. Jull G, Sterling M, Kenardy J, Beller E. Does the presence of sensory hypersensitivity influence outcomes of physical rehabilitation for chronic whiplash? A preliminary RCT. *Pain* 2007;129(2):28–34.
35. Kasch H, Qerama E, Bach F, Jensen T. Reduced cold pressor pain tolerance in non-recovered whiplash patients: a 1 year prospective study. *Eur J Pain* 2005;9(5):561–9.
36. Sterling M, Jull G, Vicenzino B, Kenardy J. Sensory hypersensitivity occurs soon after whiplash injury and is associated with poor recovery. *Pain* 2003;104:509–17.
37. Sterling M & Pedler A. A neuropathic pain component is common in acute whiplash and associated with a more complex clinical presentation. *Man Ther* 2009;14(2):173–9.
38. Rolke R, Magerl W, Cambell K, et al. Quantitative sensory testing: a comprehensive protocol for clinical trials. *Eur J Pain* 2006;10:77–88.

39. Sterling M, Carllson Y, Crommert L, Jull G. Are cervical physical outcome measures influenced by the presence of symptomatology? *Physiother Res Int* 2002;7(3):113–21.
40. Sterling M, Treleaven J, Edwards S, Jull G. Pressure pain thresholds in chronic whiplash associated disorder: further evidence of altered central pain processing. *J Musculoskeletal Pain* 2002;10(3): 69–81.
41. Jensen T & Baron R. Translation of symptoms and signs into mechanisms in neuropathic pain. *Pain* 2003; 102(2):1–8.
42. Sterling M. Testing for sensory hypersensivity or central hyperexcitability associated with cervical spine pain. *J Manipulative Physiol Ther* 2008;31:534–9.
43. Nijs J, Van Houdenhove B, Osstendorp R. Recognition of central sensitization in patients with musculoskeletal pain: application of pain neurophysiology in manual therapy practice. *Man Ther* 2010;15:135–41.
44. Ide M, Ide J, Yamaga M, Takagi K. Symptoms and signs of irritation of the brachial plexus in whiplash injuries. *J Bone Joint Surgery (Br)* 2001;83:226–9.
45. Zusman M. Mechanisms of musculoskeletal physiotherapy. *Phys Ther Rev* 2004;9:39–49.
46. Vierck C. Mechanisms underlying development of spatially distributed chronic pain (fibromyalgia). *Pain* 2006;124:242–63.
47. Schneider G, Smith A, Hooper A, et al. Minimizing the source of nociception and its concurrent effect on sensory hypersensitivity: an exploratory study in chronic whiplash patients. *BMC Musculoskelet Disord* 2010;11:29.
48. Curatolo M, Arendt-Nielsen L, Petersen-Felix S. Central hypersensitivity in chronic pain: mechanisms and clinical implications. *Phys Med Rehabil Clin North Am* 2006;17:287–302.
49. Vicenzino B, Collins D, Benson H, Wright A. An investigation of the interrelationship between manipulative therapy induced hypoalgesia and sympathoexcitation. *J Manipulative Physiol Ther* 1998;21(7):448–53.
50. Sterling M, Pedler A, Chan C, et al. Cervical lateral glide increases nociceptive flexion reflex but not pressure or thermal pain thresholds in chronic whiplash associated disorders. *Man Ther* 2010;15(2):149–53.
51. Gross A, Hoving J, Haines T, et al. A Cochrane review of manipulation and mobilization for mechanical neck disorders. *Spine* 2004;29:1541–8.
52. Buitenhuis J, de Jong P, Jaspers J, Groothoff W. Catastrophizing and causal beliefs in whiplash. *Spine* 2008;33(22):2427–33.
53. Carstensen T, Frostholm L, Oernboel E, et al. Post-trauma ratings of pre-collision pain and psychological distress predict poor outcome following acute whiplash trauma: a 12-month follow-up study. *Pain* 2008;139(2):248–59.
54. Sterling M, Pettiford C, Hodkinson E, Curatolo M. Psychological factors are related to some sensory pain thresholds but not nociceptive flexion reflex threshold in chronic whiplash. *Clin J Pain* 2008;24(2):124–30.
55. Sterling M & Kenardy J. The relationship between sensory and sympathetic nervous system changes and acute posttraumatic stress following whiplash injury – a prospective study. *J Psychosom Res* 2006;60: 387–93.
56. Hoge E, Brandstetter K, Moshier S, et al. Broad spectrum of cytokine abnormalities in panic disorder and posttraumatic stress disorder. *Depress Anxiety* 2009;26:447–55.
57. Edwards R, Kronfli T, Haythornthwaite J, et al. Association of catastrophizing with interleukin-6 responses to acute pain. *Pain* 2008;140:135–44.
58. Nijs J, Van Oosterwijck J, De Hertogh W. Rehabilitation of chronic whiplash: treatment of cervical dysfunctions or chronic pain syndrome? *Clin Rheumatol* 2009;28:243–51.
59. Sterling M, Kenardy J, Jull G, Vicenzino B. The development of psychological changes following whiplash injury. *Pain* 2003;106(3):481–9.
60. Sullivan M, Stanish W, Sullivan M, Tripp D. Differential predictors of pain and disability in patients with whiplash injury. *Pain Res Manag* 2002;7(2):68–74.
61. Vangronsveld K, Peters M, Goosens M, Vlaeyen J. The influence of fear of movement and pain catastrophizing on daily pain and disability in individuals with acute whiplash injury: a daily diary study. *Pain* 2008;139(2):449–57.
62. Bunketorp-Kall L, Andersson G, Asker B. The impact of subacute whiplash-associated disorders on functional self-efficacy: a cohort study. *Int J Rehabil Res* 2007;30(3):221–6.
63. Phillips L, Carroll L, Cassidy D, Côté P. Whiplash-associated disorders: who gets depressed? Who stays depressed? *Eur Spine J* 2010;19(6):945–56.
64. Kivioja J, Sjalin M, Lindgren U. Psychiatric morbidity in patients with chronic whiplash associated disorder. *Spine* 2004;29(11):1235–9.
65. Buitenhuis J, Spanjer J, Fidler V. Recovery from acute whiplash – the role of coping styles. *Spine* 2003;28(9):896–901.
66. Carroll L, Cassidy D, Côté P. The role of pain coping strategies in prognosis after whiplash injury: passive coping predicts slowed recovery. *Pain* 2006;124(1–2): 18–26.

67. Kuch K, Cox B, Evans R, Shulman I. Phobias, panic and pain in 55 survivors of road vehicle accidents. *J Anxiety Disord* 1994;8(2):181–7.
68. Weiss D & Marmar C. The impact of events scale – revised. In: Wilson J, Keane T (eds). Assessing psychological trauma and PTSD. New York: Guilford Press, 1997:98–135.
69. Brewin C, Rose S, Andrews B, et al. Brief screening instrument for post-traumatic stress disorder. *Br J Psychiatry* 2002;181:158–62.
70. Kori S, Miller R, Todd D. Kinesiophobia: a new view of chronic pain behaviour. *Pain Manage* 1990;3:35–43.
71. Turk D, Robinson J, Sherman J, et al. Assessing fear in patients with cervical pain: development and validation of the Pictorial Fear of Activity Scale–Cervical (PFActS-C). *Pain* 2008;139(1):55–62.
72. Sullivan M, Bishop S, Pivik J. The pain catastrophizing scale: development and validation. *Psychol Assess* 1995;7:524–32.
73. Rosenstiel A & Keefe F. The use of coping strategies in chronic low back pain patients: relationship to patient characteristics and current adjustment. *Pain* 1983;17:33–44.
74. Nicholas MK. The pain self-efficacy questionnaire: taking pain into account. *Eur J Pain* 2007;11:153–63.
75. Duffy F, Chung H, Trivedi M, et al. Systematic use of patient-rated depression severity monitoring: is it helpful and feasible in clinical psychiatry? *Psychiatr Serv* 2008;59(10):1148–54.
76. Andrew G & Slade T. Interpreting scores on the Kessler Psychological Distress Scale. *Aust N Z J Public Health* 2001;25(6):494–7.
77. George S, Fritz J, Bialosky J, Donald D. The effect of a fear-avoidance-based physical therapy intervention for patients with acute low back pain: results of a randomized clinical trial. *Spine* 2003;28:2551–60.
78. Wand B, Bird C, McAuley J, et al. Early intervention for the management of acute low back pain: a single-blind randomized controlled trial of biopsychosocial education, manual therapy, and exercise. *Spine* 2004;29(21):2350–6.
79. Buitenhuis J, DeJong J, Jaspers J, Groothoff J. Relationship between posttraumatic stress disorder symptoms and the course of whiplash complaints. *J Psychosom Res* 2006;61(3):681–9.
80. Wilson J-P & Keane T. Assessing psychological trauma and PTSD. 2nd edn. New York: Guilford Press, 2004.
81. Forbes D, Creamer M, Phelps A, et al. Treating adults with acute stress disorder and posttraumatic stress disorder in general practice: a clinical update. *Med J Aust* 2007;187(2):120–3.
82. National Health and Medical Research Council. Australian guidelines for the treatment of adults with ASD and PTSD. Canberra: NHMRC, 2007.
83. Holbrook T, Galarneau M, Dye J, et al. Morphine use after combat injury in Iraq and post-traumatic stress disorder. *N Engl J Med* 2010;362(2):110–17.
84. Strawn J & Geracioti T. Noradrenergic dysfunction and the psychopharmacology of posttraumatic stress disorder. *Depress Anxiety* 2008;25(3):260–71.
85. Jenewein J, Wittmann L, Moergeli H, et al. Mutual influence of PTSD symptoms and chronic pain among injured accident survivors: a longitudinal study. *J Trauma Stress* 2009;22(6):540–8.
86. Côté P, Hogg-Johnson S, Cassidy D, et al. Initial patterns of clinical care and recovery from whiplash injuries. *Arch Intern Med* 2005;165:2257–63.
87. Côté P, Hogg-Johnson S, Cassidy J, et al. Early aggressive care and delayed recovery from whiplash: isolated finding or reproducible result? *Arthritis Rheum* 2007;57:861–8.
88. Cassidy D, Carroll L, Côté P, Frank J. Does multidisciplinary rehabilitation benefit whiplash recovery? Results of a population-based incidence cohort study. *Spine* 2007;32:126–31.
89. Croft A. Letter to the editor. *Arthritis Rheum* 2008;15: 599–600.
90. Freeman M, Centeno C, Merskey H, et al. Letter to the editor. *Arch Intern Med* 2008;166:1239.
91. Staud R, Robinson M, Price D. Isometric exercise has opposite effects on central pain mechanisms in fibromyalgia patients compared to normal controls. *Pain* 2005;118:176–84.
92. Pape E, Hagen K, Brox J, et al. Early multidisciplinary evaluation and advice was ineffective for whiplash-associated disorders. *Eur J Pain* 2009;13(10):1068–75.
93. Williamson E, Williams M, Gates S, Lamb S. A systematic review of psyhcological factors and the development of late whiplash syndrome. *Pain* 2008;135:20–30.

CHAPTER 12
Evidence-based management of chronic whiplash associated disorders

Trudy Rebbeck

In this chapter, the evidence for the management of chronic whiplash is first discussed, with a focus on physical interventions. The chapter then focuses on how to interpret this evidence when selecting appropriate interventions for patients with chronic whiplash.

EVIDENCE BASE FOR MANAGEMENT OF CHRONIC WHIPLASH

To date, several attempts have been made at synthesising the evidence for chronic whiplash in a systematic manner. The first published guideline that included treatment options for chronic whiplash based recommendations for treatment on other chronic musculoskeletal conditions rather than on studies in chronic whiplash.[1] A UK clinical guideline for whiplash included recommendations for chronic whiplash; however, this was founded on only one trial on patients with chronic whiplash, with the remainder of the recommendations being drawn from the literature on chronic neck pain.[2] Recently, the Task Force on Neck Pain and Its Associated Disorders published recommendations on the treatment of whiplash;[3] however, their systematic review only reviewed one database (Medline) from 1980, and found only one trial utilising a chronic whiplash population. The most recent published clinical guideline for chronic whiplash made recommendations for treatment based on a wider evidence base,[4] with methodology scoring high on the Appraisal of Guidelines for Research Evaluation (AGREE) instrument.[5] The evidence for the management of chronic whiplash in this chapter is, therefore, based on the studies selected for inclusion in this recent guideline.[4]

How studies were included

Studies that formed the basis for the evidence in this chapter were initially selected from those included in the recently published guideline for chronic whiplash.[4] The literature for the guideline was searched until March 2007. In order to update the evidence, the same search criteria were applied to the same databases from March 2007 until December 2009.

Essential inclusion criteria have been described in detail elsewhere.[3, 4] Criteria for participants were: being involved in a motor vehicle crash (MVC), symptoms persisting for more than three months since the injury, and the primary complaint of neck pain. Only randomised controlled trials (RCTs) were accepted, and then rated for quality using the PEDro scale,[6] with high-quality trials satisfying a PEDro score of 8–10/10, medium-quality trials rating 4–7/10 and low-quality trials rating 1–3/10. Data, including those on populations, interventions and outcomes, were extracted. Effect sizes (mean difference [95% CI]) or relative risks (RR) (95% CI) were calculated from the primary data using an effect size calculator. Effects for pain outcomes were considered clinically significant when a mean difference of 10% was reported. This is based on previous work where effects of this size were found to be the cut-off point for patients to consider themselves to be at least 'minimally improved'.[7–9] For all other outcomes, effects were considered significant if 95% confidence intervals (CIs) did not include 1.

Thirteen trials were found that met the inclusion criteria and, therefore, formed the basis for recommendations for clinical practice in this chapter. The description of these trials is outlined in Table 12.1. The evidence has been categorised according to the intervention (Fig 12.1), namely physical interventions, psychological interventions and medical interventions.

EVIDENCE FOR PHYSICAL INTERVENTIONS

Active exercise

Active exercise has demonstrated positive effects in two trials.[10, 11] The nature of the active exercise undertaken in the first trial[10] is explained in detail

Table 12.1 Description of included randomised controlled trials for chronic whiplash

Author, Year, Title	PEDro score Quality (high/medium/low)	Included patients Setting	Intervention and control groups
Barnsley et al., 1994[24] Lack of effect of intra-articular corticosteroids for chronic pain in the cervical zygapophyseal joints.	7/10 Medium	*Patients*: 41 patients suffering chronic pain after whiplash *Setting*: Australia	*Intervention*: 21 subjects receiving corticosteroid injections into the zygapophyseal joint *Control*: 20 subjects receiving a local anaesthetic into the zygapophyseal joint
Byrn et al., 1993[23] Subcutaneous sterile water injections for chronic neck and shoulder pain following whiplash injuries.	6/10 Medium	*Patients*: 40 patients with chronic whiplash (4–6 years previously) *Setting*: Sweden	*Intervention*: 20 subjects receiving up to three sessions of injection of up to 30 pain trigger points with subcutaneous sterile water *Control*: 20 subjects receiving up to three sessions of injection of up to 30 pain trigger points with saline
Ekvall Hansson et al., 2006[14] Dizziness among patients with whiplash-associated disorder: a randomized controlled trial.	5/10 Medium	*Patients*: 29 patients with dizziness after whiplash (6 months–15 years after injury) *Setting*: Sweden	*Intervention*: 16 patients receiving vestibular rehabilitation (eye, head and trunk coordination exercises) provided by a physiotherapist *Control*: 13 subjects receiving no intervention
Fitz-Ritson, 1995[15] Phasic exercises for cervical rehabilitation after "whiplash" trauma.	4/10 Medium	*Patients*: 30 patients with chronic whiplash (>12 weeks after injury) *Setting*: Canada	*Intervention*: 15 patients receiving chiropractic therapy plus phasic exercises. Phasic exercises described as rapid eye–head–neck–arm exercises *Control*: 15 patients receiving chiropractic therapy with standard exercises
Freund et al., 2002[27] Use of botulinum toxin in chronic whiplash-associated disorder.	8/10 High	*Patients*: 28 patients with chronic whiplash *Setting*: Canada	*Intervention*: 14 patients receiving botulinum toxin injections in five points, chosen by palpation in either splenius capitis, rectus capitis, semispinalis capitis and trapezius *Control*: 14 patients receiving placebo injections in five points
Jull et al., 2007[10] Does the presence of sensory hypersensitivity influence outcomes of physical rehabilitation for chronic whiplash? A preliminary RCT.	8/10 High	*Patients*: 71 patients with chronic whiplash (3 months → 2 years (mean 12 months) after injury) *Setting*: Australia	*Intervention*: 36 patients receiving a 10-week physiotherapy package of specific motor control exercises, kinaesthetic exercises, passive joint mobilisation, education and reassurance *Control*: 35 patients receiving a self-management booklet with description of an exercise program and advice to stay active

(Continued)

Table 12.1 Description of included randomised controlled trials for chronic whiplash—cont'd

Author, Year, Title	PEDro score Quality (high/medium/low)	Included patients Setting	Intervention and control groups
Klobas et al., 2006[17] Effect of therapeutic jaw exercise on temporomandibular disorders in individuals with chronic whiplash-associated disorders.	5/10 Medium	*Patients*: 55 patients with chronic whiplash (>6 months since injury) and temporomandibular disorder *Setting*: Sweden	*Intervention*: 25 patients receiving specific jaw exercises (e.g. active and resisted mandibular movements), general rehabilitation and passive therapy *Control*: 30 patients receiving general rehabilitation and passive therapy
Lemming et al., 2005[25] The responses to pharmacological challenges and experimental pain in patients with chronic whiplash-associated pain.	7/10 Medium	*Patients*: 33 patients with chronic whiplash (>5 months) *Setting*: Sweden	*Intervention*: 33 patients receiving intravenous infusion of ketamine, lidocaine (lignocaine), morphine or placebo in random order
Lord et al., 1996[20] Percutaneous radiofrequency neurotomy for chronic cervical zygapophyseal joint pain.	9/10 High	*Patients*: 24 patients with chronic whiplash (>3 months) with confirmed facet joint pain by previous local anaesthetic blocks *Setting*: Australia	*Intervention*: 12 patients receiving radiofrequency neurotomy (temperature 80°C for 90 seconds) *Control*: 12 patients receiving placebo (temperature maintained at 37°C)
Padberg et al., 2007[28] Neck pain in chronic whiplash syndrome treated with botulinum toxin. A double-blind, placebo-controlled clinical trial.	8/10 High	*Patients*: 40 patients with chronic whiplash (>6 months) *Setting*: Netherlands	*Intervention*: 20 patients receiving botulinum injections at trigger points (muscles with clinically increased tone or tenderness, could include occipitalis–frontalis, masseter, sternocleidomastoid, splenius capitis, trapezius, semispinalis) *Control*: 20 patients receiving placebo (saline) injections at trigger points
Soderlund & Lindberg 2001[18] Cognitive behavioural components in physiotherapy management of chronic whiplash associated disorders (WAD – a randomized group study.	6/10 Medium	*Patients*: 33 patients with chronic whiplash (>3 months after injury) *Setting*: Sweden	*Intervention*: 16 patients receiving multimodal treatment plus cognitive behavioural therapy delivered by physiotherapists *Control*: 17 patients receiving multimodal treatment without cognitive behavioural therapy

Table 12.1 Description of included randomised controlled trials for chronic whiplash—cont'd

Author, Year, Title	PEDro score Quality (high/ medium/low)	Included patients Setting	Intervention and control groups
Stewart et al., 2007[11] Randomised controlled trial of exercise for chronic whiplash associated disorders.	8/10 High	*Patients*: 134 patients with chronic whiplash (3–12 months after injury) *Setting*: Australia	*Intervention*: 66 patients receiving a six-week graded and individualised active exercise program conducted with a cognitive behavioural therapy (CBT) approach, with advice provided by a physiotherapist *Control*: 68 patients receiving advice alone provided by a physiotherapist
Wicksell et al., 2008[19] Can exposure and acceptance strategies improve functioning and life satisfaction in people with chronic pain and whiplash-associated disorders (WAD)? A randomized controlled trial.	8/10 High	*Patients*: 22 patients with chronic whiplash (>3 months after injury) *Setting*: Sweden	*Intervention*: 11 patients receiving 10 sessions of CBT over eight weeks in addition to multimodal treatment (medication, acupuncture and physiotherapy) *Control*: 9 patients receiving wait list control (medication, acupuncture and physiotherapy)

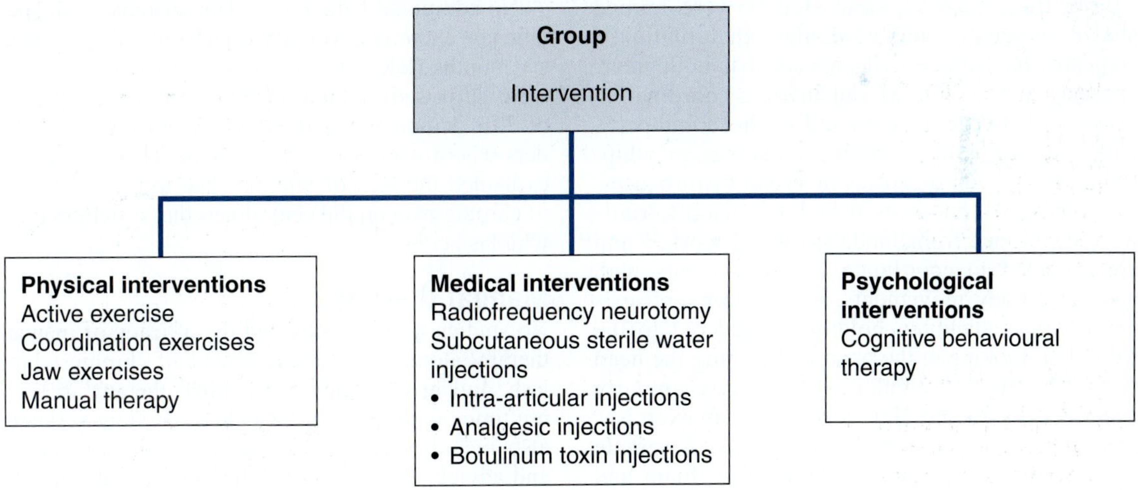

Figure 12.1 Grouping of interventions for chronic whiplash associated disorders (WAD).

elsewhere.[12] Exercises were low load in nature to avoid provocation of symptoms and were directed at rehabilitating muscle control in the cervical flexor, extensor and scapula groups of muscles, as well as retraining kinaesthetic sense (Chapters 6 and 7). Active exercise was not provided in isolation in this trial, but rather, as the authors explain, active exercise was combined with advice and manual therapy when indicated.

In contrast, the exercise undertaken in the second trial[11] was provided with the treating physiotherapists following cognitive behavioural principles, such as goal setting, shaping and reinforcement.[13] Exercises were individualised, progressive and submaximal. They were prescribed according to the functional activities outlined by the patients as being affected due to whiplash.

Both active exercise trials demonstrated small effects for the primary outcomes of both pain and disability in the short term (Table 12.2). Jull et al.[10] demonstrated a mean difference of perceived pain relief of symptoms of 2.7/10 (CI, 1.6–3.8) in the active exercise group compared with the control intervention at 10 weeks. The mean difference for disability between groups was –6% (–5.8/100 [CI, –11.4 to –0.2]). Stewart et al.[11] demonstrated a mean difference of pain intensity of –1.1/10 (CI, –1.9 to –0.3) in the active exercise group compared with the control intervention at six weeks. The mean difference for disability was 8% (–3.7/50 [CI, –6.2 to –1.2]). These reported small effects suggest that there is room for improvement in treatment outcomes with this approach, which is discussed later in this chapter.

Coordination exercises

Two trials investigated the efficacy of coordination exercises and demonstrated a positive effect in comparison to the control interventions.[14, 15] The interventions used in these studies were termed phasic exercises[15] and vestibular rehabilitation,[14] respectively. However, it appears that both interventions appear similar and involve coordination exercises between the eyes and the head and neck, with the intent of improving outcomes in whiplash patients with dizziness or visual disturbances. The phasic exercises used in Fitz-Ritson's trial[15] were developed from Janda's original work,[16] and are intended to coordinate eye movements with neck and body movements. A sample exercise is described as standing, holding a hand out to the side, then looking at the hand and turning the head to face the hand. Vestibular exercises were similarly described by Ekvall Hansson et al.[14] as exercises using eye, head and trunk movements. A sample exercise was described as 'standing on foam and turning the head from side to side'.[14] The similarities in the interventions in both of these groups have, therefore, led to these trials being discussed together in this chapter.

The effects demonstrated for coordination exercises were moderate in the 'phasic exercises trial' and small in the 'vestibular' exercise trial. Phasic exercises demonstrated a mean difference in reduction of disability at eight weeks of 24% (–24.2/100 ([CI, –29.4 to –19.0]) compared with standard exercise.[15] Vestibular rehabilitation demonstrated a mean difference of 6% (–6/100 [CI, –16.0 to 0.0]) improvement in the dizziness handicap inventory at six weeks compared with the control group.[14] It seems unusual that two studies that used similar interventions had such different effects. However, it should be noted that several methodological issues in the Fitz-Ritson trial[15] may bias the outcomes. These issues include no concealment of allocation, no blinded measurement of outcome and that the groups were not matched for age and gender. The results, therefore, should be interpreted with caution.

Therapeutic jaw exercise

One trial found no additional benefit for therapeutic jaw exercise (TJE) in patients with whiplash and temporomandibular joint (TMJ) disorder.[17] Patients were randomised to receive TJE in addition to general rehabilitation and passive therapy, or general rehabilitation and passive therapy alone. TJEs were described by the authors as aiming to improve TMJ and muscle function by improving mobility, relaxing tense muscles and improving strength and coordination. The general exercises included mobility and stabilisation exercises, as well as passive therapies, such as electrotherapy and massage.

No additional benefit was demonstrated with specific jaw exercises over general rehabilitation alone at six months (RR, 1.03 [CI, 0.67–1.59]). The authors were surprised at this outcome, given the efficacy of TJE demonstrated in RCTs of other TMJ disorders where whiplash is not present. They, therefore, explained the lack of effect as due to the influences of chronic pain on the central nervous system in their whiplash cohort.

Manual therapy

No studies have investigated the efficacy of manual therapy alone in the management of chronic whiplash. Jull et al.[10] included manual therapy in their multimodal intervention, which, as previously stated, also included active exercise, kinaesthetic exercise and advice. The effects for the multimodal program were beneficial in comparison to a self-management program. However, the effects for manual therapy alone cannot be determined.

The lack of trials investigating the effect of manual therapy on chronic whiplash may suggest an area for further research. However, given the now complex manifestation of some individuals with chronic whiplash, it would seem inadequate to address these complex manifestations with one modality alone.

Table 12.2 Effects of interventions for specific outcomes

Intervention	Trials	Intervention effects (mean difference [95% CI])*/Outcome			
		Pain	Impairment	Disability	Psychological
Physical interventions					
Active exercise	Jull et al. 2007[10]	S 2.7/10 (CI, 1.6–3.8) *Perceived relief of symptoms:* 0–10 at 10 weeks	NS 1.1 (CI, –5 to 7.2) *Range of cervical flexion and extension*	S –5.8/100 (CI, –11.4 to –0.2) Neck Pain Index (NPI) 10 weeks	NS –2.8/84 (-6.2 to 0.6) General Health Questionnaire (GHQ): 28
	Stewart et al. 2007[11]	S –1.1/10 (CI, –1.9 to –0.3) *Pain intensity:* Visual Analogue Scale (VAS) 0–10 at 6 weeks	S Mean difference unable to be calculated *Craniocervical flexion test (CCFT)*	S –3.7/50 (CI, –6.2 to –1.2) *Neck disability index (NDI):* 6 weeks	NS 2.1/68 (CI, 0.1 to 4.1) Tampa Scale for Kinesiophobia (TSK)
Coordination exercises	Ekvall Hanson et al. 2006[14]		S +2 (CI, 0.0–4.0) *Single leg balance in seconds:* at 3 months	S –4/100 (CI, –14.0 to 0.0) *Dizziness Handicap Inventory (DHI):* at 3 months	NS –3.3/75 (CI, 9.6–3) *Impact of Events Scale (IES)*
	Fitz-Ritson 1995[15]			S –24.2/100 (CI, 29.4 to –19.0) *NDI*: 8 weeks	
Manual therapy	Jull et al. 2007[10]	S 2.7/10 (1.6–3.8) *Perceived relief of symptoms:* 0–10 at 10 weeks	NS 1.1 (–5 to 7.2) *Range of cervical flexion and extension* S Mean difference unable to be calculated CCFT	S –5.8/100 (CI, –11.4 to –0.2) *NPI:* 10 weeks	NS –2.8/84 (CI, –6.2 to 0.6) GHQ 28 NS 2.1/68 (CI, 0.1–4.1) TSK NS –3.3/75 (CI, 9.6–3) IES
Jaw exercises	Klobas et al. 2006[17]	NS RR 1.03 (CI, 0.67–1.59) *Number of patients with pain on mandibular movement*			

(Continued)

Table 12.2 Effects of interventions for specific outcomes—cont'd

Intervention	Trials	Intervention effects (mean difference [95% CI])*/Outcome			
		Pain	Impairment	Disability	Psychological
Psychological interventions					
Cognitive behavioural therapy	Soderlund & Lindberg 2001[18]	NS 0.3/10 (CI, −1.3 to 1.9) *Pain intensity VAS:* 0–10 at 3 months	NS 3.0 (CI, −6.9 to 12.9) *Range of cervical extension*	NS 6.1/70 (CI, −5.4 to 17.6) *PDI:* at 3 months	S Mean differences unable to be calculated *Perceived ability to perform activities of daily living (ADLs)*
	Stewart et al. 2007[11]	S −1.1/10 (CI, −1.9 to −0.3) *Pain intensity VAS:* 0–10 at 6 weeks		S −3.7/50 (CI, −6.2 to −1.2) *NDI:* at 6 weeks	
	Wicksell et al. 2008[19]			NS −9.3/70 (CI, −21.4 to 2.8) *PDI:* at 4 months	NS −6.5 (CI, −14.1 to 1.1) *TSK* S 5.6 (CI, 0–11.2) *Satisfaction with life:* 4 months
Medical interventions					
Radiofrequency neurotomy	Lord et al. 1996[20]	S 255 days (CI, 11.6–498.4) *Return to 50% previous pain*			
Subcutaneous sterile water	Byrn et al. 1993[23]	S −1.7/10 (CI, −3 to −0.4) *Pain intensity (VAS) 0–10:* at 3 months S −2.3/10 (CI, −3.7 to −0.9) *Pain intensity (VAS) 0–10*: at 8 months	S 33 (CI, 7–59) *Total range of motion (ROM):* at 3 months		

Table 12.2 Effects of interventions for specific outcomes—cont'd

Intervention	Trials	Intervention effects (mean difference [95% CI])*/Outcome			
		Pain	Impairment	Disability	Psychological
Analgesic injections	Lemming et al. 2005[25]	NS –7.0 (CI, –17.1 to 3.1): ketamine –3.0 (CI, –13.6 to 7.6): lidocaine (lignocaine) –1.0 (CI, –10.9 to 8.9): morphine *Pain intensity VAS (0–100):* five days after test	S 31 (CI, 2.4–59.6) *Total ROM:* at 8 months		
Intra-articular steroid injections	Barnsley et al. 1994[24]	NS –0.05 (CI, –2.8 to 1.8) *Median time to return of 50% pain (days)*			
Botulinum toxin injections	Padberg et al. 2007[28]	NS –4.7 (CI, –28.2 to 13.5) *Pain intensity (VAS) 0–100:* at 12 weeks	NS –11 (CI, –40 to +17) *Total cervical ROM:* at 12 weeks		
	Freund et al. 2002[27]	S –4.1/30 (CI, –8.9 to 0.7) *Pain intensity (VAS) 0–30:* at 4 weeks	NS 35.0 (CI, 26.9 to 43.1) *Total cervical ROM:* at 4 weeks	NS 3.2/50 (CI, –1.7 to 8.1) *NDI:* at 4 weeks	

Dizziness Handicap Inventory (DHI) range: 0 (minimal handicap due to dizziness) to 100 (maximum handicap due to dizziness)
General Health Questionnaire (GHQ) range: 0 (minimal emotional distress) to 84 (maximum emotional distress)
Impact of Events Scale (IES) range: 0 (minimal post traumatic stress symptoms) to 75 (maximum post traumatic stress symptoms)
Neck Disability Index (NDI) range: 0 (0%) (minimum disability) to 50 (100%) (maximum disability)
Neck Pain Index (NPI) range: 0% (minimal disability) to 100% (maximum disability)
Pain Disability Index (PDI) range: 0 (minimal disability) to 70 (maximum disability)
Satisfaction with life range: 5 (minimally satisfied) to 35 (maximally satisfied)
Tampa Scale for Kinesiophobia (TSK) range: 17 (minimal fear associated with movement) to 68 (maximum fear associated with movement)
* S = significant; NS = not significant.

EVIDENCE FOR PSYCHOLOGICAL INTERVENTIONS

Cognitive behavioural therapy

Three trials examined the effect of cognitive behavioural therapy (CBT) approaches for patients with chronic whiplash, all reporting positive effects in comparison to the control group.[11, 18, 19] Although psychological interventions for whiplash are specifically discussed in Chapter 13, these three trials will be briefly outlined here as two of the studies were predominantly physiotherapy exercise based with adherence to principles of CBT.

The first trial, by Stewart et al.,[11] as previously mentioned, included a cognitive behavioural component in the exercise arm of treatment, with both components delivered by a physiotherapist. The elements of CBT employed were based on Nicholas and Tonkin's work,[13] and included shaping, pacing, reinforcement and goal setting. Exercise and activity in this trial were applied according to these CBT principles. Given the multimodal interventions, the benefits attributable to the CBT component cannot be separated from the active exercise component in Stewart et al.'s trial.[11] The intervention in the second trial (Soderlund & Lindberg[18]) was similar to that used by Stewart et al., in that patients in the intervention group received exercises delivered by a physiotherapist under the principles of CBT. The control group received exercises as well as other treatment modalities. However, in contrast to Stewart et al.'s trial, the effects in this trial can be attributed to the CBT element, as exercises were included in both groups. In the third trial,[19] the intervention group received individual sessions of CBT delivered by a psychologist in addition to multimodal treatment (medication, acupuncture and physiotherapy), while the control group received the multimodal treatment alone. Any effects, therefore, can be attributed to the CBT.

The effects in the studies employing a CBT approach delivered by a physiotherapist were small. Stewart et al.'s results for pain and disability have been discussed above (see also Table 12.2) and included a small effect for improvement in disability. The only positive effect reported by Soderlund and Lindberg[18] was a significant difference in the perceived ability to perform activities of daily living in the cognitive behavioural group compared to the exercise alone group (χ^2, 10.3; $P < 0.05$). There was no benefit demonstrated with CBT for short- and mid-term follow-up treatment of pain and disability outcomes (e.g. mean difference in disability at three months, 6.1/70 [CI, –5.4 to 17.6]). The effects for CBT delivered by a psychologist were not found to be significant. Although Wicksell et al.[19] reported large effects in their original data, when the mean difference between groups was calculated for this chapter, the effects for reduction in disability (using the Pain Disability Index [PDI]) were found to be insignificant (e.g. mean difference in disability, –9.3/70 [CI, –21.4 to 2.8]).

Further investigation into the role of cognitive behavioural approaches for patients with chronic whiplash is required. Two of the three studies outlined utilised a physiotherapist to deliver exercises in a manner consistent with cognitive behavioural principles, and only one study investigated CBT delivered separately by a psychologist. To date, the evidence suggests that the effect of CBT in reducing disability due to whiplash may be minimal. However, its role in managing other aspects of psychological health is discussed further in Chapter 13.

EVIDENCE FOR MEDICAL INTERVENTIONS

Radiofrequency neurotomy

One high-quality trial found a positive effect for radiofrequency neurotomy as a medical intervention compared with a control procedure.[20] In this trial, patients were included if they had previously responded to a median branch nerve block to the facet joint, thus implicating these joints as the source of neck pain in these patients. The radiofrequency neurotomy procedure was described as inserting an electrode under fluoroscopic control to the median branch of the cervical dorsal ramus of the nerve supplying the painful joint. The temperature was raised to 80°C for the neurotomy procedure, and remained at 37°C for the control procedure.

Radiofrequency neurotomy produced a large effect in terms of reduction of long-term pain (mean difference of 255 days [CI, 11.6–498.4 days] until return of 50% pain) in comparison with the control procedure. However, the authors did not comment on any other outcomes, such as pain intensity, disability or psychological outcomes despite these measures being taken at baseline.

The large effect demonstrated by radiofrequency neurotomy may need to be considered together with the costs and accessibility of this form of treatment. First, the procedure was effective with highly selected subjects (i.e. only those whose symptoms had been demonstrated, by diagnostic blocks, to arise from the lower cervical joints). Second, the trial was performed in a specialised research setting; therefore, the results may not be generalisable. The Neck Pain Task Force has also criticised this trial, commenting that responses to facet blocks were non-validated and not required to be in a pharmacological range.[21] Furthermore, no other outcomes were reported, and others that were are not statistically significant. For example, at three weeks after surgery, nine subjects in the radiofrequency group compared with six subjects in the control group reported greater than 50% pain relief.[22] Side-effects to the radiofrequency neurotomy have included long-term anaesthetic or dysaesthetic areas of skin.[22] Therefore, while radiofrequency neurotomy is recommended in the treatment of patients with chronic whiplash and confirmed facet joint involvement, caution must be applied.

Subcutaneous sterile water injections

One trial demonstrated an effect for subcutaneous sterile water injections compared with saline injections.[23] The injections were applied into tender or trigger points in the neck and shoulder. The authors explained that initially there is local pain, and that some patients are unable to tolerate this.

The effects demonstrated were small for pain effects but larger for improvement in range of motion (ROM). The mean difference between patients receiving the intervention and the control group in worst pain was –1.7/10 (CI, –3 to –0.4) at three months, and –2.3/10 (CI, –3.7 to –0.9) at eight months. The improvement in the summation of cervical ROM was also significantly different between the groups at three months (mean difference, 33 degrees [CI, 7–59]) and eight months (mean difference, 31 degrees [CI, 2.4–59.6]). Cervical ROM was measured by a Myrin goniometer. The primary authors of this trial commented that patients who are most likely to respond are those with localised musculoskeletal pain, ROM impairment and no psychological distress.

Intra-articular steroid injections

One trial investigated the use of intra-articular (zygapophyseal [Z-] joint) injections, demonstrating no benefit over local anaesthetic injections in terms of time to return of usual pain (mean difference, –0.05 days [CI,–2.8 to 1.8]).[24]

The primary authors of this trial have concluded that, on the basis of their trial, treatment of chronic whiplash with corticosteroid injections should not be recommended. Patients were carefully selected for the intervention, and only when the Z-joint was confirmed as the source of the pain. Second, the injections were administered by experienced physicians. There was no explanation by the primary authors as to what pain mechanisms may account for the lack of response. A similar lack of evidence for the use of intra-articular steroids for the management of the wider neck pain group were reported by the Task Force on Neck Pain recently.[22] Given both the Task Force finding, Barnsley et al.'s[24] conclusion and the risks associated with corticosteroid injections (e.g. exposure to radiation and infection), there is little justification for this therapy at present.

Analgesic infusions

Intravenous infusion of analgesia provided no benefit over placebo in a high-quality trial.[25] Patients were randomised to receive an intravenous infusion over 30 minutes of either morphine, lignocaine, ketamine or placebo. Lemming et al.[25] demonstrated that three different analgesics produced significant reductions in pain compared with a placebo while infusion of drugs was taking place (e.g. mean difference in morphine versus placebo, 13.0 points/100; CI, 4.4–21.6). However, no lasting effect (measured for five days post intervention) was demonstrated in the effectiveness of any drug over placebo.

Despite the lack of long-term results in this trial, the primary authors provided comment that the responders to various drugs in the short term may provide some direction for managing pain in chronic whiplash, particularly when central hyperexcitability is present. For example, there were 14 short-term responders to ketamine in the trial. Ketamine is a drug that is understood to work on the *N*-methyl-D-aspartic acid (NDMA) receptor and, therefore, responders to this drug may have a state of central hyperexcitability. Similarly, a Cochrane review of injections for mechanical neck pain reported a small effect in reducing neck pain with the use of lidocaine (lignocaine) compared with placebo in the short term.[26] Therefore, while, at present, infusion of analgesia is not recommended by current clinical guidelines for chronic whiplash,[4] there is some promise of effect for those with central hyperexcitability, and this requires further investigation.

Botulinum toxin

Two high-quality trials investigated the use of botulinum toxin injections compared with placebo, with conflicting results. In both trials, botulinum toxin injections were delivered into painful sites upon palpation (e.g. splenius capitis, trapezius).

The first trial demonstrated improvement in pain at four weeks in the botulinum toxin injection group compared with placebo (mean difference in pain at four weeks, –4.1/30 [CI, –8.9 to 0.7]).[27] However, there was no difference between groups for neck disability. Conversely, Padberg et al.[28] found no significant improvement in pain in their botulinum toxin injection group compared with placebo (mean difference in pain at 12 weeks, –4.7/100 [CI, –28.2 to 13.5]). One explanation for the differences in effect may be explained by the timing of when outcomes were measured, with Freund et al.[27] measuring outcomes at four weeks and Padberg et al.[28] at 12 weeks.

IMPLEMENTATION OF EVIDENCE IN CLINICAL PRACTICE

With a range of interventions offering positive outcomes for whiplash, clinicians could be best directed by choosing interventions based on the examination findings and the outcome desired by the patient. A thorough assessment of the whiplash patient is, therefore, necessary in order to determine the impairments present and outcomes desired, so that the intervention can be chosen accordingly. Further considerations need to be given to the cost, accessibility and risks associated with the interventions. It is most likely that clinicians will use a combination of interventions when managing patients with whiplash.

In order to provide some direction for clinicians, we have looked at the evidence in relation to the assessment findings and suggest interventions based on proposed desired outcomes. These outcomes have been broadly classified into managing pain, impairment, disability and psychological outcomes. A case vignette is provided in order to illustrate this.

CASE VIGNETTE: MARY

Mary is a 60-year-old woman who sustained an MVC 12 months ago. She complains of ongoing headaches (visual analogue pain scale [VAS], 8/10), neck pain (VAS, 7/10) and dizziness. Key findings in the physical examination include loss of cervical ROM (particularly extension and flexion), poor cervical motor control and poor cervical kinaesthetic sense. Treatment, to date, has included pain management (analgesia and anti-inflammatory drugs) and manual therapy (physiotherapy and chiropractic). Manual therapy improves symptoms for a few days, but then they return. Mary is increasingly distressed regarding her pain and is participating in life less and less. Where previously she was able to work at the desk full time, Mary is now only working at 50% of her pre-injury capacity. She has stopped her previous exercise (yoga and Pilates) as it aggravates her symptoms and she is worried she is damaging something if she continues. Her Neck Disability Index (NDI) score is 32/50, and her Tampa Scale of Kinesiophobia (TSK) score is 56.

Managing pain

Pain, and in particular neck pain and headache, are among the most common symptoms that persist into the chronic phase of whiplash.[29–32] High initial levels of pain intensity are associated with poor outcomes.[8, 33, 34] Managing pain adequately, therefore, is usually a major consideration for the patient with chronic whiplash.

The baseline management of pain recommended in acute whiplash is simple analgesia followed by non-steroidal anti-inflammatory drugs (NSAIDs).[8, 9, 35–40] These recommendations are based on expert consensus due to the limited number of trials of medication for acute whiplash associated disorders (WAD). Logically, clinicians should consider the role that these medications can continue to play in the chronic phase. Indeed, all of the trials investigating chronic whiplash stated that patients were able to continue taking pain-relieving medication. Simple analgesics should remain, therefore, as the first or baseline management of pain in chronic whiplash.

The question remains whether additional treatments have additive pain-relieving benefits, and the evidence in chronic whiplash can inform the clinician here. There is evidence to show that the interventions of active exercise, sterile water injections and radiofrequency neurotomy were all effective in reducing pain in patients with chronic whiplash. Pragmatically, clinicians should consider the risk, costs and benefits in applying these interventions. Given that active exercise is the least invasive and most accessible intervention, it is reasonable to offer this as the next line of pain management.

In our case study, Mary has ongoing pain and has been offered manual therapy in the acute phase of her condition, with some effect, but the pain has persisted into the chronic phase. She has not yet been prescribed an exercise approach, so offering her an exercise-based approach would be reasonable. It has been demonstrated that following a 10-week neck-specific exercise approach, patients reported a reduction in levels of pain and disability that were just clinically relevant—10.4% on the Northwick Park Neck Pain Index.[10] Similarly, the more general exercise approach can also reduce pain by a similar effect (e.g. mean reduction was 2 points on a 10 point scale over six weeks). This interpretation of the evidence may direct the clinician to offering patients an exercise-based approach in order to further manage chronic pain after whiplash.

More invasive methods have shown a capacity to reduce pain; however, the effect needs to be considered against the risk. Sterile water injections, for example, reduced pain by a similar magnitude to general exercise (namely, 1.7–2.3/10). However, given the greater risks (including infection and increase in pain) associated with sterile water injections, this risk may not be worth the benefit (i.e. no greater benefit than general exercise). A similar consideration applies to radiofrequency neurotomy. The greatest effect in reducing pain of all the interventions was found to be provided by radiofrequency neurotomy.[20] However, given the risks (previously discussed) and the indications (only indicated for those patients who responded to median branch blocks), this may be an intervention only offered as a last resort. The authors of this trial agree, and suggest that radiofrequency neurotomy should only be offered to those who have failed to respond to conservative management.[20]

Clearly, there is room for improving pain management in individuals with chronic whiplash, and, therefore, alternative approaches may need to be considered. Interventions worth consideration may be opioids and corticosteroids. Epidural corticosteroids have shown significant effects in reducing chronic neck pain associated with radiculopathy;[22, 26] however, such an approach has not yet been studied in a similar subgroup (WAD grade III[41]) of patients with whiplash. It was noted that non-responders to active exercise were those with both mechanical and cold hyperalgesia,[10] which may be indicative of augmented central pain-processing mechanisms. Lemming et al.[25] suggest that patients with augmented central pain-processing mechanisms do respond (albeit only in the short term) to intravenous opioid analgesic infusion. This, therefore, may suggest that patients with a central hyperexcitability component to their pain may need more aggressive pain management in order to improve outcomes. More complex pain management is outlined in Chapter 5.

Reducing disability and improving impairment

In general, impairments present in patients with chronic whiplash appear to improve when the intervention directly addresses that particular impairment. In Mary's example, her assessment revealed impairments in cervical motor control and postural control. Mary's impairment in cervical motor control, such as craniocervical flexion control, is likely to improve when specifically targeted, compared to when she just exercises unsupervised.[10] Similarly, her inability to maintain single leg balance is likely to improve with specific exercises targeting this impairment, compared to a more general exercise approach.[14] Of note is that disability also reduced in patients in both of these trials that addressed the specific impairments.[10, 14] While it remains unclear as to whether the impairment changes can account for the concurrent changes in disability, clinicians can be confident that by applying treatment targeting specific impairments, concurrent reduction in disability is likely to be obtained.

Changing Mary's cervical ROM is an interesting debate, when the evidence is considered. Reduction in cervical ROM in the acute phase of whiplash is associated with long-term disability.[4] This would suggest that improving cervical ROM may also improve disability, and many clinicians target improvement of cervical ROM in their treatment plans. ROM exercises are considered part of the first-line management of patients with acute whiplash,[4] and these exercises are often continued into the chronic phase. In both the active exercise trials, patients were permitted to continue with cervical ROM exercises.[10, 11] Therefore, it would seem reasonable that cervical ROM exercises should continue if restricted ROM is still present in patients with chronic whiplash.

The evidence, however, in this case would suggest that sterile water injections provided the greatest effect in improving cervical ROM,[23] in comparison to the other interventions, such as specific exercise and botulinum toxin injections.[12, 28] However, clinicians should interpret these findings with caution. First, it is likely that a similar effect was found with specific exercise. The authors of the specific exercise approach reported improvements in cervical ROM in both of their groups of a similar magnitude to that reported by the author who used subcutaneous sterile water injections (i.e. approximately 31 degrees versus approximately 33 degrees). Second, the authors of the sterile water injection trial measured ROM with a Myrin goniometer, rather than more reliable instruments, such as the cervical range of motion device (CROM) and electromagnetic measurement of ROM (Fastrack system), which were used in the studies that failed to find a change. Lastly, Byrn et al.[23] did not measure disability in their trial; hence, the improved range of cervical ROM with the intervention of sterile water injections cannot be interpreted as also providing outcomes of reduced disability for their patients. Pragmatically, therefore, clinicians may prefer to offer their patients a specific exercise approach or at least continue ROM exercises in order to address this impairment.

In order to provide Mary with confidence that her self-reported disability may improve, clinicians can be directed by the evidence. Disability was significantly reduced with the interventions of active exercise and coordination exercises. Active exercise had a small effect on reducing disability related to neck pain, as measured by self-reported disability questionnaires.[11, 12] Coordination exercises reduced dizziness-related disability[14] and self-reported neck disability,[15] respectively. The later trial by Fitz-Ritson[15] reported a large effect (mean difference, approximately 24%)

in the reduction of disability, which is significantly greater than that in the other three trials (reporting mean differences of between 6% and 8%). While this may suggest that the intervention in Fitz-Ritson's trial is more beneficial, the methodological flaws in this trial (previously discussed) may mean that the actual effect is somewhat less than reported. In contrast, when the intervention in trials did not directly target disability (e.g. with Padberg et al.'s trial on botulinum toxin[28]), no effects for disability were reported.

Clinicians can be encouraged by the above findings and choose one of the forms of exercise (i.e. either active or coordination) and be confident that some reduction in disability will be obtained. While there is no clear recommendation on which form of exercise to choose, the authors of the trials provide some direction. For example, coordination exercises improved disability in whiplash patients with dizziness. In addition, Stewart et al.[11] noted that responders to general exercise were those with higher levels of baseline disability (i.e. those who usually have the poorest prognosis[7, 33, 34]). This suggests that by selecting such patients, treatment effects may improve. In Mary's case, she demonstrated both high levels of disability (e.g. NDI, 32/50) and dizziness, and, hence, would be well suited to either approach.

In practical terms, it is most likely that clinicians should progress from a more specific exercise approach to a general approach. Progression from a specific to a general approach hypothetically should have an additive effect on reducing disability levels. This combination approach is being proposed by the primary authors of the original trials.[42]

Changing beliefs

The evidence provides the clinician with some direction in managing patients' beliefs about their condition. CBT, an intervention that directly targets patients' beliefs about their condition, has demonstrated positive effects on those beliefs.[18] However, to date, CBT has not demonstrated significant effects in reducing pain and disability. It would appear, therefore, that clinicians should use the principles of CBT when changing belief systems are considered integral to a successful outcome. The psychological management of whiplash is discussed further in Chapter 13.

SUMMARY

In summary, the evidence base for the management of chronic whiplash is growing, and is able to provide the clinician with some options to assist managing their patients. Exercise programs addressing specific impairments and progressing to addressing more general functional goals appear to have evidence in reducing pain and disability. These should be offered as first-line management. CBT appears to be important in addressing beliefs systems, particularly if they are dominant in the patient's pain presentation.

More invasive options with a higher associated risk are emerging as further options to manage pain, including sterile water injections and radiofrequency neurotomy. These should be offered if the less-invasive options are ineffective and the patient is identified as appropriate for such interventions (e.g. an identified painful facet joint is a prerequisite for success with radiofrequency neurotomy).

However, as outlined above, by applying the available evidence to manage a patient like Mary, the approach is conservative and Mary is unlikely to fully recover with this approach. The major issue is that the effects for the reduction in pain, disability and impairment are minimal to moderate in most studies, leaving room for improvement.

The question arises, therefore, what is likely to provide a larger effect for a patient like Mary? The primary authors of the studies have provided some direction. There is increasing consensus among authors that those who are not responding to current treatment approaches are those with higher levels of pain with elements of central hyperexcitability. Such a presentation is often accompanied by considerable psychological distress. Accordingly, researchers are investigating more complex interventions encompassing multiprofessional approaches involving all aspects of care.

Finally, the efficacy of all treatments over a longer term follow-up needs to be investigated. Only one trial investigated the effects of treatment in the long term (i.e. >12 months).[12] In this trial, no effect for the intervention was demonstrated at 12 months. Clearly, future trials need to examine the effect of their therapies over the long term, in order for cost-effective decisions to be made.

ACKNOWLEDGMENTS

The author would like to acknowledge the primary authors of the recent systematic review and clinical guidelines from which the recommendations for the treatment of chronic whiplash in this chapter were made. These include Dr Mark Stewart, Professor Ian Cameron and Dr Jim Stewart.

References

1. Scholten-Peeters GG, Bekkering GE, Verhagen AP, et al. Clinical practice guideline for the physiotherapy of patients with whiplash-associated disorders. *Spine* 2002;27(4):412–22.

2. Moore A, Jackson A, Jordan J, et al. Clinical guidelines for the physiotherapy management of whiplash associated disorder. London: Chartered Society of Physiotherapy, 2005.
3. Hurwitz EL, Carragee EJ, van der Velde G, et al. Treatment of neck pain: noninvasive interventions: results of the Bone and Joint Decade 2000–2010 Task Force on Neck Pain and Its Associated Disorders. *Spine* 2008;33(4 Suppl):S123–S152.
4. TRACsa. Clinical guidelines for best practice management of acute and chronic whiplash-associated disorders. Canberra: National Health and Medical Research Council of Australia, 2008.
5. The AGREE Collaboration. Appraisal of Guidelines for Research and Evaluation (AGREE) Instrument. London: St George's Hospital Medical School, 2001. Available at:www.agreecollaboration.org.
6. PEDro: Physiotherapy Evidence Database. PEDro scale: how are trials rated? Available at: http://www.pedro.org.au/english/faq/#question_five.
7. Scholten-Peeters GGM, Verhagen AP, Bekkering GE, et al. Prognostic factors of whiplash-associated disorders: a systematic review of prospective cohort studies. *Pain* 2003;104(1–2):303–22.
8. Barnsley L & Barnsley L. An evidence-based approach to the treatment of acute whiplash injury. *Pain Res Manage* 2003;8(1):33–6.
9. Conlin A, Bhogal S, Sequeira K, Teasell R. Treatment of whiplash associated disorders – part 1: non invasive interventions. *Pain Res Manage* 2005;10(1):21–32.
10. Jull G, Sterling M, Kenardy J, et al. Does the presence of sensory hypersensitivity influence outcomes of physical rehabilitation for chronic whiplash? A preliminary RCT. *Pain* 2007;129(1–2):28–34.
11. Stewart M, Maher C, Refshauge K, et al. Randomised controlled trial of exercise for chronic whiplash associated disorders. *Pain* 2007;128:59–68.
12. Jull G, Sterling M, Falla D, et al. Whiplash, headache and neck pain. Research based directions for physical therapists. Edinburgh: Elsevier, 2008.
13. Nicholas M & Tonkin L. Persisting pain: using cognitive behavioural therapy principles for activity-based pain management. In: Refshauge K, Gass E, eds. Musculoskeletal physiotherapy Clinical science and evidence-based practice. Oxford: Butterworth Heinemann, 2005.
14. Ekvall Hansson E, Mansson NO, Ringsberg KA, et al. Dizziness among patients with whiplash-associated disorder: a randomized controlled trial. *J Rehabil Med* 2006;38(6):387–90.
15. Fitz-Ritson D. Phasic exercises for cervical rehabilitation after "whiplash" trauma. *J Manipulative Physiol Ther* 1995;18(1):21–4.
16. Janda V. Muscles, central nervous motor regulation and back problems. In: Korr IM, ed. Neurobiologic mechanism in manipulative therapy. New York: Plenum Press, 1977.
17. Klobas L, Axelsson S, Tegelberg A, et al. Effect of therapeutic jaw exercise on temporomandibular disorders in individuals with chronic whiplash-associated disorders. *Acta Odontol Scand* 2006;64(6):341–7.
18. Soderlund A & Lindberg P. Cognitive behavioural components in physiotherapy management of chronic whiplash associated disorders (WAD) – a randomized group study. *Physiother Theory Pract* 2001;17(4): 229–38.
19. Wicksell R, Ahlqvist J, Bring A, et al. Can exposure and acceptance strategies improve functioning and life satisfaction in people with chronic pain and whiplash-associated disorders (WAD)? A randomized controlled trial. *Cogn Behav Ther* 2008;37(3):169–82.
20. Lord SM, Barnsley L, Wallis BJ, et al. Percutaneous radio-frequency neurotomy for chronic cervical zygapophyseal-joint pain. *N Engl J Med* 1996;335(23):1721–6.
21. Nordin M, Carragee EJ, Hogg-Johnson S, et al. Assessment of neck pain and its associated disorders: results of the Bone and Joint Decade 2000–2010 Task Force on Neck Pain and Its Associated Disorders. *Spine* 2008;33(4 Suppl):S101–S122.
22. Carragee EJ, Hurwitz EL, Cheng I, et al. Treatment of neck pain: injections and surgical interventions: results of the Bone and Joint Decade 2000–2010 Task Force on Neck Pain and Its Associated Disorders. *Spine* 2008;33(4 Suppl):S153–S169.
23. Byrn C, Olsson I, Falkheden L, et al. Subcutaneous sterile water injections for chronic neck and shoulder pain following whiplash injuries. *Lancet* 1993;341(8843):449–52.
24. Barnsley L, Lord SM, Wallis BJ, et al. Lack of effect of intraarticular corticosteroids for chronic pain in the cervical zygapophyseal joints. *N Engl J Med* 1994;330(15):1047–50.
25. Lemming D, Sorensen J, Graven-Nielsen T, et al. The responses to pharmacological challenges and experimental pain in patients with chronic whiplash-associated pain. *Clin J Pain* 2005;21(5): 412–21.
26. Peloso PMJ, Gross A, Haines T, et al. Medicinal and injection therapies for mechanical neck disorders. *Cochrane Database Syst Rev* 2007;(3):CD000319.
27. Freund BJ & Schwartz M. Use of botulinum toxin in chronic whiplash-associated disorder. *Clin J Pain* 2002;18(6 Suppl):S163–S168.

28. Padberg M, de Bruijn SF, Tavy DL, et al. Neck pain in chronic whiplash syndrome treated with botulinum toxin. A double-blind, placebo-controlled clinical trial. *J Neurology* 2007;254(3):290–5.
29. Barnsley L, Lord SM, Bogduk N. Whiplash injury. *Pain* 1994;58:283–307.
30. Sturzenegger M, Di Stefano G, Radanov B, Schnidrig A. Presenting symptoms and signs after whiplash injury: the influence of accident mechanisms. *Neurology* 1994;44:688–93.
31. Malik H & Lovell M. Soft tissue neck symptoms following high energy road traffic accidents. *Spine* 2004;29:E315–E317.
32. Rodriquez A, Barr K, Burns S. Whiplash: pathophysiology, diagnosis, treatment, and prognosis. *Muscle Nerve* 2004;29:768–81.
33. Côté P, Cassidy JD, Carroll L, et al. A systematic review of the prognosis of acute whiplash and a new conceptual framework to synthesize the literature. *Spine* 2001;26(19):E445–E458.
34. Kamper SJ, Rebbeck TJ, Maher CG, et al. Course and prognostic factors of whiplash: a systematic review and meta-analysis. *Pain* 2008;138(3):617–29.
35. Conlin A, Bhogal S, Sequeira K, Teasell R. Treatment of whiplash associated disorders—Part 2: Medical and surgical interventions. *Pain Res Manage* 2005;10(1):33–40.
36. Lundmark H & Persson AL. Physiotherapy and management in early whiplash-associated disorders (WAD) – a review. *Adv Physiother* 2006;8(3):98–105.
37. Magee D, Oborn-Barrett E, Turner S, Fenning N. A systematic overview of the effectiveness of physical therapy intervention on soft tissue neck injury following trauma. *Physiother Canada* 2000;52: 111–30.
38. McClune T, Burton AK, Waddell G, et al. Whiplash associated disorders: a review of the literature to guide patient information and advice. *Emerg Med J* 2002;19(6):499–506.
39. Seferiadis A, Rosenfeld M, Gunnarsson R, et al. A review of treatment interventions in whiplash-associated disorders. *Eur Spine J* 2004;13(5):387–97.
40. Verhagen AP, Scholten-Peeters GGM, van Wijngaarden S, et al. Conservative treatments for whiplash. *Cochrane Database Syst Rev* 2007;(2):CD003338.
41. Spitzer W, Skovron M, Salmi L, et al. Scientific monograph of Quebec task force on whiplash associated disorders: redefining 'whiplash' and its management. *Spine* 1995;20(8 Suppl):S1–S73.
42. Michaleff Z, Sterling M, Jull G, et al. A randomised controlled trial of a comprehensive exercise programme for chronic whiplash. *BMC Musculoskelet Disord* 2009;10:149.

CHAPTER 13
Psychological management of chronic whiplash associated disorders

Jan Jaspers, Jan Buitenhuis, Gerbrig Versteegen, Peter de Jong

This chapter discusses the theoretical starting points and current evidence base for psychological approaches to the management of chronic whiplash associated disorders (WAD). Management of acute and subacute whiplash has been discussed in Chapter 11. The clinical presentation of chronic WAD has been described in Chapter 2. Chronic WAD is a serious problem. The results of a recent systematic review and meta-analysis indicate rapid improvement in pain and disability in the first three months but, beyond this, there is little, if any, improvement.[1] Although recovery rates across the 38 cohorts that were included in this meta-analysis were highly variable, in most studies 15–20% of people develop chronic complaints.[2] But the numbers vary up to 42%, which is probably due to variations in the measurement of recovery and sample characteristics.[3]

First, this chapter describes the dominant theory-derived interventions of chronic whiplash. Special attention is paid to two theoretical models: the fear-avoidance (FA) model and the post-traumatic stress disorder (PTSD) model. Overlap with Chapter 8 will be as limited as possible.

Second, the evidence for these interventions is evaluated by reviewing the available treatment outcome studies. The number of randomised controlled trials (RCTs) is very limited and most studies assessed the efficacy of multimodal rather than focused treatments. This approach renders it difficult to evaluate the relative efficacy of the various components that are part of these treatments (e.g. graded activity and exercise therapy). It is also difficult to differentiate the relative contribution of physiotherapy and cognitive behavioural interventions. So, some overlap with Chapter 12 will be inevitable.

The chapter ends with a discussion of the general guidelines that can be derived from the limited empirical database and the limitations of evidence-based treatment for chronic WAD.

THEORY-DERIVED PSYCHOLOGICAL INTERVENTIONS

Fear-avoidance interventions

In clinical practice, the chronic whiplash syndrome is often considered a specific form of a chronic pain syndrome, not essentially different from chronic low back pain or functional syndromes. One of the most influential models in the context of chronic low back pain is the so-called fear-avoidance (FA) model. The FA model promises to aid understanding about how acute whiplash may develop into chronic complaints.[4, 5] In Chapter 8, the FA model was reformulated to better understand chronic WAD. In this causal beliefs–anxiety (CBA) model, the role of culturally embedded (dysfunctional) causal attributions of whiplash symptoms is more prominent than in the FA model (see Fig 8.1 in Chapter 8).

The review of psychological determinants in Chapter 8 suggests that, in comparison with chronic low back pain, attributional bias and pain catastrophising may be more influential than kinesiophobia in the development and maintenance of chronic WAD. This is an important conclusion with clinical implications. The CBA model implies that realistic attributions of neck pain will result in uncomplicated recovery. The results of a recent study support this assumption: early expectations for recovery of WAD (a few weeks after the accident) were an important prognostic factor for recovery; those who expected to get better soon recovered over three times as quickly as those who expected that they would never get better.[6]

Most importantly for the present context, the CBA model provides a helpful starting point for specific cognitive and behavioural interventions, known as cognitive behavioural therapy (CBT). Importantly, CBT does not refer to a unitary treatment but rather includes a wide range of different interventions. *Cognitive restructuring* is of primary importance in order to change attributional bias and pain catastrophising.

Pain catastrophising refers to an exaggerated negative orientation towards actual or anticipated pain. The habitual tendency to make catastrophic interpretations of pain is associated with a heightened pain experience and heightened disability, independent of the level of actual physical impairment.[7] Causal attributions or illness beliefs can be defined as the patient's ideas about the origin or cause of the symptoms or illness experienced. The causal beliefs of the patient are very relevant in relation to the persistence of complaints when an organic cause has not been verified, as in chronic WAD. These illness perceptions or cognitive representations directly influence behaviour parameters and the emotional response.[8]

Dysfunctional causal beliefs in WAD can be defined as the attribution of the cause of acute neck complaints to severe, neural or irreparable causes. At the chronic stage of WAD, somatic or organic beliefs, in general, can be considered dysfunctional. The tendency to attribute neck complaints to irreparable or severe causes may elicit catastrophic interpretations of potentially benign muscular symptoms.

The first step in the CBT intervention, *cognitive restructuring*, involves identifying the dysfunctional causal attributions by assessing in which situations these attributions occur, assessing the concrete contents of the attribution (e.g. 'This pain means something must be broken in my neck') and establishing the emotions that arise from the attribution. Registration of these situations, cognitions and emotions in daily life is often the first homework assignment in CBT for the patient with chronic WAD. In the second step, the dysfunctional beliefs are evaluated and defined by asking questions like: 'What evidence is there for this attribution?' and 'Does this attribution help you to feel better?'. The third step is to formulate a more realistic and/or helpful attribution and evaluate the effect of this reformulation on the emotional state.

This cognitive approach is often followed by so-called behavioural experiments, aimed at testing the dysfunctional attribution. Catastrophic predictions of what would happen if the patient should perform some avoided movement or behaviour can be refuted in this way. This exposure in vivo to the threatening behaviour is often more convincing than cognitive restructuring alone.

Patients with chronic WAD often show a wide range of avoidance behaviour, especially concerning movements of the head and neck (as a result of kinesiophobia, see Fig 8.1), but also concerning all kinds of physical and social activities. As with other functional syndromes, the pain and other complaints have become a central focus in life and have consequences for many aspects of functioning. CBT for functional syndromes not only focuses on causal attributions for symptoms, but also on these consequences for normal functioning.[9] These consequences may vary from affective and cognitive consequences (e.g. depression, problems with attention and concentration), behavioural consequences (e.g. avoidance behaviour), physical consequences (e.g. increased muscle tension, loss of physical condition) to social and professional consequences (e.g. social isolation, loss of job).

The primary goal of CBT for functional syndromes mostly is not to reduce pain or other symptoms, but to reduce or redress these invalidating consequences. That is why interventions like *graded activity* and *physical exercises* fit well in a cognitive behavioural approach for patients with chronic WAD.

Formulating concrete treatment goals in dialogue with the patient is an essential element before starting CBT. After thoroughly drawing up an inventory of the specific consequences of chronic WAD for the patient, the therapist and patient can decide which consequences will be tackled and what will be the concrete goals (e.g. full return to work or resume earlier sporting activities).

Psycho-education or *patient education* is an often-applied intervention in patients with acute WAD, although the effectiveness of this intervention is unclear.[10] Psycho-education is an important intervention for patients with chronic WAD. It can be the first step in altering dysfunctional attributions and it provides a rationale for CBT. An individualised version of the CBA model can be explained and discussed, resulting in a better understanding of the course and maintenance of chronic WAD for the patient.

Within the context of CBT, recently developed approaches, such as *acceptance and commitment therapy* and *mindfulness-based interventions,* have been successfully applied to chronic pain. The relative efficacy of these types of interventions in the treatment of chronic WAD have recently been evaluated,[11] and will be discussed in the next section.

A case description is given on page 137 to illustrate the CBA model.

Post-traumatic stress disorder interventions

Another promising model that seeks to explain the psychological effects of traffic accidents is the PTSD model. The essential feature of PTSD is the development of characteristic symptoms following exposure

CASE A

John was involved in a rear-end motor vehicle crash (MVC) about a year ago. His car was only two months old and was written off. He experienced no significant injuries, only neck pain. His general practitioner advised him to take a few days rest and to be careful moving his head and neck.

When pain persisted, John wondered whether there was some damage to the spine. He returned to his office job quickly but avoided sudden movements of the neck and kept his head in the same position as much as possible: moving increased the pain. In the course of time he worried about if the pain would last, if he could not do his work properly and in the end he would lose his job. Because of the pain he did not sleep well, could not concentrate on his job and made mistakes he never made before. He stopped playing soccer and missed contact with his sporting friends. He noticed that he was irritated quickly and his mood was low. One year after the accident John consulted a Pain Clinic.

to an extreme traumatic stressor involving direct personal experience of an event that involves actual or threatened death or serious injury, or other threat to one's physical integrity; or witnessing an event that involves death, injury or a threat to the physical integrity of another person; or learning about unexpected or violent death, serious harm, or threat of death or injury experienced by a family member or other close associate. PTSD is an anxiety disorder which consists of three symptom clusters: re-experiencing, avoidance and hyperarousal symptoms. Symptoms of re-experiencing are, for example, sudden unexpected memories of the car accident or dreaming about the accident. Avoidance of the place of the car accident may occur as well as avoiding talking about the incident. Hyperarousal symptoms include intensified jumpiness or being hyperalert, especially when driving a car.

Research has provided evidence to indicate that post-traumatic stress symptoms are related to WAD. Hyperarousal symptoms, especially, have been shown to be involved in patients with chronic WAD.[12] However, there is evidence that the other symptom clusters may be involved as well.[13] The co-occurrence of anxiety disorders (especially PTSD) and chronic pain syndromes (especially WAD) has recently been the subject of some debate. Some theorists propose that there might be a reciprocal relationship, with PTSD and WAD influencing one another in a mutual maintaining way.[14] This mutual maintenance model holds that physiological, affective and behavioural components of PTSD maintain or exacerbate symptoms of pain and, similarly, that cognitive, affective and behavioural components of chronic pain maintain or exacerbate symptoms of PTSD. A recent empirical examination of the model in a longitudinal study of injured accident victims yielded support for a mutual maintenance of pain intensity and PTSD symptoms in the first half year after the accident.[15] Across the second half year, PTSD symptoms impacted significantly on pain but not vice versa. So, over time no reciprocal relationship was found. The mutual maintenance model has been extended, suggesting that some maintenance factors denote a shared vulnerability for developing both conditions.[16] This shared vulnerability model stresses three predisposing factors in the development of both disorders: psychological vulnerability (e.g. high anxiety sensitivity), confrontation with traumatic life events (e.g. a traffic accident), and a lowered physiological threshold for alarm reactions (e.g. sympathetic dysregulation, hyperalgesia). So, co-occurring PTSD and chronic WAD are most likely to develop in cases where vulnerable people are exposed to a car accident that is both traumatic and painful, wherein reminders of the trauma and sensations of pain can serve as triggers for further alarm reactions.

The potential role of the stress response system in understanding the aforementioned alarm reactions is stressed in the theoretical model of McLean et al.,[17] who reformulated the FA model, incorporating the hypothesised role of the stress response system in the development of aberrant pain and/or emotional processing after an MVC. Recent research on the relationship between sensory and sympathetic nervous system changes and post-traumatic stress reaction following WAD showed that this relationship was mediated by pain and disability levels.[18] Therefore, interpretation of this relation is difficult and warrants further investigation.

There are several clinical implications of the co-occurrence of chronic WAD and PTSD. Primarily, PTSD and subclinical post-traumatic stress symptoms warrant clinical attention. Patients with chronic WAD do not always report post-traumatic stress symptoms spontaneously, so active exploration of these symptoms should occur.

Several evidence-based interventions are available for the treatment of PTSD. Trauma-focused CBT and eye movement desensitisation and reprocessing (EMDR) are highly effective treatments for PTSD.[19,20] *Imaginal exposure* is the most applied trauma-focused CBT intervention for PTSD. The patient is systematically and repeatedly confronted with the anxiety-provoking memories of the traumatic events by telling the therapist in a structured way about the traumatic events. At first, exposure to these memories can evoke anxiety and other negative emotions, but after repeated confrontation the emotional reactions decrease. Repeated exposure to the trauma memory can also be accomplished by letting the patient write a narrative of the traumatic events. So, *structured writing about the trauma* is another trauma-focused CBT intervention that may prove useful. In general, these interventions have a positive effect on all three clusters of symptoms of PTSD.[21, 22] In some cases, however, avoidance behaviour, especially avoidance of driving a car, can persist.[23] Then, *exposure in vivo* is a necessary additional intervention to free the patient of this fear to participate in driving.

EMDR is another highly effective intervention for PTSD, specifically when exposure is included in the treatment protocol.[24] EMDR utilises dual attention tasks to help the patient process the traumatic event and involves focusing on negative trauma-related memories, emotions and thoughts while engaging in a task involving some form of bilateral stimulation, such as eye movements, hand tapping or tunes, until distress has reduced and belief in more positive trauma-related thoughts has increased.[20]

A CBT intervention that is less frequently applied to PTSD and/or chronic pain is *interoceptive exposure* (i.e. exposure to anxiety-provoking bodily sensations). This intervention is highly effective for panic disorder, as it helps to modify the catastrophic idea that particular bodily sensations are predictive of a heart attack. Recently, interoceptive exposure has been added to trauma-focused interventions to reduce both PTSD symptoms and fear of pain.[25] In this study, interoceptive exposure preceded trauma-focused interventions. The rationale was that interoceptive exposure would decrease anxiety sensitivity (one of the predisposing factors in the shared vulnerability model), a determinant of both PTSD and chronic pain. Interoceptive exposure is the first intervention aimed at reducing both PTSD and chronic pain by focusing on a shared predisposing factor. Exposure in vivo has been applied to both PTSD and chronic WAD too, but for the reduction of different kinds of avoidance behaviour. Avoidance behaviour in PTSD mostly concerns driving a car or avoiding (other) situations that evoke traumatic memories. Avoidance behaviour in chronic WAD mostly concerns situations that evoke neck pain.

A case description is given below to illustrate the PTSD model.

CASE B

Maria was involved in a rear-end MVC two years ago. She was waiting for traffic lights to change, with cars in front of her and cars on the left and the right of her. Suddenly she saw, in the rear-vision and side mirrors of her car, a huge truck approaching quickly. She could only think: 'This truck will crash my car and I will be dead'. She believes she will never forget the clash when the truck hit her car. In the first months after the accident the image of the truck reappeared in dreams about the accident and in flashbacks during daytime. For more than a year she avoided the place of the accident, driving many miles extra to reach her workplace. After two years loud noises still startle her and bring back memories from the accident. When driving her car she is hyperalert: she drives very carefully, constantly looking for potential danger; when she spots a truck behind her, tension rises and she tries to lose it at full speed.

EVIDENCE-BASED PRACTICE

This section provides an overview of the relevant treatment outcome studies. Although chronic WAD is a considerable health problem, the number of published RCTs is very limited. Psychological interventions that are common in the treatment of chronic WAD vary from patient education to multimodal treatment. Most outcome studies have evaluated the efficacy of multimodal rather than focused treatments. This approach makes it difficult to evaluate the relative efficacy of the various components that are part of these treatments. Moreover, outcome studies are limited to the effects on chronic WAD, and no RCTs include the effects on both chronic WAD and PTSD.

The methodological quality of the efficacy studies is poor: Seferiadis et al.[26] assessed the quality of 26 RCTs, of which most studies were on interventions in the acute phase. These studies were assessed on 15 criteria for methodological quality. The three most prevalent shortcomings were lack of information on patient and/or care provider blinding, lack of information on concealment of treatment allocation and lack of description of adverse effects. For chronic WAD, Seferiadis et al.[26] recommend combined CBT and physiotherapy interventions on the basis of three low-quality RCTs. As described below, some additional RCTs for psychological interventions have been published recently, but the number and quality of the studies is still limited.

Psycho-education

As mentioned before, patient education or psycho-education is an effective part of the multimodal treatment of patients with chronic WAD. Studies on the effect of (psycho-) education are only available for patients with acute and subacute WAD, and the results are disappointing: no effect for patient education (mostly advising to keep active) has been found.[10] However, in most outcome studies psycho-education is limited (e.g. an educational pamphlet versus oral advice once).[27] In clinical practice, especially in the multimodal programs, psycho-education is more elaborate. Moreover, it seems important to consider the context in which education is given. Education as an isolated intervention or in a medical–somatic context may even have a negative effect.

The effect of early multidisciplinary evaluation and advice, four weeks or more after the injury, has been assessed.[28] The intervention consisted of a thorough clinical examination by a general practitioner and comprehensive testing by a physiotherapist. The examination lasted approximately 2.5 hours. In addition, 50% of patients were examined by a rehabilitation physician and 30% by a neurologist. Results were summarised in a report, which also included advice on treatment and self-management, and a prognostic evaluation. The report comprised reassurance that the prognosis was good and a recommendation of an early return to normal physical activity. For 27% of the patients, no additional therapy was recommended. Mostly, manual therapy or regular physiotherapy and exercises were advised. The study showed a significantly increased risk of chronic neck pain among those who received the intervention compared to those who did not. In interpreting these unexpected results, the authors state that the patients may have misinterpreted the thorough examination as a support for their worries of being seriously injured. Moreover, the frequent referral to manual therapy and physiotherapy may have further enhanced the patients' somatic attributions and search for somatic solutions for their complaints instead of finding other ways to cope and live with their pain.

Although no studies on the effects of psycho-education in patients with chronic WAD are available, this study indicates that (psycho-) education should be formulated in such a manner that the intervention does not strengthen dysfunctional causal attributions.

Multimodal treatment

Many multidisciplinary and multimodal treatment programs for chronic pain have been developed, some for groups of patients with different kinds of chronic pain, some for specific groups (e.g. chronic back pain). The composition of these programs varies, with some emphasising physical rehabilitation and others psychological aspects of pain. The latter are mostly CBT programs. These treatments include a wide variety of interventions: psycho-education, goal setting, graded activity training, pacing of activities, applied relaxation, cognitive techniques, social skills training, drug reduction methods, contingency management of pain behaviours and planning of return to work.[29] In clinical practice, patients with chronic WAD are often offered this kind of evidence-based treatment in a mixed group of patients with chronic pain. In general, these CBT programs have modest positive effects on pain, disability and mood.[30]

One of the first specific interventions for chronic WAD described in the literature is an integrated physiotherapy/cognitive behavioural approach.[31] These authors evaluated this approach in three experimental single case studies. Psychological and physical functional analyses were used to describe the problem areas and as a basis for the management of WAD. The results showed that the combination of physiotherapeutic exercises and the behavioural application of such exercises in daily activities decreased pain intensity.

An early multimodal treatment program for chronic WAD (over six months) has been developed.[32] The program is a daily, four-week, outpatient multimodal program to restore a normal pattern of daily functioning, including complete return to work. Decreasing pain symptoms was not a direct goal of the program. The physical training according to operant learning principles (graded activity) was combined with group sessions where patients' dysfunctional beliefs regarding symptoms and disability were discussed. The occupational therapist assisted the patient in the process of returning to work. The study was an uncontrolled pre- and post-treatment design, including a six-month follow-up period. Results of 26 patients were evaluated: symptoms improved significantly on nearly all self-report measures of pain, disability and psychological functioning. At follow-up, 65%

realised complete return to work, with 92% achieving complete or partial return to work; also, medical service utilisation decreased significantly in these patients.

The outcomes of another early multimodal rehabilitation program for patients with chronic WAD were less positive.[33] In this uncontrolled study it was found that the 90 patients enrolled in the group program were satisfied with the program and experienced several benefits of it on retrospective evaluation, but the prospective data (pre-, post-, six-month follow-up measures) showed no significant improvements. However, differences in program content, outcome measures and participants, may, in part, explain the inconsistent outcomes.

More recent descriptions of a multimodal treatment for patients with chronic WAD include those of Sullivan et al.[34] and Adams et al.[35] The treatment program used, the Progressive Goal Attainment Program (PGAP), is a standardised, manual-driven intervention that aims to maximise activity and return to work. For 10 weeks, patients meet individually with the PGAP clinician (physiotherapist or occupational therapist) on a weekly basis for approximately one hour. Activity scheduling and graded activity were used as techniques to reduce catastrophic thinking, fear of movement and perceived disability. So, clearly, this intervention was based on the FA model. Disability reduction was the primary goal of the intervention, not pain management or pain reduction. The PGAP is designed to be an addition to existing medical and physiotherapy interventions. In the studies of Sullivan et al.[34] and Adams et al.,[35] all patients were also participating in a functional restoration physiotherapy program and were being followed by a primary care physician. Sullivan et al.[34] compared a PGAP plus physiotherapy group with a group that underwent physiotherapy alone. Adams et al.[35] compared the effects of PGAP for a subacute (four to 12 weeks), an early chronic (three to six months) and a chronic (six to 18 months) group. Sullivan et al.[34] found that participation in PGAP plus physiotherapy resulted in a higher return-to-work rate (75%) than did participation in physiotherapy alone. PGAP was relatively more effective for patients who initially scored high on the psychosocial risk factors of pain catastrophising, fear of movement or reinjury, and perceived disability. Adams et al.[35] found that return to work rates were 80%, 72% and 32% for the subacute, early chronic and chronic groups, respectively. In the chronic group, pre-treatment scores on pain catastrophising and fear of movement were significantly higher than in the two other groups. The magnitude of treatment-related reductions in catastrophising, fear of movement and pain intensity was comparable over groups, but in the chronic group change in self-reported disability was lowest. These findings emphasise the importance of early intervention.

Specific interventions

Thus far only a few treatment outcome studies have focused on specific theory-derived interventions. An excellent example is a recent study that was based on the FA model.[36] Using a replicated single-case crossover phase design in eight patients, this study compared the relative efficacy of a more general intervention of 'graded activity' versus a more specific intervention of 'graded exposure in vivo'. This meant that four patients first received the graded activity intervention followed by the graded exposure in vivo intervention and that, for the other four patients, the sequence was the other way around. Daily measures of pain catastrophising, fear of movement and reinjury, fear of pain, and pain intensity were gathered.

Graded exposure in vivo consisted of individually tailored practice tasks based on a graded hierarchy of fear-eliciting activities and/or movements. The exposure took the form of a series of behavioural experiments in which dysfunctional beliefs were explicitly being challenged (e.g. 'If I lift up my child, then nerves in the neck will rupture and my muscles will get blocked'). Graded activity consisted of a gradual increase of activity, where activity is no longer pain-contingent but time-contingent.

The results showed decreasing levels of pain catastrophising, fear of movement and reinjury, fear of pain, pain intensity and disability, and improvements in physical activity level only when graded exposure in vivo was introduced, and not in the graded activity condition. These differential effects of both interventions are in accordance with the FA model. It is remarkable that during the graded exposure in vivo intervention, a sudden improvement occurred in the sessions in which exposure to personally relevant activities was undertaken. Although the authors call the effective intervention 'graded exposure in vivo', it is clear that cognitive restructuring takes place and that it is an essential aspect of the intervention, so the cognitive component of the intervention should not be underestimated. Thus, it is important to distinguish between the therapeutic method and the proposed theoretical mechanism of change.

Another RCT evaluating a specific theory-derived intervention was based on a new development in CBT—acceptance and commitment therapy (ACT).[11] An important difference between ACT and regular CBT is that ACT does not aim at changing dysfunctional cognitions, but rather at accepting these cognitions as 'nothing more than a thought'. The most important goal in ACT, in contrast to symptom reduction, is to improve functioning by increasing psychological flexibility, defined as a capacity to act in accordance with personal values in the presence of negative private experiences, such as pain or distress.[37] Wicksell et al.[11] compared two groups, which both continued to receive treatment as usual, but in addition were randomly assigned to a wait-list condition (n = 9) or to the ACT intervention group (n = 11). The intervention was conducted individually and consisted of 10 sessions over eight weeks. The intervention started with pain education followed by a thorough assessment of individual values in important life domains. Subsequently, behaviourally oriented goals were generated (i.e. what behaviours are needed to act in line with individual values). Next, previous strategies to reduce pain and distress were evaluated, emphasising both short- and long-term effects as well as the impact on functionality and individual values. The therapist then introduced the idea of acceptance of a certain amount of pain and distress to enable engagement in behaviours towards an increase in valued life. After this shift in perspective, patients were encouraged to perform gradual values-based exposure to increase values-directed behaviours.

After treatment, significant differences in favour of the treatment group were seen in the primary outcome variables of pain disability, and life satisfaction, and in the secondary outcome variables of fear of movements/reinjury, depression and psychological inflexibility in relation to pain. These positive effects were maintained at seven-months follow-up. No change was seen in pain intensity, anxiety and post-traumatic stress symptoms.

In comparing CBT in the study of De Jong et al.[36] and ACT in the study of Wicksell et al.[11] we learn that both treatments are effective, although not all outcome measures in these studies were the same. ACT has been described as a novel treatment, but it has also been argued that ACT is not an entirely different approach and that it is fully compatible with CBT.[38]

Finally, we describe the study of Wald et al.,[25] which evaluated the effect of interoceptive exposure preceding trauma-related exposure therapy on both PTSD and chronic musculoskeletal pain (over six months) arising from an MVC on five female patients. Four 90-minute sessions of interoceptive exposure preceded eight sessions of trauma-related exposure. These eight sessions consisted of four sessions of imaginal exposure to traumatic events followed by four sessions of exposure in vivo. Exposure occupied 60 minutes of each of the eight sessions, and patients were asked to complete 60 minutes daily of exposure homework between sessions.

Four patients reported a reduction in PTSD symptoms after treatment, and three no longer met the diagnostic criteria for PTSD. Interoceptive exposure was associated with larger reductions in anxiety sensitivity than trauma-related exposure, as hypothesised. Both interventions were associated with a reduction in PTSD symptoms, but the effect of trauma-related exposure was larger, especially on avoidance behaviour. Pain symptoms lessened slightly during interoceptive exposure and then kept practically unchanged following trauma-related exposure. At three-months follow-up, pain ratings had generally returned to pre-treatment levels. The disappointing results for pain are not well understood. Wald et al.[25] suggest that other interventions should be added, such as a graduated physical exercise program or cognitive restructuring or other CBT interventions. These results do not support the shared vulnerability model and, as described further in the next section, these results have clinical implications for the treatment of the co-occurrence of PTSD and chronic WAD.

REMAINING ISSUES AND FUTURE PROSPECTS

The results of the study of Wald et al.,[25] the only study to our knowledge that evaluated an intervention aimed at both chronic pain and PTSD symptoms, show that it is probably unattainable to develop one focused intervention for the co-occurrence of chronic WAD and PTSD. The important clinical question is how treatment for this co-occurrence should be designed (i.e. which syndrome should be focused on first). For a number of reasons we prefer to treat PTSD first. It is a good clinical rule that, in the case of co-morbidity, it is preferable to choose the evidence-based treatment with the best results first. An early success in treatment not only strengthens the working alliance, which may be important in tackling the more difficult problems later, but also the relief of symptoms in the treated disorder will mostly give some relief in symptoms in the other disorder. In this case, results for treating PTSD seem to be better than those for treating chronic WAD. Of course, this point of view should be stated with some caution, because these results are based on treatment of no co-occurring disorders. But there also are theoretical reasons for treating PTSD first. The important role of anxiety in chronic pain is acknowledged in the shared vulnerability model.[16] Moreover, the results of the study of Jenewein et al.[15] point out that after six months, PTSD symptoms impacted significantly on pain but not vice versa. So, lowering anxiety by treating PTSD, especially a decrease of hyperarousal symptoms, might well have a beneficial effect on pain.

Although the available studies concerning the treatment of chronic WAD are promising with regard to the efficacy of the available interventions, the present evidence is not yet sufficiently specific and elaborate to formulate detailed clinical guidelines. As in other functional syndromes, in patients with chronic WAD the primary goal of treatment should be improvement of functioning; reduction of pain is only secondary. In any case, it seems essential to focus on the dysfunctional causal attributions for pain and other symptoms. Treatment should be personalised as the results of De Jong et al.[36] and Wicksell et al.[11] strongly suggest. Both a graded exposure in vivo intervention (De Jong et al.[36]) and a gradual values-based exposure intervention (Wicksell et al.[11]) seem successful in tackling dysfunctional cognitions, although in quite a different way.

Other interventions often used in the treatment of chronic pain and functional syndromes are less successful, unless there are clearcut goals of treatment, like return to work.[32, 34] Therefore, it is the question of whether the usual interventions for chronic pain (i.e. graded activity) can be applied in the case of chronic WAD. Nijs et al.[2] state that there is consistent evidence for altered central pain-processing mechanisms and central sensitisation in patients with chronic WAD. They warn that physical rehabilitation may aggravate symptoms in some patients. They recommend staying below the pain threshold and the use of low-load exercises and low-velocity mobilising techniques in connection with central sensitisation.[2] In multimodal CBT programs, time-contingent exercise therapy is often used. Nijs et al.[2] suppose that a time-contingent approach teaches the patient to ignore pain aggravations, which is likely to sustain the process of central sensitisation. Therefore, CBT programs should be adapted in such a way that exercise intensity and duration stay below the pain threshold. Thus far, there is no evidence for this hypothesis, but it seems worthwhile to evaluate this.

CONCLUSION

In conclusion, some of the factors that are critical in the development of chronic WAD appear hard to change.[39] Therefore, it seems important not only to focus on the reduction of symptoms but also on reducing the invalidating consequences of these complaints.[9] Many patients with chronic WAD typically attribute their symptoms to physical causes. These patients are often highly resistant to psychological evaluation and treatment. So for these cases, special attention to motivational techniques (e.g. motivational interviewing[40]) may be necessary to enhance treatment success and to prevent early dropout.

References

1. Kamper SJ, Rebbeck TJ, Maher CG, et al. Course and prognostic factors of whiplash: a systematic review and meta-analysis. *Pain* 2008;138:617–29.
2. Nijs J, Van Oosterwijck J, De Hertogh W. Rehabilitation of chronic whiplash: treatment of cervical dysfunctions or chronic pain syndrome? *Clin Rheumatol* 2009;28:243–51.
3. Poorbaugh K, Brismée J-M, Phelps V, et al. Late whiplash syndrome: a clinical science approach to evidence-based diagnosis and management. *Pain Pract* 2008;8:65–89.
4. Vangronsveld K, Peters ML, Goossens ME, et al. Applying the fear-avoidance model to the chronic whiplash syndrome. *Pain* 2007;130:258–61.
5. Nieto R, Miró J, Huguet A. The fear-avoidance model in whiplash injuries. *Eur J Pain* 2009;13:518–23.
6. Carroll LJ, Holm LW, Ferrari R, et al. Recovery in whiplash-associated disorders: do you get what you expect? *J Rheumatol* 2009;36:1063–70.
7. Severeijns R, Vlaeyen JW, Van den Hout MA, et al. Pain catastrophizing predicts pain intensity, disability, and psychological distress independent of the level of physical impairment. *Clin J Pain* 2001;17: 165–72.
8. Petrie KJ & Weinman J. Why illness perceptions matter. *Clin Med* 2007;6:536–9.
9. Speckens AEM, Spinhoven P, Hawton KE, et al. Cognitive behavioural therapy for medically unexplained symptoms: a pilot study. *Behav Cogn Psychother* 1996;24:1–16.
10. Haines T, Gross AR, Burnie S, et al. A Cochrane review of patient education for neck pain. *Spine J* 2009;9: 859–71.
11. Wicksell RK, Ahlqvist J, Bring A, et al. Can exposure and acceptance strategies improve functioning and life satisfaction in people with chronic pain and whiplash-associated disorders (WAD)? A randomized controlled trial. *Cogn Behav Ther* 2008;37:169–82.
12. Buitenhuis J, De Jong PJ, Jaspers JPC, et al. Relationship between posttraumatic stress disorder symptoms and the course of whiplash complaints. *J Psychosom Res* 2006;61:681–9.

13. Sterling M, Kenardy J, Jull G, et al. The development of psychological changes following whiplash injury. *Pain* 2003;106:481–9.
14. Sharp TJ & Harvey AG. Chronic pain and posttraumatic stress disorder: mutual maintenance? *Clin Psychol Rev* 2001;21:857–77.
15. Jenewein J, Wittmann L, Moergeli H, et al. Mutual influence of post traumatic stress disorder symptoms and chronic pain among injured accident survivors: a longitudinal study. *J Trauma Stress* 2009;22(6):540–8.
16. Asmundson GJG & Katz JK. Understanding the co-occurrence of anxiety disorders and chronic pain: state of the art. *Depress Anxiety* 2009;26:888–901.
17. McLean SA, Clauw DJ, Abelson JL, et al. The development of persistent pain and psychological morbidity after motor vehicle collision: integrating the potential role of stress response systems into a biopsychosocial model. *Psychosom Med* 2005;67: 783–90.
18. Sterling M & Kenardy J. The relationship between sensory and sympathetic nervous system changes and posttraumatic stress reaction following whiplash injury – a prospective study. *J Psychosom Res* 2006;60: 387–93.
19. Bisson JI, Ehlers A, Matthews R, et al. Psychological treatments for chronic post-traumatic stress disorder. Systematic review and meta-analysis. *Br J Psychiatry* 2007;190:97–104.
20. Ponniah K & Hollon SD. Empirically supported psychological treatments for adult acute stress disorder and posttraumatic stress disorder: a review. *Depress Anxiety* 2009;26:1086–109.
21. Schoutrop MJ, Lange A, Hanewald G, et al. Structured writing and processing major stressful events: a controlled trial. *Psychother Psychosom* 2002;71: 151–7.
22. Van Emmerik AA, Kamphuis JH, Emmelkamp PM. Treating acute stress disorder and traumatic stress disorder with cognitive behavioral therapy or structured writing therapy: a randomized controlled trial. *Psychother Psychosom* 2008;77:93–100.
23. Mayou R & Bryant B. Consequences of road traffic accidents for different types of road user. *Injury* 2003;34:197–202.
24. Forbes D, Creamer M, Phelps A, et al. Australian guidelines for the treatment of adults with acute stress disorder and post-traumatic stress disorder. *Aust N Z J Psychiatry* 2007;41:637–48.
25. Wald J, Taylor S, Chiri LR, Sica C. Posttraumatic stress disorder and chronic pain arising from motor vehicle accidents: efficacy of interoceptive exposure plus trauma-related exposure therapy. *Cogn Behav Ther* 2010;39(2):104–13.
26. Seferiadis A, Rosenfeld M, Gunnarsson R. A review of treatment interventions in whiplash-associated disorders. *Eur Spine J* 2004;13:387–97.
27. Kongsted A, Qerama E, Kasch H, et al. Education of patients after whiplash injury. Is oral advice any better than a pamphlet? *Spine* 2008;33:E843–E848.
28. Pape E, Hagen KB, Brox JI. Early multidisciplinary evaluation and advice was ineffective for whiplash-associated disorders. *Eur J Pain* 2009;13:1063–70.
29. Johansson C, Dahl J, Jannert M, et al. Effects of a cognitive-behavioral pain-management program. *Behav Res Ther* 1998;36:915–30.
30. Eccleston C, Williams AC, Morley S. Psychological therapies for the management of chronic pain (excluding headache) in adults. *Cochrane Database Syst Rev* 2009; (2):CD007407.
31. Söderlund A & Lindberg P. An integrated physiotherapy/cognitive-behavioural approach to the analysis and treatment of chronic whiplash associated disorders, WAD. *Disabil Rehabil* 2001;23:436–47.
32. Vendrig AA, Van Akkerveen PF, McWorther KR. Results of a multimodal treatment program for patients with chronic symptoms after a whiplash injury of the neck. *Spine* 2000;25:238–44.
33. Sterner Y, Löfgren M, Nyberg V, et al. Early interdisciplinary rehabilitation programme for whiplash associated disorders. *Disabil Rehabil* 2001;23:422–9.
34. Sullivan MJL, Adams H, Rhodenizer T, et al. A psychosocial risk factor-targeted intervention for the prevention of chronic pain and disability following whiplash injury. *Phys Ther* 2006;86:8–18.
35. Adams H, Ellis T, Stanish WD, et al. Psychosocial factors related to return to work following rehabilitation of whiplash injuries. *J Occup Rehabil* 2007;17:305–15.
36. De Jong JR, Vangronsveld K, Peters ML, et al. Reduction of pain-related fear and disability in post-traumatic neck pain: a replicated single-case experimental study of exposure in vivo. *J Pain* 2008;9:1123–34.
37. Hayes SC, Strosahl KD, Wilson KG. Acceptance and commitment therapy: an experiential approach to behavior change. New York: Guilford Press, 1999.
38. Hofmann SG & Asmundson GJ. Acceptance and mindfulness-based therapy: new wave or old hat? *Clin Psychol Rev* 2008;28:1–16.
39. Williams E, Williams M, Gates S, et al. A systematic literature review of psychological factors and the development of late whiplash syndrome. *Pain* 2008;135: 20–30.
40. Ang D, Kesavala R, Lydon JR, et al. Exercise-based motivational interviewing for female patients with fibromyalgia: a case series. *Clin Rheumatol* 2007;26(11):1843–9.

CHAPTER 14
COMPENSATION AND HEALTH OUTCOMES

Luke B. Connelly and Natalie Spearing

INTRODUCTION

Insurance provides cover, in the form of financial compensation, against a range of losses, including those arising from personal injury. Insurance is regulated by legislation and the principles of case law, and in many jurisdictions it is mandatory for some parties, such as road users and employers (and others), to purchase insurance.[1] Common examples include compulsory third-party (personal injury—auto) insurance, and workers' compensation insurance, both of which provide compensation to eligible injured parties. While the rationale for specific legislative and regulatory arrangements governing personal injury compensation for injuries varies between jurisdictions, there is common concern for the health and wellbeing of individuals following an injury. Consequently, the question of whether or not compensation and/or the associated processes could affect health outcomes is of interest to academics, clinicians and legislators, and has been examined in some depth primarily in clinical journals (hereinafter, 'the literature').

Other things being equal, relieving some or all of the costs of treatment—as most compensation schemes do—should improve the wellbeing of injured people. Compensation schemes usually embody such an insurance function: by alleviating the financial burden of medical expenses that are associated with the treatment of an injury, injured individuals are protected from expenses that, otherwise, would represent 'random deductions'[2] from their incomes/wealth. In circumstances where there is no 'scheme' or insurance, but the law establishes a right to compensation for harm, similar principles apply when reparation is made. Similarly, compensation for the lost income, pain, suffering and other adverse effects of an injury should also, other things being equal, leave injured parties better off than they would have been if no compensation were available. However, there are also reasons that the availability of compensation could lead to actual or perceived reductions in health, relative to the situation in which compensation were not provided. Indeed, a negative correlation between compensation and health outcomes has been observed in the empirical literature and has led researchers to pose a hypothesis that may be expressed as follows:

> H_0: Injury compensation payments cause the health outcomes for injured individuals to be worse, on average, than they would have been had compensation not been available.

For brevity, throughout this chapter H_0 is referred to as the hypothesis that compensation is 'bad for health'.

How can this hypothesis above be tested? The counterfactual cannot be observed: the outcome that would have prevailed if individuals had not been compensated cannot actually be known. Similarly, the effect of compensation on those who did not receive it is unknown. Thus, in order to test H_0, the influence of compensation on health has to be inferred by comparing the health outcomes of, say, uncompensated and compensated groups. Comparisons of non-randomly allocated groups are problematic for a variety of reasons that have been acknowledged in the literature on compensation and health. To date, though, writers in this literature have, in our view, paid insufficient attention to the implementation of econometric or statistical strategies that may minimise the chance that such comparisons are biased.[3]

The purpose of the chapter is to explore the reasons that an inverse association between compensation and health outcomes could be observed in practice. It considers the circumstances under which compensation processes and/or outcomes could genuinely lower health outcomes by comparison with the counterfactual. The primary emphasis, though, is on the reasons that the evidence may appear to support the hypothesis that compensation is bad for health, even if compensation and related processes have a zero, or positive, effect on health. The rationale for this focus is that little attention has been paid to these possibilities in the existing literature, which too often proceeds from the observation of a negative empirical correlation between compensation and health outcomes to the causal interpretation that there is a perverse relationship between compensation and health. This is a serious issue, because the results from this literature have already been used to recommend changes to the apparatus of compensation schemes,[4] including limits to some types of compensation. The prevailing sentiments are exemplified in the following quote:

> 'There is now convincing evidence that when an injured patient receives compensation, their long-term outcomes are worse.'[5]

We believe this to be a heroic claim given the assumptions it entails. This chapter lays out the reasons that researchers and policy-makers should be considerably more circumspect about the meaning of research findings to date. Based on the flaws in the existing literature and their implications for the quality of the evidence, this chapter concludes that policy interventions to limit compensation on the basis that compensation is bad for health are built on a shaky premise.

Although many of the problems that are addressed in this chapter have serious econometric or statistical consequences, it is beyond the scope and purpose of this chapter to describe them and their solutions. (Some suggestions for further reading on the related statistical issues are, however, provided at the end of the chapter.) Rather, the chapter concentrates on outlining the conceptual issues in a non-technical way and providing an overview of the empirical work on this question to date. While some of the examples in this chapter are taken from the health and compensation literature generally, our particular focus is on the literature concerning compensation and health outcomes following a whiplash injury.

This chapter first outlines and defines some compensation-related concepts and the relationships between them. It then provides a discussion of measurement problems that are related to these compensation-related concepts and relationships. The chapter then addresses another set of conceptual and measurement issues that are associated with trying to measure health and improvements in health, along with the question of what may motivate people to misrepresent their underlying, true health state.

COMPENSATION AND RELATED CONCEPTS

This section defines some important compensation-related concepts and some of the relationships between them.

First, it is important to define precisely what is meant by the terms 'compensation', 'compensation scheme' and 'litigation'. These terms are used routinely in this literature, often interchangeably, but are seldom actually defined. In this chapter, the following definitions are invoked:

> **Compensation:** Reparation, in cash or in kind (e.g. the provision of medical treatment) for the losses that arise due to an injury or harm.
>
> **Compensation scheme:** The laws and legal processes that govern how compensation claims are made, defended and paid.
>
> **Litigation:** The 'conduct of legal proceedings by parties before a court'.[6]

Note that the term 'compensation scheme', as defined, is general enough to encompass common law provisions, even where no insurance mandate exists. Finally, note that litigation itself is rare, as most legal actions are settled out of court.[1] Indeed, in many jurisdictions, the proportion of matters that proceed to court is extremely small.

Conceptual representation of a compensation scheme and related concepts

Figure 14.1 is a conceptual representation of compensation processes and outcomes. It is a stylised representation of a *compensation scheme* and it builds upon the distinctions that Wright and Melville[7] have made in relation to litigation per se. The purpose of Figure 14.1 is to provide a way of thinking about the distinction between concepts that are poorly described in the literature. The distinction between these concepts is directly germane to attempts to test the hypothesis that compensation is bad for health.

Figure 14.1 should be read from left to right, and top to bottom. The largest rectangle in Figure 14.1 is labelled '(i) Incidents (compensable and non-compensable injuries)'. Rectangle (i) represents all injuries that occur in a particular jurisdiction, irrespective of how or where they occur, who causes them and whether or not they are compensable. The second-largest rectangle, which is marked '(ii) Legal incidents (compensable injuries)', represents the subset of incidents to which legal rights to compensation are attached. The size of this subset, relative to the incident rate of injuries per se, depends upon the laws and institutions that are in place in a given jurisdiction. For example, in Figure 14.1, it is assumed that not all incidents (injuries, in this case) are legal incidents

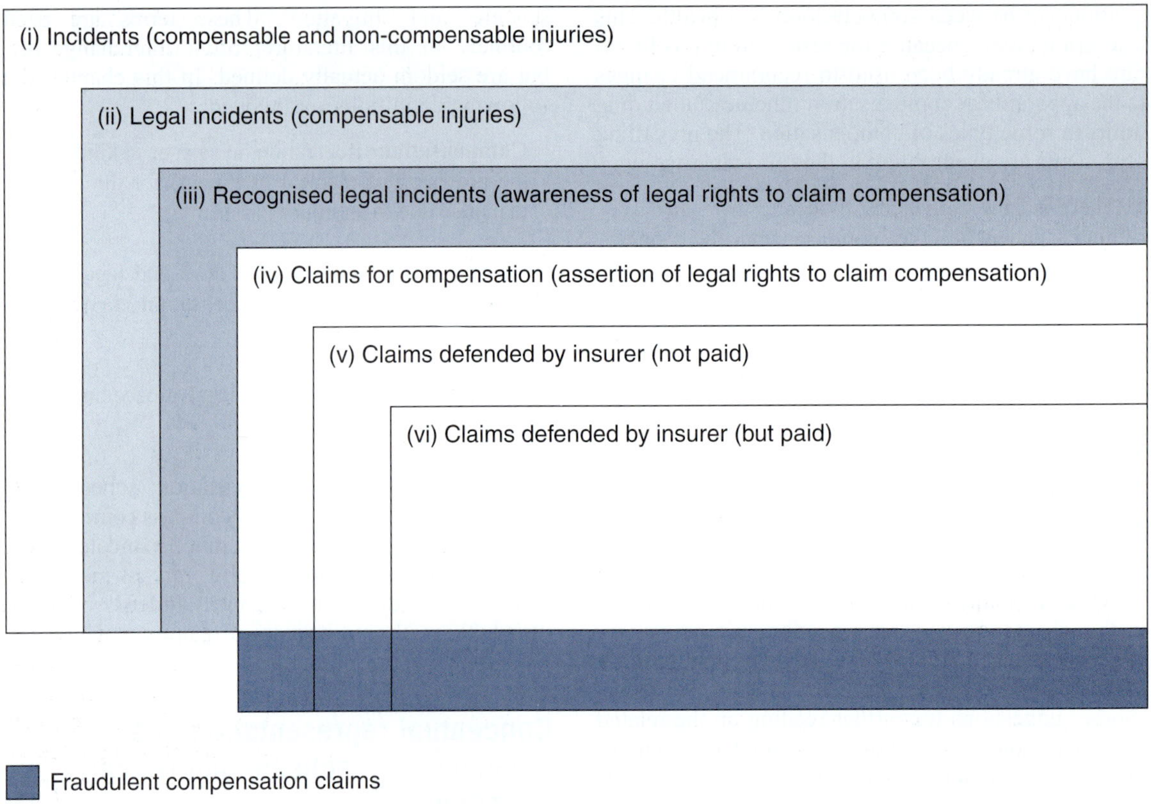

Figure 14.1 Compensation schemes and related concepts.

(i.e. compensable injuries). Thus, (ii) provides one way of considering the scope of a compensation scheme.

The next rectangle that sits within (i) and (ii) is marked '(iii) Recognised legal incidents (awareness of legal right to claim compensation)'. This area represents the subset of legal incidents that are recognised as such by the injured party. In other words, it is assumed that some individuals who have compensable injuries are not aware of their legal right to make a compensation claim.

The rectangle that is marked (iv) represents the proportion of recognised rights that are asserted (i.e. the number of claims for compensation). The part of (iv) that lies outside (i) and is shaded blue indicates claims for injury compensation where no injury exists (i.e. fraudulent claims). Note that individuals could also mistake genuine injuries as compensable ('Legal incidents') when they are not and make claims for them; however, for simplicity, these phenomena are not depicted in Figure 14.1. Within the assertions of legal rights (iv), (v) represents the claims for damages that are defended (e.g. by the insurer) and, among these, (vi) represents claims that are defended but nevertheless do result in compensation. Claims that are defended and where no compensation is paid are depicted by the area of (v) that is shaded blue. Finally, note that Figure 14.1 implicitly assumes that some fraudulent cases are successfully defended, but that others are paid.

Definitional considerations (compensation, litigation and lawyer involvement)

One point to be taken from Figure 14.1 is that litigation, compensation, lawyer involvement and other related legal processes and terms are all quite distinct—despite the prevailing tendency to aggregate them, as described in detail by Grant and Studdert.[3] Studies in the health literature often use these terms as if they are interchangeable.

Treating 'compensation/litigation', for example, as a single, homogeneous category is problematic. Litigation and compensation are not synonymous and, indeed, litigation is neither a necessary nor a sufficient condition for the payment of compensation. Similarly, in the empirical literature the involvement of lawyers sometimes appears to be erroneously equated with litigation or, indeed, compensation itself. Although lawyer involvement obviously is common in litigated cases, in some jurisdictions self-representation may constitute a significant proportion of claims for compensation, especially for smaller claims.

Thus, it is not sensible to treat compensation, litigation, lawyer involvement and other terms associated with personal injury compensation as homogeneous concepts. For example, returning to Figure 14.1, if compensation, litigation and lawyer involvement were treated as synonymous, into which group would the latter two categories fit? Unfortunately, the answer is 'probably both', because some individuals who are uncompensated will have pursued a compensation claim, retained a lawyer and engaged in (unsuccessful) litigation of their case. Similarly, a number of compensated individuals may have pursued a successful claim without lawyer involvement. Irrespective of whether a lawyer is involved or not, litigation in this context is uncommon. For example, in Queensland, Australia, only about 3–4% of motor accident compensation cases are litigated,[8] with the vast majority of cases being settled out of court.[1]

COMPENSATION: EMPIRICAL CONSIDERATIONS

Selection bias and confounding have been acknowledged as common problems in research on compensation and whiplash recovery.[9, 10] Additionally, as the research is comprised of non-randomised studies, it is not possible to determine whether there is a causal relationship between compensation and health.[11, 12]

Figure 14.1 shows how compensation payments are preceded by a claims process that is governed by the law, institutional arrangements and, crucially, the choices that parties to a harm make. That process usually commences only if injured parties recognise their legal right to seek compensation and then assert that right by making a claim. Whether and how much compensation is actually paid, if this occurs, then depends upon the legal and institutional framework and processes that are in place and the decisions of the individuals who are subject to them. Not only are compensation payments not randomly nor (usually) automatically allocated, but the entitlement to compensation also varies across jurisdictions and schemes. The non-random nature of the allocation of compensation payments and the systematic differences in the ways that different compensation schemes operate have important ramifications for comparisons between the groups in Figure 14.1, both across and within compensation schemes. The specific issues that are implied for empirical studies that seek to test the hypothesis (H_0) that compensation is bad for health primarily involve problems related to selection bias and confounding, which will now be outlined.

Sample selection bias and confounding

It is generally not feasible to randomise the allocation of compensation for experimental purposes. Thus, differences that are observed between compensated and uncompensated individuals, for example, may be due to the treatment, that is, compensation, and due to selection effects. The latter term refers to differences that are not due to the treatment itself, but to factors that vary systematically between those people who seek and those who do not seek compensation. Selection bias may be thought of as an error in the way that individuals are 'assigned' to the intervention and control groups.[12] Selection bias can lead to confounding as it creates differences between these groups, and the validity of between-group comparisons hinges on whether the groups are composed in a manner that allows for appropriate comparison.[13] While it is possible to apply statistical techniques to control for the effects of observed factors, such as age and gender, which may differ between the groups, observational (non-randomised) studies in the clinical literature often do not address the potential for unobserved differences to confound the results.

Sampling problems are not limited to primary studies. Systematic reviews that have investigated the prognostic impact of compensation on whiplash recovery have not searched specifically for compensation-related studies, and thus it is unclear whether the samples of primary studies included in the reviews are truly representative of the existing research.[14–16] Moreover, systematic reviews are also subject to the methodological limitations inherent in the primary research on this topic. Attempts to consider the effects of compensation on health are complicated further by authors pooling the results of studies that concern different types of compensation schemes and/or legal processes. The heterogeneity problem is outlined below. Examples of the ways in which the problems of selection bias and confounding may affect the results of studies examining the association between compensation and health status are provided in the following sections.

Cross-jurisdictional scheme comparisons ('apples and oranges' problem)

One of the distinctions in Figure 14.1, between areas (i) and (ii), is particularly relevant to attempts to compare individuals' health outcomes across different compensation schemes. Whether this is the primary purpose of the study (e.g. to compare health outcomes in one jurisdiction versus another), or is simply an incidental aspect of the sample design (e.g. to test H_0, the health outcomes of claimants and non-claimants are measured using studies performed in various jurisdictions), there are important empirical implications. Essentially, differences between schemes may create an 'apples and oranges' problem that makes inter-jurisdictional comparisons and the policy conclusions that may be based on them problematic.

A review of the law of negligence highlighted the variation in personal injury compensation laws and schemes in Australia.[17] This review described how, for example, the amount of compensation for similar injuries differs depending upon which injury compensation law is applicable, as these laws vary according to where and how an injury occurs. Liability rules, the recovery of legal costs, discount rates, award payment structures such as lump sum or periodic payments, and other aspects of scheme design also vary. Such variations are also evident in the laws and processes governing compensation for road traffic injuries, and these differ between and even within some countries, notably, Australia,[17] the United States[18] and Canada.[19] Thus, regional comparisons and broad conclusions about the effects of compensation and the related legal processes on health status are limited in their validity because laws and legal processes differ across jurisdictions.[20] In addition, it is unclear which, if any, of the features of compensation scheme design may have an impact on health status as there has been little attempt by researchers to describe these characteristics, let alone attempt to relate their hypothesis to them in a lucid manner. While it is outside the scope of this chapter to present a survey of different compensation schemes, their heterogeneity is demonstrable[17] and noteworthy.

To illustrate this point, consider a simplified example wherein the health outcomes of claimants in jurisdictions A and B are compared. Suppose that jurisdiction A has a compensation scheme in which all injuries are compensable (i.e. (ii) and (i) are equal sets), but jurisdiction B's compensation scheme covers only injuries that are sustained by workers at work. Now, suppose that data on the *populations* of claimants from both jurisdictions are available. After controlling for injury severity, age and gender, suppose that the health outcomes in jurisdiction B are, on average, found to be considerably better than those in jurisdiction A. What conclusions may be drawn from this kind of evidence?

Clearly, the claimant populations of jurisdictions A and B are likely to differ because the definition of (ii) differs between jurisdictions. So, it would be fairly surprising if the characteristics of the injuries and the subjects from these two jurisdictions were not also systematically different. If systematic differences between the two compensation groups correlate with their prognosis for recovery, this could constitute a serious problem. The analyst may be able to observe and account for some such characteristics, such as injury severity, age and gender, but if there are unobserved differences between the groups that are systematically related to the outcome following injury, the comparison will be biased. For example, if workers who are injured in the workplace receive quicker or higher quality treatment than individuals who are injured in other circumstances—but these aspects of the system are not measured—one risks misattributing the apparently superior outcomes in jurisdiction B to its limited scope of compensation, even if the result is purely due to selection bias. Indeed, the selection bias problem could be strong enough to conclude that compensation is bad for health even if the converse is true.

This problem can, of course, be mitigated in a number of ways. For example, by restricting the analysis to workers injured in the workplace in both jurisdictions A and B, the extent of bias may be reduced; but what if the compensation schemes in jurisdictions A and B also differ substantially? If, for example, the compensation available to workers in jurisdiction A were less generous, less immediate, of lower quality and provided via a more adversarial claims system, the result could persist even when the sample is limited in this way. Unfortunately, few empirical studies consider such issues, let alone control for them. Typically, compensation is treated as a binary variable where subjects are classified as either 'compensated' or 'not compensated'; details of the size of the 'dose' among compensated individuals (i.e. the quantum of compensation) and the 'route' by which it is administered (e.g. the legal process and other features of the particular scheme) are infrequently available or described.

Within-jurisdiction scheme comparisons ('apples and oranges' problem)

To illustrate the foregoing points about selection bias within one compensation scheme, let us return to our previous hypothetical example but now suppose that one is interested in a comparison of the health outcomes of claimants and non-claimants in jurisdiction A only. Now consider Figure 14.1 and recall that the health outcomes of claimants are represented by area (iv). Which group of non-claimants in Figure 14.1 should be chosen for the intended comparison? Note that three approaches are possible as one could compare the health outcomes of claimants with one or more of at least three distinct groups:

1. non-claimants who recognised their right to claim but chose not to do so (i.e. those individuals who are represented by area (iii) minus area (iv))
2. non-claimants who were entitled to claim but did not recognise their right to do so (i.e. those individuals who are represented by area (iii) minus area (ii))
3. non-claimants who did not have a legal right to claim (i.e. those individuals who are represented by area (i) minus area (ii)); or, any combination of 1 through 3.

Which of these groups is of interest, for the purpose of testing H_0?

Reverse causality

Suppose, for argument's sake, that one chose to compare the health outcomes of claimants in (iv) with the health outcomes of non-claimants in (iii) who knew of their legal right to pursue a claim. Suppose that, controlling for observable factors, the health outcomes for non-claimants in (iii) were, on average, better than those of claimants in (iv). Does this constitute evidence for the hypothesis that compensation is bad for health?

Although such a result could be interpreted as evidence in support of H_0, it is also consistent with a competing hypothesis, namely:

> H_1: Individuals with worse health outcomes and prognoses are, all else being equal, more likely to pursue a claim for compensation.

The hypotheses H_0 and H_1 are both consistent with a positive correlation between compensation and poor health outcomes.

A similar reverse causality argument applies to studies of the effect of lawyer involvement on claim duration and other outcomes. Several studies show that lawyer involvement[18, 21] and frequent visits to health professionals[18, 22] are associated with longer periods before claim settlement. Other studies have examined the impact of lawyer involvement on whiplash symptoms such as pain.[23, 24] However, drawing a causal interpretation about the effects of lawyers on health status by concluding that lawyers are 'bad for health' from such correlations is not sensible. These studies are subject to the same concerns about selection and reverse causality issues that have been outlined thus far. Teasell,[25] for example, has argued that lawyer involvement may be a marker of injury severity, so one should expect a positive correlation between lawyer involvement and claim duration for that reason. Remarkably, such concerns have not prevented authors in this literature from drawing a causal interpretation of the correlations between legal representation and various measures of claim and health outcomes.

Selection bias and changes to compensation scheme design

The problem of controlling for the qualitative aspects of the way a compensation scheme operates has tempted researchers to compare health outcomes across different compensation schemes, including before-and-after studies of natural experiments arising from fundamental changes to compensation schemes.

The sample selection issues that were outlined above, however, also create serious problems for studies of this kind. Changes to 'scheme design' can affect any or all of the elements of Figure 14.1, including the relative magnitudes of (ii) through (iv). Before-and-after studies that seek to compare the health status of claimants and non-claimants before and after a change (e.g. a reduction) in the availability of compensation, should attempt to take account of the fact that the sample selection problem will, itself, likely be affected by the scheme changes. For example, an across-the-board reduction in compensation payments would be expected to reduce the size of (iv) relative to (iii). If H_1 is true, the group that is discouraged from pursuing a compensation claim by the reduction in compensation awards is likely to have, on average, better outcomes/prognoses than the group that persists with claims. This would tend to exaggerate the difference in average health status for claimants and non-claimants after the scheme change, because the claimant pool's average prognosis/health outcome falls as individuals with better outcomes/prognoses are discouraged from making claims.

Thus, empirical studies that consider changes in scheme design are also subject to these sample selection issues. For example, a study in New South Wales by Cameron et al.[26] examined the effects of a suite of legislative changes, which included the abolition of financial compensation for pain and suffering in minor claims, on the health status of individuals with whiplash injuries. They found that health outcomes were better among those exposed to the altered scheme with its less generous compensation provisions; however, the problem with attributing an outcome improvement to this change per se is that the change in provisions is likely to have affected the decision to claim itself (i.e. the size of area (iv) in Figure 14.1), so that sample selection bias in the pre–post comparison cannot be discounted.

A study conducted in Saskatchewan by Cassidy and colleagues,[21] which found that longer claim duration was associated with poorer health status regardless of scheme design, and propensity to claim decreased when compensation for pain and suffering was eliminated (i.e. compensation benefits were reduced), is subject to similar limitations. Importantly, the study populations in the studies by Cameron et al.[26] and Cassidy et al.[21] also were comprised solely of people who received compensation. Without a control group of uncompensated subjects, or some other mechanism to control for selection bias, it is not possible to say whether even the observed correlations are due to a causal effect, selection bias or both.

Selection bias and treatment

Another type of selection problem may arise due to practitioners' choices with respect to claimants and non-claimants. If, for example, institutional arrangements are such that workers' compensation claimants are subject to a lower price–cost margin (e.g. if the fees paid are lower for workers' compensation claimants, or the costs of treating them are higher say, due to greater paperwork and transactions costs), some of the most skilled practitioners may avoid treating compensable patients. Lower skilled practitioners, on the other hand, may be attracted to the treatment of compensable patients as the fees they command are likely to be lower, and the price–cost margin may be higher for workers' compensation claimants than for other patients. Consequently, an adverse selection of treating practitioners may lead to relatively poorer health outcomes for compensable patients. Conversely, a favourable selection of practitioners (which may be induced via a higher price–cost margin, for example) may result in better health outcomes for compensable patients.

Propensity to claim

The recognition of a compensable injury, itself, seems unlikely to occur at random. Additionally, among individuals who do recognise their right to pursue compensation, the decision to do so is unlikely to be random. Rather, individuals who recognise their legal rights may vary from those who do not in a systematic way, such as by educational level. Furthermore, when the right to claim is recognised, the conditional probability of pursuing a claim may also be related to systematic differences, such as income or education, for example, and to other variables that are not observed by the researcher. Indeed, there is now considerable literature that shows this to be the case (see, for example, Dunbar and Sabry[27]).

If systematic differences of this kind exist, and the variables that affect the recognition and assertion of legal rights are correlated not only with the decision to claim but also with health status, a sample selection or sample bias issue may arise when comparisons between claimants and non-claimants are made.

The potential strength of sample selection problems should not be underestimated. There is evidence from studies conducted in no-fault settings, where there are presumably fewer impediments to obtaining compensation compared to fault-based schemes, that the proportion of eligible claims actually asserted is relatively small. For example, a study of American automotive workers found that only 25% of people who were eligible for workers' compensation for work-related musculoskeletal conditions actually filed a claim and the strongest predictor of claiming was the severity of the injury.[28] Similarly, under New Zealand's universal no-fault scheme, only 2.9–4.8% of eligible people claimed compensation for medical injuries arising from hospital-based adverse events. Conceptually, this coincides with (iv) in Figure 14.1 being 2.9–4.8% of the size of (i), where medical injuries are concerned. In this study, those least likely to assert a claim tended to be older, poorer, or of Māori or Pacific Island ethnicity.[29] Hence, these studies provide evidence that selection bias is likely to be an important empirical phenomenon.

HEALTH: THE CONCEPT AND ITS MEASUREMENT

Thus far, the question of how health itself is measured in this literature has not been addressed. This section addresses that question by considering self-reported and other indicators of health status and the problems that are associated with their use to test the hypothesis that compensation is bad for health.

Health can be defined as follows:

Health: 'is a state of complete physical, mental and social well-being and not merely the absence of disease or infirmity.'[30]

Self-reported health status

The existing empirical literature depends heavily on comparisons between the self-reported health states of compensated and uncompensated individuals. While there are problems with the way in which compensation is measured, as described earlier, the reliance on self-reported health status is a further complication: there is reason to suspect that self-reported whiplash injuries are subject to systematic measurement error, as opposed to random error (chance).

At the heart of the problem is the inherently latent nature of the variable of interest—health. Latent variables are not directly observable and, therefore, their impact must be assessed using other variables ('indicators') that are observable. Clinical indicators of the underlying health state may include blood pressure, cholesterol level, absence or presence of a fracture, and so on. The foregoing examples are positive measures, meaning that they are verifiable or falsifiable. Not all aspects of health can, however, be captured with such indicators.

Whiplash injuries and their sequelae constitute a particularly good example of these problems. There is no gold standard diagnostic test for whiplash. Imaging techniques[31] and physical examination[32, 33] cannot currently verify or falsify claims of whiplash associated disorder (WAD) and, hence, the diagnosis relies almost exclusively on self-reports. Consequently, there is the potential for the condition to be reported when it does not exist, or for the symptoms of a bona fide injury to be exaggerated when compensation is available. Furthermore, the extent of measurement errors that arise for this reason is unquantifiable in the absence of a valid and reliable diagnostic test.

Self-reported health status data often constitute the best available measures of the underlying health state of interest. A critical question, though, is whether or not differences in self-reported health status may be taken to reflect differences in the underlying, latent, health states. In the case of individuals who are and are not pursuing compensation claims, the question is whether there is any reason to suspect systematic differences in reported health states between claimants and non-claimants. If claimants systematically understate their latent health status—and they may have financial incentives to do just that—any observed differences in the health status of claimants and non-claimants may be partly or wholly attributable to systematic differences in measurement error rather than systematic differences in health per se.

Moral hazard, self-reported health status and whiplash

When individuals are insured against the losses that are associated with some risk, such as a motor vehicle crash (MVC), the expected cost of such incidents to them is reduced. This reduction in the expected cost of the insured event may, itself, have behavioural consequences. Individuals may take less care to prevent the loss occurring, and/or consume more services (e.g. repair services) if the event does occur, than would be consumed in the absence of insurance. This behaviour under insurance is the phenomenon of moral hazard,[2, 34] which can arise when insured parties hold more information about their loss prevention behaviour than their insurer.

The possession of insurance may affect behaviour in a way that increases the likelihood of the insured event (*ex ante* moral hazard) and/or increases the size of the loss after an event occurs (*ex post* moral hazard).[35] Individuals with compensable whiplash injuries generally have more information about the consequences of their injury than their insurer (e.g. injured parties have superior information about their true health states). Thus, the potential for *ex post* moral hazard arises because there is an opportunity for the insured to overstate the adverse consequences of their whiplash injuries on health-related quality of life, productivity and so on, and to receive greater compensation benefits as a result. In other words, hypotheses of malingering behaviour in the literature on compensation and health are aligned with the economic theory of behaviour under insurance.

While it is generally accepted that whiplash causes acute injury and short-term neck pain,[36] there is still considerable debate as to whether or not compensation is associated with the chronic whiplash symptoms that are seen in between 15%[37] and 42% of whiplash cases.[20] Reports that whiplash is virtually unheard of in countries where no compensation is available,[38–40] and that placebo rear-end collisions induce acute neck pain and psychological distress,[41] have fuelled speculation that the self-reported health status of whiplash claimants may not reflect the actual health state. This speculation is arguably the result of the unverifiable nature of the injury itself and the concomitant reliance on self-reports of pain and disability. That is, the diagnosis relies on self-reported health status rather than the presence of discernible pathology.[42] Without pathoanatomical evidence of an injury, the possibility of claims for entirely or partially exaggerated injuries arises,[43] as does a concern that compensation for whiplash injuries leads to (presumably, unwarranted) compensation-seeking behaviour.[20]

Empirical studies provide some insight into claiming behaviour in the context of financial compensation. These show that the number of claims involving whiplash injuries increases when benefits are higher, such as, for example, in fault-based schemes where compensation may be sought for pain and suffering in addition to recompense for lost income and medical costs.[19, 21] Similarly, in the (generally) no-fault workers' compensation setting, an increase in compensation benefits has been shown to increase the number of claims and, more specifically, to increase the number of claims involving unverifiable injuries, such as sprains and strains.[44, 45]

Thus, there is evidence that asymmetric information of the kind that exists in relation to whiplash injuries, coupled with the potential for higher compensation benefits, increases the propensity to claim regardless of the scheme design. This may be characterised as evidence of *ex post* moral hazard. Regardless of whether the injury is 'real' or not, individuals will inevitably evaluate whether the marginal benefit of making a compensation claim is greater than the marginal cost of doing so.[46]

It has also been proposed that lawyers and health professionals may reinforce or enable *ex post* moral hazard in eligible claimants in order that they themselves might benefit from injury compensation payments.[47, 48] This may be viewed as a form of moral hazard on the part of suppliers, who, as a result of the information they hold, determine the nature and extent of services provided. Few studies have attempted to quantify this effect (as distinct from perfect agency), let alone considered the effects of related actions on health outcomes. The methodological problems in this literature again make it impossible to tell whether there is any substance to theories about the (allegedly iatrogenic) roles that some health professionals and some lawyers may play.

The frequency of pain simulation (or exaggeration) in a medicolegal context is unknown,[49] and the inherent difficulties in objectively verifying the soft tissue injuries typically suffered in road crashes arguably makes motor vehicle insurance fraud relatively inexpensive to perpetrate and costly to deter[50] and detect. Insurers, where permitted, attempt to curb such behaviour via the design features of insurance contracts, such as co-payment provisions, thresholds and caps on benefits, premium discounts or penalties, and through claims monitoring and audits.

Verifiable injuries

A strategy that some authors have used in an attempt to address the problem of hidden information about the underlying health state is to concentrate on compensation and health outcomes for verifiable injuries. Although there is less room to dispute an individual's eligibility for compensation when there is (presumably) verifiable evidence of an injury, the problem of moral hazard is not completely obviated by such designs. Individuals who are in the process of pursuing a compensation claim may still have an incentive not to reveal their true health state as the amount of damages may be inversely related to their recovery and prognosis. This could also occur, though, if individuals systematically understated their true health states, not as an attempt to defraud other parties, but as a rational strategy to win a settlement that approximates their true loss. Furthermore, even though such studies may use health states or injuries that are verifiable (e.g. fractures visible upon diagnostic imaging), the health state measures still tend to be self-reported.

One such study, a meta-analysis,[51] concluded that postoperative health outcomes were worse among people who received compensation compared to those who did not. Nonetheless, the quality of the 129 studies included in this meta-analysis was not appraised, most (75%) were not controlled studies, the measurement of health outcomes varied across studies and the method of dichotomising them as 'satisfactory' or 'unsatisfactory' is open to question, and conceptually different features, such as 'workers' compensation' and 'litigation', were pooled.[52] Thus, although this study contains a number of potential sources of bias in addition to the problems of selection bias and reverse causality described in this chapter, it is heralded as 'convincing evidence' that 'compensation' is associated with worse health outcomes.[5]

Use of proxy measures

Another approach to measuring the association between compensation and health has been to identify proxy measures of health status that are based on objective data—usually obtained from insurer or employer records—rather than to rely on self-reported data. The types of measures that have been used as health status (or inverse health status) proxies include the duration of compensation claims, time away from work, return-to-work and so on. While these data are objective and routinely collected (in contrast to data on health outcomes), their relationship with the underlying variable of interest—health—is questionable.

In a well-known study, Cassidy and colleagues attempted to link whiplash symptoms to claim duration,[21, 53] equating quicker claim resolution with faster recovery and concluding, henceforth, that switching to a no-fault scheme where claim duration is generally shorter will hasten recovery from whiplash. Freeman and colleagues[54] argue that this outcome could reasonably be expected, as claim durations for individuals with worse health outcomes and prognoses could be expected to be longer. The observation of a correlation between longer claim durations for individuals with poor health outcomes is consistent with the claim that compensation is bad for health, but it is also consistent with the hypotheses of selection bias (i.e. individuals with poor outcomes may be more likely to claim) and reverse causality (i.e. worse health outcomes lead to longer claim durations for those who do claim). The study by Cassidy and colleagues[21, 53] has also been criticised for, among other things, omitting consideration of reopened claims under the no-fault system (amounting to 28% of claims) in their analysis. The size of this omission implies that individuals subject to such a system may not have recovered to the extent implied. Merskey and Teasell[55] argue that claim files are commonly reopened in response to complaints from claimants that their case was closed even though their symptoms persist.

Proxy measures of health, such as claim duration, are generally unsuitable for research on the hypothesis that compensation is bad for health. Many variables other than the latent health state are likely to influence decisions about the duration of compensation claims[54] and the duration of absence from work.[56] For example, in some jurisdictions, workers' compensation payments fall from 100% income replacement to a fraction (say, 60% income replacement) after a certain period of time (e.g. three months). It would not be surprising to find that individuals return to work more quickly in such jurisdictions than in jurisdictions where the income replacement is more generous. It would, however, be erroneous to draw the conclusion that individuals in the jurisdiction with less generous compensation provisions returned to work sooner because they recovered more quickly. Rather, the motivation for earlier returns-to-work (i.e. a 40% income cut) may be purely financial and, perhaps in some cases, clinically premature.

For related reasons, the rate of recovery that is inferred from claims data may also be very different from that which is inferred from self-reported symptoms or disability.[57] Thus, the use or non-use of proxy measures for health may have an influence on the research findings and, in turn, decisions about the design of compensation laws. The conflicting results among systematic reviews of whiplash recovery present a case in point. Those reviews in which the authors have accepted claim duration as a proxy for recovery[14, 16] have concluded that compensation/legal factors/insurance constitute impediments to recovery. By contrast, the review by Scholten-Peeters et al.,[15] which excluded studies using proxy measures, found strong evidence of no association between compensation/litigation and health outcome measures.

However, in one recent study, a proxy measure was used as part of a clever design that avoids the pitfalls that can be associated with duration proxies. Leth-Petersen and Rotger[58] examined the long-term earnings of whiplash injury claimants in an attempt to discern whether compensation-seeking behaviour explained claims of chronic whiplash symptoms. The interesting aspects of this study's design are that: in Denmark, all such claims are assessed by an independent board of medical consultants and experts; and, in the event that a payment of compensation is made, it is irrevocable, so there is no financial incentive to remain out of the labour market. The latter characteristic, in particular, means that in the long run, individuals face strong incentives to return to their full income earning capacity (although the authors also acknowledge the possibility that the payment of compensation could enable compensated individuals to buy more leisure time and, hence, reduce their labour supply). Leth-Petersen and Rotger[58] compared pre-collision and post-collision earnings and found that individuals who were granted compensation experienced persistent reductions in earnings—long after their claims were settled—relative to earnings without whiplash exposure and this was true even when there was a strong financial incentive to not reduce earnings. These authors concluded that their evidence suggests that '… moderate whiplash injuries tend to be chronic, and that compensation-seeking behaviour is not the main explanation [of poorer health outcomes] for this group [of whiplash claimants]'.[58]

CONCLUSIONS

This chapter has highlighted several complex problems that are associated with trying to examine the effects of compensation on health. One source of difficulty, in the extant literature, is confusion about fundamental questions such as how best to define and measure compensation. Another problem is that good measures of health that cannot be manipulated for financial gain are difficult to identify. This problem is particularly acute for potentially compensable conditions, like whiplash injuries, that are not objectively verifiable. Additionally, because a range of factors is likely to influence the decision to make a claim for compensation, thereby affecting the constitution of the samples (e.g. compensated and uncompensated subjects) that are compared, there is a very real danger of bias in studies that make such comparisons without any attempt to control for sample selection problems. Each of these problems is serious. Individually and together, their impact is to limit the internal and external validity of the existing research on the question of whether compensation is bad for health.

As experimental research on this topic is unlikely to be feasible, the problems that have been outlined in this chapter are likely to persist. Yet the situation is far from hopeless: clever and purposeful study designs can limit the severity of these problems. Furthermore, when these problems cannot be eliminated by design, they should be addressed statistically, using the appropriate methods to control for the statistical consequences of reverse causality, sample selection and so on. This is a topic upon which we—and, we are sure, many others—will have much more to say.

RELEVANT INDEX TERMS

Index terms that are applicable to the issues discussed on compensation include: endogeneity, endogenous variable, exogenous variables, reverse causality, unobserved heterogeneity, sample selection, sample selection model, treatment effects, Heckman correction, and two-part model (2PM).

Index terms that are applicable to the discussion of health as a latent variable include: limited dependent variables, binary dependent variables, ordered dependent variables, discrete choice, probit, logit, ordered probit, ordered logit.

ACKNOWLEDGMENT

The authors gratefully acknowledge the helpful comments provided by Genevieve Grant, LLB, Melbourne Law School and Melbourne School of Population Health, The University of Melbourne, on an earlier draft of this chapter. The responsibility for any remaining errors rests with the authors.

References

1. Latimer P. Australian business law. 19th edn. Sydney: CCH Australia, 2000.
2. Arrow KJ. Uncertainty and the welfare economics of medical care. *Am Econ Rev* 1963;LIII:941–73.
3. Grant G & Studdert DM. Poisoned chalice? A critical analysis of the association between personal injury compensation processes and adverse health outcomes. University of Melbourne Legal Studies Research Paper No. 442. 2009. Online. Available at: http://ssrn.com/abstract=1520788.
4. NSW Parliament. Legislative Council. General Purpose Standing Committee No. 1: Inquiry into personal injury compensation law. Report 28. 2005. Online. Available at: http://www.nsw.gov.au/.
5. Cameron P & Gabbe B. The effect of compensation claims on outcomes after injury. *Injury* 2009;40(9): 905–6.
6. Butt P & Nygh P, eds. Butterworth's Encyclopaedic Australian Legal Dictionary Online. Online. Available at: http://www.lexisnexis.com.au/aus/products/catalog/current_htm/BEALD%20ONL.asp?productid=BEALD%20ONL&jurisdiction=0&category=27&medium=0&author=&title=&;overview=; June 2010.
7. Wright T & Melville A. Hey, but who's counting? The metrics and politics of trends in civil litigation. In: Prest W & Anleu S, eds. Litigation: past and present. Sydney: University of New South Wales Press, 2004.
8. Queensland Government Motor Accident Insurance Commission (MAIC). Statistical information 2009–10. Brisbane: Queensland Government. Online. Available at: http://www.maic.qld.gov.au/forms-publications-stats/pdfs/maic-stat-info-1209-1jul-31dec09.pdf.
9. Freeman MD, Croft AC, Rossignol AM, et al. A review and methodologic critique of the literature refuting whiplash syndrome. *Spine* 1999;24(1): 86–96.
10. Kwan O & Friel J. A review and methodologic critique of the literature supporting 'chronic whiplash injury': part I – research articles. *Med Sci Monit* 2003;9(8):RA203–15.
11. Levy H & Meltzer D. The impact of health insurance on health. *Annu Rev Public Health* 2008;29: 399–409.
12. Grimes D & Schulz K. Bias and causal associations in observational research. *Lancet* 2002;359:248–52.
13. Grimes D & Schulz K. Compared to what? Finding controls for case-control studies. *Lancet* 2005;365:1429–33.
14. Côté P, Cassidy JD, Carroll L, et al. A systematic review of the prognosis of acute whiplash and a new conceptual framework to synthesize the literature. *Spine* 2001;26(19):445–58.

15. Scholten-Peeters G, Verhagen A, Bekkering G, et al. Prognostic factors of whiplash-associated disorders: a systematic review of prospective cohort studies. *Pain* 2003;104:303–22.
16. Carroll L, Holm L, Hogg-Johnson S, et al. Course and prognostic factors for neck pain in whiplash-associated disorders (WAD): results of the Bone and Joint Decade 2000-2010 Task Force on Neck Pain and Its Associated Disorders. *Spine* 2008;33(4S):83–92.
17. Australian Government. Review of the Law of Negligence report. 2002. Online. Available at: http://revofneg.treasury.gov.au/content/review2.asp.
18. Rolph JE. Automobile accident compensation. Volume I: Who pays how much how soon? R-3050ICJ. Santa Monica: RAND Institute for Civil Justice, 1985.
19. Spitzer WO, Skovron ML, Salmi LR, et al. Scientific monograph of the Quebec Task Force on Whiplash-Associated Disorders: redefining 'whiplash' and its management. *Spine* 1995;20(8 Suppl):1S–73S.
20. Barnsley L, Lord S, Bogduk N. Whiplash injury. *Pain* 1994;58(3):283–307.
21. Cassidy D, Carroll L, Côté P, et al. Effect of eliminating compensation for pain and suffering on the outcome of insurance claims for whiplash injury. *N Engl J Med* 2000;342(16):1179–86.
22. Borchgrevink GE, Kaasa A, McDonagh D, et al. Acute treatment of whiplash neck sprain injuries: a randomized trial of treatment during the first 14 days after a car accident. *Spine* 1998;23:25–31.
23. Gun RT, Osti OL, O'Riordan A, et al. Risk factors for prolonged disability after whiplash injury: a prospective study. *Spine* 2005;30(4):386–91.
24. Dufton JA, Kopec JA, Wong H, et al. Prognostic factors associated with minimal improvement following acute whiplash-associated disorders. *Spine* 2006;31(20):E759–65.
25. Teasell RW. Compensation and chronic pain. *Clin J Pain* 2001;17(4S):S46–S51.
26. Cameron ID, Rebbeck T, Sindhusake D, et al. Legislative change is associated with improved health status in people with whiplash. *Spine* 2008;33(3):250–4.
27. Dunbar FC & Sabry F. The propensity to sue: why do people seek legal actions? *Business Econ* 2007;42(2):31–42.
28. Rosenman KD, Gardiner JC, Wang J, et al. Why most workers with occupational repetitive trauma do not file for workers' compensation. *J Occup Environ Med* 2000;42(1):25–34.
29. Bismark MM, Brennan TA, Davis PB, et al. Claiming behaviour in a no-fault system of medical injury: a descriptive analysis of claimants and non-claimants. *Med J Aust* 2006;185(4):203–7.
30. World Health Organization. WHO definition of health. Preamble to the Constitution of the World Health Organization as adopted by the International Health Conference, New York, 19–22 June, 1946; signed on 22 July 1946 by the representatives of 61 States (Official Records of the World Health Organization, no. 2, p. 100) and entered into force on 7 April 1948. Online. Available at: http://www.who.int/about/definition/en/print.html/.
31. Elliott J, Noteboom JT, Flynn TW, Sterling M. Characterization of acute and chronic whiplash-associated disorders. *Orthop Sports Phys Ther* 2009;39(5):312–23.
32. Australian Acute Musculoskeletal Pain Guidelines Group (AAMPGG). Evidence-based management of acute musculoskeletal pain. 2004. Canberra: NHMRC. Online: Available at: http://nhmrc.gov.au/publications/synopses /cp94syn.htm.
33. King W, Lau P, Lees R, et al. The validity of manual examination in assessing patients with neck pain. *Spine* 2007;7(1):22–6.
34. Pauly MV. The economics of moral hazard: comment. *Am Econ Rev* 1968;58:531–7.
35. Shavell R. On moral hazard and insurance. *Q J Econ* 1979;93(4):541–62.
36. Radanov BP, Sturzenegger M, Di Stefano G. Long-term outcome after whiplash injury. A 2-year follow-up considering features of injury mechanism and somatic, radiologic, and psychosocial findings. *Medicine* 1995;74(5):281–97.
37. Bogduk N & Teasell R. Whiplash: the evidence for an organic etiology. *Arch Neurol* 2000;57: 590–1.
38. Ferrari R, Kwan O, Russell AS, et al. The best approach to the problem of whiplash? One ticket to Lithuania, please. *Clin Exp Rheumatol* 1999;17(3):321–6.
39. Schrader H, Obelieniene D, Bovim G, et al. Natural evolution of late whiplash syndrome outside the medicolegal context. *Lancet* 1996;347(9010): 1207–11.
40. Balla JI. The late whiplash syndrome: a study of an illness in Australia and Singapore. *Cult Med Psychiatry* 1982;6(2):191–210.
41. Castro WH, Meyer SJ, Becke ME, et al. No stress—no whiplash? Prevalence of 'whiplash' symptoms following exposure to a placebo rear-end collision. *Int J Legal Med* 2001;114(6):316–22.
42. Sterner Y & Gerdle B. Acute and chronic whiplash disorders—a review. *J Rehabil Med* 2004;36(5): 193–209.
43. Ferrari R. Myths of whiplash. *Surgeon* 2003;1(2):99, 101–3.

44. Fortin B & Lanoie P. Substitution between unemployment insurance and workers' compensation. *J Public Econ* 1992;49:287–312.
45. Dionne G & St-Michel P. Workers' compensation and moral hazard. *Rev Econ Stat* 1991;73:236–44.
46. Cummins JD & Tennyson S. Moral hazard in insurance claiming: evidence from automobile insurance. *J Risk Uncertain* 1996;12(1):29–50.
47. Ferrari R & Russell A. Epidemiology of whiplash. *Ann Rheum Dis* 1999;58:1–5.
48. Kwan O, Ferrari R, Friel J. Tertiary gain and disability syndromes. *Med Hypotheses* 2001;56:77–84.
49. Mendelson G & Mendelson D. Malingering pain in the medicolegal context. *Clin J Pain* 2004;20(6):423–32.
50. Loughran D. Deterring fraud: the role of general damage awards in automobile insurance settlements. *J Risk Insur* 2005;72(4):551–75.
51. Harris I, Mulford J, Solomon M, et al. Association between compensation status and outcome after surgery: a meta-analysis. *JAMA* 2005;293:1644–52.
52. Spearing NM & Connelly LB. Is compensation "bad for health"? A systematic meta-review. *Injury* 2010;41(7):683–92.
53. Côté P, Hogg-Johnson S, Cassidy JD, et al. The association between neck pain intensity, physical functioning, depressive symptomatology and time-to-claim-closure after whiplash. *J Clin Epidemiol* 2001;54(3):275–86.
54. Freeman M, Centeno C, Merskey H, et al A. Greater injury leads to more treatment for whiplash: no surprises here (letter). *Arch Intern Med* 2006;166:1238–9.
55. Merskey H & Teasell RW. Comment: Effect of eliminating compensation for pain and suffering on the outcome of insurance claims. *N Engl J Med* 2000;343(15):1119.
56. Baldwin M, Johnson W, Butler R. The error of using returns to work to measure the outcomes of health care. *Am J Indust Med* 1996;29:632–41.
57. Rebbeck T, Sindhusake D, Cameron I, et al. A prospective cohort study of health outcomes following whiplash associated disorders in an Australian population. *Inj Prev* 2006;12:93–8.
58. Leth-Petersen S & Rotger GP. Long-term labour market performance of whiplash claimants. *J Health Econ* 2009;28:996–1011.

Further reading

Readers who are interested in the statistical consequences of, and solutions to, the problems outlined are encouraged to refer to the following sources:

Angrist JD & Pischke JS. Mostly harmless econometrics. Princeton: Princeton University Press, 2009.

Greene WH. Econometric analysis. 6th edn. Upper Saddle River, NJ: Prentice Hall, 2008.

Wooldridge JM. Econometric analysis of cross section and panel data. Cambridge, MA: MIT Press, 2002.

Wooldridge JM. Introductory econometrics: a modern approach. 4th edn. Mason, OH: Thomson South-Western, 2009.

CHAPTER 15
Whiplash and the law

Ian Freckelton S.C.

Compensation law has intersected with whiplash injuries in a number of ways. None have been comfortable. Claims arising from what are described as whiplash associated disorders (WAD) constitute one of the issues that generate fundamental disagreement between plaintiff and defence lawyers when civil claims are made for pecuniary compensation. As whiplash injuries a number of years after a traumatic incident are generally not radiologically demonstrable, and are principally ligamentous or soft tissue injuries, they are an example of the experience of pain which often cannot be proved empirically and, thus, may, in principle, be psychogenic, embellished or fabricated.

The law deals with facts that can be proved by admissible evidence, not speculation. It is dyadic. A fact is either proved or not proved in court. A failure to prove, on the balance of probabilities, an injury that is the subject of a compensation application results in the plaintiff/claimant losing the case and paying the costs of the defendant/s (save in the United States, where the 'costs rule' does not apply). Because of the exigencies of proof for fact-finding, the law is mistrustful of, and does not grapple easily with, phenomena (such as whiplash) that cannot be visualised, objectively validated and/or measured. These considerations influence the conduct of litigation involving whiplash injuries, decision-making about them and the formulation of statutory policies about the compensability of such injuries.

This chapter outlines how the legal system, in a number of contexts, has dealt with the award of compensation for whiplash injuries and the potentially counter-therapeutic effects of the legal system for those who sustain whiplash injuries and seek compensation for them. It concludes by briefly exploring the human rights repercussions of a statutory experiment in Alberta, Canada, to curtail the compensability of whiplash and what it designated to be other 'minor injuries'.

THE TEST FOR COMPENSABILITY

The orthodox position for determining compensation in personal injury cases was summarised by McHugh J in *Nominal Defendant v Gardikiotis [1995] HCA 56;* (1996) 186 CLR 49 at 54:

> When a defendant has negligently injured a plaintiff, the common law requires the defendant to pay a money sum to the plaintiff to compensate that person for any damage that is causally connected to the defendant's negligence and that ought to have been reasonably foreseen by the defendant when the negligence occurred. The sum of money to be paid to the plaintiff is that sum which will put the plaintiff, so far as is possible, 'in the same position as he would have been in if he had not sustained the wrong for which he is now getting his compensation'.

In some situations there are multiple incidents or aetiologies that resulted or may have resulted in the ultimate symptomatology experienced by a patient (e.g. see *Amaca Pty Ltd v Ellis* [2010] HCA 5). The law is that where the negligence of a defendant causes an injury and the plaintiff subsequently suffers a further injury, where the further injury results from a subsequent accident that would have occurred had the plaintiff been in normal health, but the damage sustained is greater because of aggravation of the earlier injury, the additional damage resulting from the aggravating injury is treated as caused by the defendant's negligence (see *State Government Insurance Commission v Oakley* (1990) Aust Torts Reps 81-003 at 67,577; *Gerada v Fitzgerald* [2008] ACTSC 56 at [107]). Thus, a tortfeasor (a person or entity committing a tort, namely a civil wrong, such as negligence) is regarded as responsible for the extent to which the tortfeasor worsens the state of a victim.

Identifying the damage

It is pain and suffering and loss of amenity of life, as well as economic sequelae, caused by a tort (usually arising from a breach of care, but also on occasion by intentional acts) which are compensated by the civil courts. They need to be established by admissible evidence on the balance of probabilities. Thus, proof of the existence and the extent of an injury, as well as what caused it, are subjected to forensic scrutiny, including assessment of expert evidence,[1] to ascertain the legitimacy of a plaintiff's claims of injury.

A difficulty that arises with asserted whiplash injuries is that, frequently, whiplash cases come to court without clear concomitants of objectively measurable physical injury. As Underwood J put it in *Hoare v Pritchard* [1997] TASSC 94 at p1: 'The plaintiff suffered a "whiplash" injury to her cervical spine. As is so often the case with this injury, there is neither clinical nor radiological evidence of physiological damage'. This can raise the 'index of suspicion' and result in judicial cynicism in the face of expert evidence from medical practitioners who hold legitimately differing views about the ongoing symptomatology of the plaintiff and its aetiology or aetiologies.

There have been many expressions of judicial approach on the subject. Frequently, defendants over the past decade have called neurologists, general surgeons and neurosurgeons to opine that, in the absence of objective radiological evidence, it is unlikely that a plaintiff's traumatic injury, which was initially a whiplash injury, could be causing the ongoing impairment asserted by the plaintiff unless such pain is psychiatric in nature or is the subject of malingering. By contrast, plaintiffs have tended to call general practitioners, chiropractors, osteopaths, physiotherapists, rehabilitation physicians and pain management practitioners to contend that their whiplash injuries have resulted in an ongoing restriction of movement, functionality and an experience of pain. The ideological divide between such camps of health practitioners has been deep. However, an end to this unfortunate difference of approach may be signalled in *Guerrero v Fukuda*, 2008 CanLII 49158 (ON SC) at [3]-[5], where Little J of the Ontario Supreme Court observed that:

> ... we have transcended the era when whiplash, due to the fact that it is often without objective findings, was equated with faking. A whole specialty in medicine now exists dealing with physical medicine and rehabilitation. This is sometimes referred to as physiatry. Experts in this field are relied upon by litigants often. They do not rely upon the expert for treatment or rehab but rather to determine whether or not the expert believes pain exists. Pain, and its degree of severity, are subjective and can exist without any objective finding. Calling an expert to say that no objective finding equals no pain is no longer acceptable. That same expert will often *treat* the pain that exists even though it is without objective findings.

Typical case example

The decision of the Tasmanian Supreme Court in *Luttrell v McLennan* [2005] TASSC 79 remains orthodox for Australian law. The 43-year-old employed plaintiff was driving her motor vehicle, which came to a halt in heavy traffic. The defendant negligently drove into the rear of her vehicle, causing what she asserted was a whiplash injury. She sued for damages. She was admitted to hospital, examined in an outpatients' department and released on the same day with a cervical collar. After the accident she maintained that she was unable to return to full-time employment. She asserted that she continued until the trial to experience pain and discomfort on the left side of her neck, the left shoulder, the left arm, the left hand, and the ring finger and little finger of the left hand. She developed a tendency to lift the left shoulder to make herself more comfortable. According to her account, her level of pain and discomfort fluctuated but were exacerbated by exertion, or by repeated minor physical movements while maintaining a fixed physical position. Since the accident she was prescribed anti-inflammatory medication and pain killers. In the aftermath of the accident, she asserted, her symptoms interfered with:

- her ability to undertake physical activity with her grandchildren
- her capacity to undertake housework
- her ability to undertake activities associated with horses.

She gave evidence that her symptoms and their consequences, particularly the loss of full-time employment, caused her considerable frustration and distress, but she did not assert a specific psychological or psychiatric abnormality.

The plaintiff received treatment from a variety of medical practitioners, including family doctors, rheumatologists, anaesthetists, pain management specialists and others. Her principal witness diagnosed her as having suffered a whiplash injury which led to an ongoing chronic pain condition. The principal witness for the defence, by contrast, opined that the plaintiff had no objectively demonstrable physical injury and that it was the legal process and her attitude that were precluding her from rejoining the workforce.

Justice Blow preferred the evidence of the plaintiff's medical experts and expressed concern about the inclination of the main defence expert to trespass outside his area of expertise into the domains of psychiatry and psychology. He accepted that most patients who suffer whiplash find that their symptoms resolve relatively quickly but found that this fact did not mean that the plaintiff did not continue to suffer from such symptomatology or that the symptoms which she did still experience had another aetiology. He ordered damages of A$323,000 for the plaintiff.

Credibility dilemmas

A corollary of the absence of objective evidence in many whiplash cases is that courts are propelled into assessing the credibility of the plaintiff's account, recognising that litigants will have a financial motivation either to fabricate or to exaggerate (deliberately or unintentionally) in order to optimise the financial outcome from their compensation litigation. A result is that the assertions of plaintiffs both to courts and to forensic assessors, and even to treaters, have come to be examined with particular care to evaluate consistencies and their obverse. This raises the issue of both the reliability of the history and narrative of plaintiffs and the probative value of the opinions held by professionals who give evidence to the court. Such opinions, inevitably, are heavily dependent upon what they are told by treaters' and third-party assessors' patients, as well as upon the symptoms that they identify. When the presentation of patients to third-party assessors and even to those providing them with treatment is taking place in the shadow of the courts and patients are aware that everything that they do or say may be the subject of the drawing of inferences, there is the risk of distortion.

Such distortion has a number of components. There is the risk that a plaintiff may consciously or unconsciously embrace a sick role in order to enhance their claim. Litigation tends, in most jurisdictions, to be a once and for all exercise, with plaintiffs having just the one opportunity to prove their case. This can propel unscrupulous plaintiffs to fabricate or deliberately exaggerate and it can also encourage genuine plaintiffs to focus more upon their state of unwellness or pain than upon what they can do to relieve their symptomatology and recover. To this extent the litigation phenomenon can militate against wellness, inhibit recovery and be counter-therapeutic.

In addition, there is the risk that in what is a stressful situation, in order to communicate effectively their symptomatology, patients may over-describe or over-emphasise their experience of pain and their levels of impairment. This can arise from a concern that without such a presentation, their real experience may be discounted or not adequately taken into account by treaters, assessors and fact-finders alike.

As well, there is always the potential for plaintiffs to attribute to a specific incident a variety of the adverse aspects of their lives, resulting in excessive allocation to the one perhaps tortious incident (e.g. a traumatic motor vehicle injury) a range of symptoms which, strictly speaking, may not be clinical sequelae and may have independent aetiologies. This is a question of causation in which indirect connections and influences can complicate what might otherwise have been a more straightforward clinical course. Disentangling the strands of causation is ultimately more of a legal exercise than a medical one but the vicissitudes of what can be unhappy lives, made worse by a traumatic injury, can be difficult to unravel, especially in the environment of litigation.

In *Vlad v TAC* [2002] VCAT 1298 at [63] a number of these issues arose. Member Preuss of the Victorian Civil and Administrative Tribunal heard extensive expert evidence about a variety of conditions said to be suffered by an applicant for compensation. Ultimately, she rejected key evidence for the applicant for compensation, holding that the expert's evidence carried little weight:

> ... having regard to the fact that he obtained an inaccurate history from the applicant as to his past medical history. In this regard, the applicant told Dr V that, prior to the accident, he had no persistent headaches or lower back pain, contrary to Dr B's evidence. Further, Dr V based his opinion in part on the assumption that the applicant lost consciousness at the time of the accident. This was not the initial history he obtained from the applicant and, in fact, the evidence does not establish any loss of consciousness.

In the search for yardsticks to evaluate plaintiffs' credibility, a number of factors can be resorted to by courts, either covertly or explicitly. There is the risk of what Perlin,[2] in another context, has called 'pretextuality', in which assumptions and ideological positions significantly influence decision-making. The hint that this is occurring can emerge from the language employed by decision-makers. Thus, in a case in the Australian Capital Territory (*Spasovska v Nominal Defendant* [2005] ACTSC 2 at [49]), Master Harper found that 'the plaintiff comes from a cultural and ethnic background where it is common to find an abnormal perception of pain and abnormal emotional reaction to trauma and injury ... Queanbeyan has a large ethnic Macedonian community'. He appeared to attach significance to this factor—detrimentally to the interests of the plaintiff. Another way in which such 'moral biases' can affect the deliberative process can be in the expectation that injured plaintiffs will make active attempts to 'recover' and 'rejoin the workforce' to return to 'breadwinner' status for their families, rather than become resigned to their pain or to 'assume a sick role'.

Ongoing symptomatology

A challenge for plaintiffs is to prove the continuing symptomatology of whiplash injuries in light of the fact that the preponderance of clinical opinion is that most such injuries improve relatively quickly. This issue was summed up by the NSW Court of Appeal in *Werner v Krahe* [2002] NSWCA 168 at [12]:

> ... whiplash injuries to the neck, generally speaking, resolve and become symptom free with the passage of time, some quickly and some more slowly. Some lead to chronic pain and disability. There are marked differences in the severity and duration of pain occasioned by such injuries.

A risk exists that because most whiplash injuries resolve within two years, decision-makers will approach their fact-finding task unduly critically or cynically when litigants assert ongoing symptomatology in the absence of radiological corroboration. From time to time, witnesses for defendants/insurers refer to literature asserting that in countries which do not have schemes for compensation, whiplash injuries resolve promptly, in an attempt to bolster the argument that a plaintiff is either malingering or engaging in an attempt to hoodwink the decision-maker/s (e.g. see *Horvath v Rajic* [2001] QDC 358). However, this tactic is generally found by courts to be of limited assistance when decisions need to be made in specific cases.

The risk of undue suspicion on the part of decision-makers can manifest in terms of assessment of credibility or the drawing of adverse inferences from the nature of the traumatic incident asserted to have precipitated the injury. An article by Freeman et al.[3] is commonly cited on behalf of plaintiffs (e.g. see *Nash v Berton* [2001] SASC 94):

> ... One of the more frequently disputed conditions in the medical literature in recent decades is the constellation of symptoms comprising acute whiplash and its chronic iteration, late whiplash (collectively known as whiplash syndrome). The primary reason for the dispute stems from the fact that the validity of whiplash syndrome often is a key issue in litigation arising from the alleged etiology of the whiplash, i.e., a motor vehicle crash in which the injured party is not at fault. The judge and/or jury in such cases are asked to weigh opposing medical and scientific evidence supporting both the plaintiff's position that whiplash injuries and their sequelae are real and the defense position that the injuries are manufactured or greatly exaggerated. ... As a result of the current literature review, it was determined that there is no epidemiologic or scientific basis in the literature for the following statements, whiplash injuries do not lead to chronic pain, rear impact collisions that do not result in vehicle damage are unlikely to cause injury and whiplash trauma is biomechanically comparable with common movements of daily living.

The psychogenic issue

A recurrent issue that arises in the course of whiplash litigation is whether the injuries asserted are to be regarded as physical or psychiatric/psychological. From the defendant's perspective, if the injuries fall into the latter category, there is the risk that they are being exaggerated or even fabricated. At the very least, courts tend to regard non-somatic injuries with greater suspicion than those that are either physical or caused by physical difficulties. In a number of jurisdictions, the barriers for compensation are higher for non-somatic injuries than for purely physical injuries. Thus, a diagnosis such as 'whiplash injury' that has 'developed into' or 'now manifests as' chronic pain syndrome, fibromyalgia, regional pain syndrome or abnormal illness behaviour (or even 'whole body vibration syndrome': see Decision No: 2009-888, 2009 CanLII 55051 (AB WCAC)) can prompt particular hesitation in judges. In such a scenario, there is a causation issue about the relationship between, first, the initial incident and the whiplash injury and, then, between the whiplash injury and the later presenting symptomatology. Unusual vulnerability of plaintiffs—who might not be accounted as of 'ordinary robustness' or 'normal fortitude'—can emerge to impede plaintiffs' claims for what becomes more a question of either a primary or a secondary psychiatric injury than a physical injury. This can be overt or can be an indirect prejudice to which appeal is made by defendants.

In 1994 the International Association for the Study of Pain defined two types of chronic regional pain syndrome (CRPS), the first associated without an observable lesion (CRPS type 1) and the second associated with an observable nerve lesion (CRPS type II). In *Bell v Accident Compensation Corporation* [2007] NZACC 12, a case dealing with whiplash injuries that allegedly had developed into a regional pain syndrome, Judge Ongley observed (at [29]) that:

> Remembering which is which, Type 1 or II, has proved a problem, so the customary nomenclature

> has been to add a basic diagnostic term to the phrase, to distinguish those who have a clear origin. Thus the broad term 'chronic regional pain syndrome' is used where no disease or injury has been diagnosed as the origin.
>
> This option is not available to psychiatrists. They are asked to specify their diagnosis in terms of DSM-IV, the Diagnostic and Statistical Manual of Mental Disorders, of the American Psychiatric Association. They must always specify a cause (p 499 DSM-IV) for the pain syndrome, the possibility that one cannot be identified has not been left open to them.
>
> Thus the term 'pain syndrome', when used without a qualifying phrase, has no signs and is without an underlying medical diagnosis. It can only be based on what the patient tells you, not on observation.

He concluded that the opinions of various of the experts called on behalf of the plaintiff rested:

> … strongly on the foundation that the [plaintiff] suffered a severe whiplash injury, a proposition for which there is no evidence apart from the appellant's history given some years later in support of a claim. Until Dr W examined the [plaintiff], there was no documented association between the whiplash and pain symptoms which reached a severe level some five years after the motor vehicle accident. None of the doctors had earlier drawn such a conclusion. (at [35])

The plaintiff lost.

Such issues are exacerbated if expert assessors do not personally examine the person claiming to have the whiplash injury or if they provide no clinical findings to justify their diagnosis, instead basing it upon electroencephalogram (EEG) analysis, psychological testing and the history as provided by the claimant. This can result in their views being given little or no weight (e.g. see Decision No: 2009-888, 2009 CanLII 55051 (AB WCAC)).

CANADIAN TRANSPORT ACCIDENT COMPENSATION

A number of legislative attempts have been made to reduce the compensability of WAD and, thereby, disincentives that have been asserted by some to exist for persons to recover quickly from such injuries. This is often said to be done in order to preserve the viability of insurance schemes in the motor vehicle context.

In this regard, the compensation scheme related to motor vehicle accidents in Canada is described below, with a particular emphasis upon the system in force in Alberta and the legal controversies (including those in relation to human rights) that have latterly attended it.

In Canada, the provinces have different systems with respect to compensation for transport accidents, including for whiplash injuries (see *Morrow v Zhang* [2008] 5 WWR 285 at [58]ff). There are two principal categories: the supplementation of the common law tort system, and its replacement. The first category includes the add-on no-fault schemes under which an insured driver is entitled to some first-party no-fault benefits, but under which the right to sue negligent third parties is preserved. The second category includes threshold and pure no-fault schemes. Under threshold schemes, there is total exclusion or a limitation of tort actions below some defined threshold, either 'verbal' or 'monetary'. A verbal threshold relates to the type or severity of the injury. Thus, when there is a verbal threshold, the injury must meet certain criteria in order to trigger the right to sue. Finally, in pure no-fault schemes, in return for first-party benefits, the right to sue in tort is extinguished.

The provinces of Manitoba, Quebec and Saskatchewan have a publicly run pure no-fault regime. For these provinces, in return for relatively generous first-party no-fault benefits, motor vehicle accident victims forgo the right to sue negligent drivers for their injuries. The Quebec regime includes scheduled no-fault impairment benefits, to which claimants are entitled, in addition to economic losses: *The Manitoba Public Insurance Corporation Act*, CCSM c. P215; *The Automobile Accident Insurance Act*, RSS 1978, c. A-35; *Automobile Insurance Act*, RSQ, c. A-25). In Saskatchewan, residents can also opt out of the regime and choose the tort coverage instead of the no-fault coverage.

The provinces of Newfoundland and Labrador, Nova Scotia, Prince Edward Island, New Brunswick, Ontario and Alberta have adopted a threshold no-fault system of motor vehicle accident insurance. In Newfoundland and Labrador, there is no threshold, but there is a C$2500 deductible for pain and suffering (*Automobile Insurance Act*, RSNL 1990, c. A-22, s. 39.1; *Automobile Insurance Regulations*, NLR 81/04, s. 6). The provinces of Nova Scotia, New Brunswick and Prince Edward Island have C$2500 caps on recovery for non-pecuniary losses that are tied to a definition of minor injury. This means that recovery in tort systems for pain and suffering damages is restricted to a cap (*Insurance Act*, RSNS 1989, c. 231, ss. 5 (na) and 113B; *Automobile Insurance Tort Recovery Limitation Regulations*, NS Reg 182/2003, s. 3; *Insurance Act,* RSNB 1973, c. I-12, s. 265.21 and 267.9; *Injury Regulation – Insurance Act*, NB Reg 2003-20, s. 4; *Insurance Act*, RSPEI 1988, c. I-4, s. 254.1). In Ontario, the right to sue for pain and suffering is permitted only if a threshold is met: where the injured person dies or sustains permanent and serious disfigurement or if the injured person sustains an impairment of important physical, mental or psychological function. In these cases, the right to sue is subject to a C$30,000 deductible (C$15,000 if a *Family Law Act*, RSO 1990, c. F-3 claim). In British Columbia and the three territories, the regime in place is an add-on no-fault system that provides for a range of first-party no-fault benefits and an unconstrained right to sue negligent third parties for pain and suffering (*Insurance (Vehicle) Act*, RSBC 1996 c. 231; *Insurance (Vehicle) Regulation*, BC Reg 447/83; *Insurance Act*, RSY 2002, c. 119; *Schedule of Benefits*, Y OIC 1988/90; *Insurance Act*, RSNWT 1988, c. I-4; *Insurance Act (Nunavut)*, RSNWT 1988, c. I-4, as duplicated for Nunavut by s. 29 of the *Nunavut Act*, SC 1993, c. 28).

In 2004, Alberta passed innovative legislation that was stated to be drafted to address concerns from insurers and the public, including the rising cost of motor vehicle insurance premiums and an increase in uninsured drivers. One of the legislative reforms was the *Minor Injury Regulation*, AR 123/2004 (MIR), which, among other things, imposed a C$4000 cap on non-pecuniary damages for minor injuries as defined under the MIR. This specifically included WAD. The MIR was enacted as part of a scheme of legislation that included protocols for diagnosing and treating 'minor injuries', increases in certain medical benefits, and caps on motor vehicle insurance premiums for all Albertans.

The Alberta approach

The question of whether the Alberta approach is consistent with the Canadian Charter of Human Rights and Freedoms arose in *Morrow v Zhang* (2008) 5 WWR 285, where Wittmann ACJ was called upon to analyse the changes made by the MIR and to evaluate its repercussions. He observed that in the years leading up to 2008, the private passenger class of motor vehicle insurance for all coverages had come to represent about 75–80% of the total motor vehicle insurance in Alberta as measured by premium volume. In Alberta, car insurance has been compulsory since 1972, with each vehicle being required to carry a basic coverage of a minimum of C$200,000 third-party liability coverage, no-fault accident or 'Section B coverage' for medical, funeral expense and death, total disability benefits, as well as uninsured motorist coverage (*Insurance Act*, ss. 608, 627, 629 and 640). Premiums for compulsory coverage are determined by the Alberta Automobile Insurance Board (AIB).

In the late 1980s to the mid 1990s, Alberta experienced 'a hard market' in motor vehicle insurance (where there is not strong competition among insurers and where premiums tend to rise) but from the mid-1990s to 2001, the property casualty insurance market in Canada, including Alberta, was in a period of soft market. From that time, markets in Canada, including Alberta, entered into another hard market period, which peaked approximately in 2003. During that period, private passenger motor vehicle insurance premiums rose quite sharply in Alberta. Motor vehicle insurance became less available as the insurance markets tightened, and property casualty insurance profitability significantly improved. Many Albertans who had previously been insured through the conventional markets were denied coverage and had no choice but to turn to non-standard insurance companies.

In March 2003, 'Bill 33' was tabled in Alberta. It would have implemented tort reforms to address, among other things, basing loss of income awards on net, rather than gross income in the calculation of damages for lost income. The government was faced with significant opposition and decided to conduct further consultations on a broader range of possible options to address problems in the mandatory motor vehicle insurance regime, rather than to proceed with Bill 33. The options it considered included: not making any changes to the existing system, a no-fault insurance scheme, caps on claims, deductibles, public delivery (either tort, no-fault or both), increased accident benefit limits and caps on premiums. An analysis of insurance systems in other provinces was completed at this time.

In Alberta, in the mid-1990s up to approximately 1999, bodily injury costs increased. However, from 1999 to 2001 there was a decrease, and then, from 2001 to 2002 there was another increase. Bodily injury costs decreased from 2002 to 2005. To the extent that, overall, there was an increase in such costs in Alberta, as well as in other Canadian provinces, it was regarded as attributable to increasing amounts awarded for non-pecuniary damages. As well, the proportion of claims that were specifically for minor soft tissue injuries appeared to be significant (at [78]).

In 1991, the AIB undertook a study in order to determine whether there was a problem with premium instability and, if there was, whether the cure was to modify its tort and no-fault features.[4] The study outlined problems related to the rise in awards for non-pecuniary damages. It found that 47.7% of compensation for third-party liability claims consisted of non-pecuniary damages, and that this figure rose to 83.1% for claims under C$10,000, and was 57.1% for claims over C$10,000 up to C$75,000. However, it was only 18.2% for claims over C$75,000 (*Morrow v Zhang* (2008) 5 WWR 285 at [82]). The AIB study observed that, since 1985, loss costs had increased dramatically and concluded that the main reason for the increase in claims costs was the increase in bodily injury loss costs and that most of these costs resulted from non-pecuniary damage claims.

The AIB opined that, when compared to other traffic accident claims, minor injury victims, in particular those asserting whiplash injuries, were overcompensated on the tort side of the system and that claimants with catastrophic injuries were undercompensated. It examined two methods that could flatten or reduce future premium costs. The first method was a series of government measures, which would reduce severity and frequency of accident costs. The second method was a mechanism to adjust the amount of monetary compensation, which would control premium increases. The AIB recommended the implementation of tort reforms, including a limitation upon the right of recovery for non-pecuniary damage claims under a deductible of C$10,000 or a restriction of tort rights to only the most serious injury claims. It also suggested that the government consider the possibility of a full no-fault system (*Morrow v Zhang* (2008) 5 WWR 285 at [84]).

The concern regarding the increase of non-pecuniary damages was also shared by other provinces. In fact, non-pecuniary damages appear to have been a significant part of bodily injury loss costs in New Brunswick, Nova Scotia and Newfoundland. Studies conducted by the Insurance Bureau of Canada (IBC) in New Brunswick and Nova Scotia, with a sample of claims closed in 2001, showed that for claims of C$20,000 or less, about 80% of total settlement amounts were for pain and suffering. These results appear to be very similar to the Alberta situation when compared to the 1991 or 2006 closed claim study. In New Brunswick, soft tissue injury claims only, with no other injuries, were found to represent 61% of all bodily injury and 39% of the money paid out. Also, when considering all claims, 61% of the total settlement amount was for pain and suffering. The closed claim study conducted in Nova Scotia concluded that 67% of all claims settlement amounts were for pain and suffering. In addition, soft tissue injury claims accounted for 70% of all bodily injury insurance claims, as well as 56% of the money paid out (*Morrow v Zhang* (2008) 5 WWR 285 at [85]-[86]).

The analysis of Alberta claims closed in April and May of 2004 showed that non-pecuniary damages were even more significant in Alberta, when compared to the 1991 closed claim study.[4] Indeed, the 2006 closed claim study revealed that 70.8% of the total settlement amounts were for pain and suffering. It also indicated that 62% of the claimants made claims only for soft tissue strains or sprains of the neck, back or other body parts and received 43% of the total settlement amounts.

In November 2003, Bill 53, which was the enabling legislation for the Alberta insurance reforms, was introduced (*Insurance Amendment Act, 2003 (No 2),* SA 2003, c. 40). It came into force on 1 October 2004 (see *Morrow v Zhang*, 2009 ABCA 215). A key component was the capping of general damages for pain and suffering at C$4000 with respect to 'minor injuries', which were defined as sprains, strains and minor WAD caused by an accident arising from the use or operation of a motor vehicle, that did not result in 'serious impairment' (*Morrow v Zhang* (2008) 5 WWR 285 at [93]). The scheme does not limit claims for economic loss incurred following a motor vehicle accident.

Before the insurance reforms, there were no protocols with respect to minor injuries, and the maximum amount recoverable for medical and rehabilitation costs was set at C$10,000. The new scheme increased this amount. Expert evidence before Wittmann ACJ was that the increase under Section B had proved to be a positive change. However, he noted that:

> … the benchmark study conducted pre reform in anticipation of the introduction of reforms to Section B, as well as the post reform studies, specifically show that Minor Injury victims generally claimed or received significantly less than $10,000 for medical and rehabilitation loss costs.' (at [95])

Expert evidence before him established that in the first 12 weeks after the reforms, the cost per treatment rose, which might have been expected considering that some providers may have seen an opportunity to raise their charges. The second post-reform study showed this situation then moderated, probably because fee guidelines were introduced.

Following the implementation of the regulations, the scheme was subject to review and follow-up studies. Wittmann ACJ found that:

> the portion of claimants not receiving health services in the first 12 weeks following their injury declined from almost 10% (in the benchmark study conducted pre reform) to 2.6% in the second post reform study. Similarly, for the first 26 weeks following the injury the two studies indicated a decline from 5.9% in the benchmark study to 2.1% in the second post reform study. The average medical rehabilitation cost for the first 12 weeks for those claimants who received care was $841 in the second post reform study, representing a 15% increase from the benchmark study. The average number of healthcare visits in the first 12 weeks following injury increased for each successive study, from 11.5 in the benchmark study to 13.5 in the second post reform study. Finally, the costs per treatment decreased by more than 13.5%. The number of claims that remained open following 26 weeks decreased from 71% in the benchmark study compared with 41.5% in the second post reform study. (at [100])

He found that the evidence established that, in the years preceding the insurance reforms, the government of Alberta had good reason to be concerned about the significance of non-pecuniary damages with respect to bodily injury costs. However, he noted that it was also apparent that motor accident premiums in Canada did not vary solely as a function of bodily injury costs, such as those generated by claims for WAD. There were other significant factors that influenced the rates, including the cyclical nature of the insurance market which, if not regulated, would affect premiums differently depending on whether the period is a soft market or a hard market.

The discrimination controversy

In a series of cases the Alberta insurance reforms have been challenged on the basis of their being said to constitute an illegitimate form of discrimination against people suffering soft tissue injuries. In *Morrow v Zhang* (2008) 5 WWR 285 it was contended before Wittman ACJ (at first instance) that the reforms also breached section 7 of the Canadian Charter of Rights and Freedoms, which states that 'Everyone has the right to life, liberty and security of the person and the right not to be deprived thereof except in accordance with the principles of fundamental justice'. The plaintiffs contended that the scheme affected people who suffer soft tissue injuries in two adverse ways: by removing their right to sue tortfeasors for damages for pain and suffering exceeding C$4000 and by the cap having a negative effect in practice on the ability of the right to choose, in an unfettered manner, what medical treatment is appropriate following a motor vehicle crash. Claimants who failed to comply with the scheme's regulations without a 'reasonable excuse', they asserted, and were later diagnosed as 'seriously impaired', as defined in the MIR, could suffer financial consequences. They argued that this feature of the MIR interferes with soft tissue injury victims' physical integrity and their ability to control their own body, and removed the physicians' discretion. Put another way, they contended that the MIR could not coerce injury victims into medical treatment by imposing a 'potential financial penalty' without infringing section 7 of the Charter. Wittmann ACJ, however, found that these arguments were misconceived on the basis that section 7 does not protect the civil right to bring an action for personal injury and that there is no general constitutional right to counsel. He also found no deprivation of the plaintiffs' right to security.

More significantly, it was also argued by the plaintiffs that the scheme breaches section 15 of the Charter, which provides that 'Every individual is equal before and under the law and has the right to the equal protection and equal benefit of the law without discrimination and, in particular, without discrimination based on race, national or ethnic origin, colour, religion, sex, age or mental or physical disability'. Wittmann ACJ found that the essence of the MIR scheme was to treat minor accident victims differently and less beneficially than other accident victims. He accepted that minor injury victims:

> … particularly those suffering whiplash associated disorder, are subjected to stereotyping and prejudice. In sum they are often viewed as malingerers who exaggerate their injuries or their effects in an effort to gain financially. The fact that these injuries are often not objectively verifiable may contribute to this perception. (at [205])

He noted too (at [206]) that the existence of this stereotype was aptly demonstrated in an excerpt from

Alberta Hansard, 7 April 2004, where MLA Masyk stated, in the context of a debate concerning Bill 204 Insurance (*Accident Insurance Benefits Amendment Act, 2003*):

> Mr. Speaker, it's noted at some point that when somebody gets in an accident, they open the glove box and there is already an inflatable collar. We have to discourage these things. This law suit based system for compensating auto injuries allows claimants to seek payment for uneconomic damages such as pain and suffering. So the rule of thumb is for lawyers and the claimant to calculate these losses at two or three times the claimant's economic losses. Economic losses are things like lost wages and medical expenses. Since pain and suffering awards are measured as a multiple of medical and wage losses, there's a powerful incentive to inflate one's claim of economic damages and pursue legal action. This should give all members a better idea of why insurance premiums have been going through the roof of late.

He found that by limiting the amount of non-pecuniary damages available to those suffering from minor injuries, the legislature had effectively categorised that group of injury victims as less worthy of non-pecuniary damages:

> The basis of this distinction is the type of injury from which they suffer. In limiting non-pecuniary damages in relation to the complainant group, the MIR effectively signals that the pain and suffering resulting from these medically unverifiable injuries are less deserving of damages than that caused by other injuries. As a result, the MIR perpetuates the unfortunate stereotype that I find exists in relation to Minor Injury victims. (at [215])

He found it to be discriminatory within the meaning of section 15 of the Charter and that a reasonable person in the circumstances of the claimant group would conclude that the distinction created by the cap was demeaning to the dignity of those in the claimant group (at [258]). He also found there to be evidence that without the ability to sue for non-pecuniary general damages beyond the cap, the claimant group may have a reduced ability to retain legal counsel, as lawyers are often retained on a contingency basis (at [259]). In sum, this meant that the severity of the consequences of the cap on the claimant group were more than trivial and were, as a matter of law, discriminatory.

His finding in this regard required him to consider within the meaning of section 1 of the Charter whether the breach of section 15(1) was reasonable and demonstrably justified. He accepted that maintaining affordable mandatory insurance was a 'pressing and substantial objective' of the legislature (at [299]). He concluded that it was reasonable for the Crown to perceive that:

> … an insurance crisis existed or was imminent and that mandatory automobile insurance was becoming inaccessible to many Albertans at the time that the Insurance Reforms were implemented. (at [310])

He accepted that insurance premiums had been reduced since the reforms and that mandated reductions had decreased compulsory motor vehicle insurance rates by 18%. However, he found that the blanket cap on all sprains, strains and WAD of a minor nature had targeted a group of people that was the subject of pejorative stereotyping. This led him to allow the constitutional challenge and strike down the MIR.

Wittman ACJ's decision was appealed to the Court of Appeal of Alberta (*Morrow v Zhang*, 2009 ABCA 215). His decision was reversed: Rowbotham J for the court found that Wittmann ACJ erred in inadequately assessing the reform package of insurance reforms and excessively concentrating on the MIR. She rejected the proposition that the comparator group for the purposes of assessing discrimination was individuals with MIR-defined soft tissue injuries, who have been diagnosed as having a 'serious impairment' as a result of their injuries (at [72]).

Justice Rowbotham found that it was the type and severity of the injury that formed the basis for comparison: soft tissue injury as compared to other types of motor vehicle injury. In addition, the benefit withheld by the MIR scheme was the ability to claim compensation in excess of C$4000 for non-pecuniary damages, including an individual assessment of pain and suffering. She concluded that the comparator group proposed by the plaintiffs was inadequate because it ignored the fact that victims with injuries other than soft tissue injuries were not subject to the cap, even if their injuries resolved quickly. She observed that:

> The medical evidence in this case demonstrates that patients experiencing [Whiplash Associated Disorder] I and II strains and sprains can be as, or more, seriously affected as victims of other injuries such

> as uncomplicated bone fractures and minor brain injuries. Some soft tissue injuries take longer to heal. (at [75])

However, she found that the comparator group proposed by the plaintiffs could have no, or very few, members. She was prepared to defer to the trial judge's finding that soft tissue injury claimants had been subjected to stereotyping. However, she concluded that Wittmann ACJ had inadequately taken into account the measures in the scheme which promoted and assisted treatment.

The position of the Crown at the appeal (at [108]) was that the legislation, which in part reduced the financial entitlements of whiplash victims, had a panoply of legislative purposes, including:

- increasing accessibility and affordability of mandatory motor vehicle insurance
- creating a fairer system of setting premiums for mandatory motor vehicle insurance
- addressing problems identified with the diagnosis, treatment and no-fault benefits available for sprains, strains and WAD
- seeking to control rising claims costs attributable to sprains, strains and WAD to stabilise premiums over the long term
- ensuring those with sprains, strains and WAD who had functional limitations that were not expected to improve substantially would be exempted from the cap
- strengthening the role of and increase regulatory control of the board
- addressing the solvency concerns of the insurance companies.

Justice Rowbotham accepted that if the legislation did no more than place a cap on non-pecuniary damages, it might perpetuate the stereotype of the soft tissue injury claimant but found 'this legislation recognizes that those who suffer soft-tissue injuries require early, affordable treatment' (at [102]). This led her to conclude that Wittmann ACJ erred in failing to analyse the scheme as a whole and, thus, had inappropriately determined that it was discriminatory. She accepted the submissions from the Crown that the scheme had a number of different purposes and concluded that Wittmann ACJ had overemphasised the purpose relating to a reduction in premiums.

She found that the needs of claimants were first and foremost medical diagnosis and treatment, preferably by a medical practitioner of choice:

> There should be compensation for out of pocket expenses, including lost income. In accordance with our current common law tort system, there should be a recognition of pain and suffering and loss of amenities of life. (at [117])

She found that the legislative scheme addressed each of these issues and concluded that the scheme was adequately responsive to the actual needs and circumstances of claimants, such as those with WAD, before the court.

CONCLUSIONS

Whiplash claims present the courts and policy-makers with dilemmas that have no easy solution. They are unusual in the calendar of injuries argued in the litigation context in that, like psychiatric injuries, the reliability of patients' claims of pain and impairment is not easily evaluated. Generally, the symptomatology presenting at court is not corroborated by objective evidence, in the form of radiological or comparable information. This propels the courts into subjective assessments of credibility and difficult exercises in discernment between medical opinions based upon clinical assessments that inevitably vary somewhat and, sometimes, considerably. All too often there is scope for assumptions of ideologically based approaches to contaminate the fact-finding exercise.

Not surprisingly, then, a number of legislatures have endeavoured to limit WAD claims. As the saga surrounding the new version of the compensation for motor vehicle accidents in Alberta attests, this can generate concerns about whether those with WAD are being unfairly stigmatised and unreasonably made the subject of discrimination. The Alberta scheme constitutes one form of legislative response. There are others. However, what is apparent is that both courts and legislatures experience particular concern in relation to the potential for false positive errors to be made in assessing whiplash claims that persist beyond the 'normal' clinical course of pain arising from minor traumatic injuries to the neck. While insurance reforms by legislatures in this context are said to be designed to maintain insurance schemes' viability and to enhance the incentives for prompt recovery for whiplash victims, the reality is that the elephant in the corner is the concern that a significant percentage of those pressing their whiplash claims in litigation are either exaggerating or malingering their injuries.

ACKNOWLEDGMENT

The author acknowledges, with gratitude, the assistance of Dr Patricia Molloy.

References

1. Freckelton I & Selby H. Expert evidence: law, practice, procedure and advocacy. 4th edn. Sydney: Thomson-Reuters, 2009.
2. Perlin M. The hidden prejudice: mental disability on trial. Washington, DC: American Psychological Association, 2000.
3. Freeman M, Croft AC, Rossignol AM, et al. A review and methodologic critique of the literature refuting whiplash syndrome. *Spine* 1999;24(1):86–96.
4. Alberta Automobile Insurance Board. A Study of Premium Stability in Compulsory Automobile Insurance by the Alberta Automobile Insurance Board for the Minister of Consumer and Corporate Affairs of the Government of Alberta. Edmonton, Alberta: AAIB, 1991.

CHAPTER 16
Malingering and symptom magnification in whiplash associated disorders

Brian McGuire

WHY STUDY MALINGERING IN THE AREA OF WHIPLASH?

The relevance of considering malingering in the clinical assessment of a person with any injuries or complaints arises from the co-occurrence of two necessary factors:

1. an injury (either physical or psychological) has occurred as a result of a specified event, and
2. there is an incentive (financial or otherwise) to complain of symptoms.

Symptoms of whiplash associated disorders (WAD) clearly meet these two fundamental criteria, since:

1. the injuries arise after a specified event (almost always a motor vehicle crash [MVC]), and
2. almost all developed societies have insurance systems that compensate for injuries arising from such accidents.

In the case of whiplash-associated injuries, it is now well established that even low-impact MVCs may result in a range of physical and psychological complaints.[1–3] The most common complaints after whiplash are of increased pain and decreased range of neck movement, but a range of other symptoms may develop, including sensorimotor deficits, psychological and psychiatric sequelae (e.g. anxiety about driving, post-traumatic stress disorder and depression) and a broad spectrum of cognitive complaints, including reduced memory function and attentional problems. While the development of chronic pain is well documented after whiplash, the possible psychological consequences of MVCs are related to the severity of the accident.[4] In the case of whiplash injury, a serious impact is not a prerequisite and so reactive psychological disorders, such as post-traumatic stress disorder (PTSD), are not commonly associated with whiplash per se, but with the subjective psychological impact of the accident in which the whiplash injury occurred.

The precise extent and nature of whiplash-associated cognitive complaints is also controversial. The controversy regarding the presence of cognitive complaints arises from the question—can a whiplash injury cause brain damage without direct trauma to the head? There is a proposed mechanism by which acceleration–deceleration forces may cause 'neuronal shearing' and there is evidence confirming the presence of generalised cognitive impairment after whiplash, but there is no compelling evidence that the forces exerted in a whiplash injury are sufficient to cause damage to the brain. The evidence that neuropsychological function is compromised may have alternative explanations, such as the impact of chronic pain, the effects of medication or the influence of psychological disorders, such as reactive depression and PTSD in more serious accidents.[5] Studies that adequately examine these competing explanations have yet to be carried out.

For the reasons outlined above, the current discussion will focus on malingering of pain symptoms, as there is incontrovertible evidence that chronic pain can occur after whiplash injury. It is inconceivable that all chronic pain claimants after whiplash are malingerers, so the challenge for clinicians is to differentiate genuine chronic pain from malingered chronic pain.

While the relationship between whiplash and cognitive impairment is still unclear, a good deal of the methodological advancement in the identification of malingering has been in the domain of cognitive impairment. This chapter considers some of the advances in the identification of malingered cognitive impairment, as these methodologies have implications for the identification of malingered pain.

It is important from the outset to clarify that, although there is a perception among healthcare professionals that malingering is a common occurrence in those claiming compensation for pain,[6] there is little evidence to support this view. The history of doubt and scepticism about symptom veracity when compensation is a factor has perhaps been immortalised in the phrase 'compensation neurosis', coined by

Rigler,[7] who noted the high level of disability among injured railway workers, and the concept of 'accident neurosis' defined by Miller[8]—a 'a state of mind, born out of fear, kept alive by avarice, stimulated by lawyers and cured by a verdict'.

Although perhaps less extreme views are held at present, there is a persisting belief by some that compensation and disability are intimately related.[9–11] However, a meta-analysis suggests that malingering may actually only be present in between 1.25% and 10.4% of people with chronic pain, although this conclusion is based on very limited evidence.[6] Indeed, the explicit fabrication of symptoms in the absence of a genuine injury is rare. Furthermore, it may be argued that all clinical complaints should be treated equally. We know from extensive clinical and research experience that a multitude of variables may individually or in combination influence:

1. the manner in which people experience symptoms
2. the way in which people report symptoms to health professionals and others
3. individual responses to social, cultural and environmental cues when ill or injured
4. the course of an illness
5. the likelihood of responding to treatment
6. the extent to which a person will recover.

All of these trajectories occur in a range of health conditions. The presence of a medicolegal context on top adds another layer of complexity but is not the sole determinant of a claimed chronic pain problem. Indeed, considering all of these contributing factors, it could be argued that inconsistency in pain onset, presentation and course is perhaps the norm. This is not a new observation—Hackett[12] eloquently identified many of the intra-individual factors that influence pain experience. More recently, it has been noted that the current definition of chronic pain from the International Association for the Study of Pain (IASP)[13] uses a reference standard of 'normal' pain, but argued that that there is no agreement, either statistical or empirical, about what constitutes 'normal' pain.[14] From the perspective that variability in pain experience is, in fact, normal, it may be further argued that the efforts of clinicians should be focused on assisting people to recover functioning to the greatest extent possible, rather than seeking to apply labels such as malingering.

Having made the argument that variability in pain is the norm, there can be little doubt that some deliberate symptom fabrication and deception does occur, and many clinicians are required to provide reports for legal purposes and/or to provide an opinion about the veracity of the claimant. This chapter aims to outline the state of our knowledge to assist the clinician in arriving at an informed opinion about claimant veracity—or whether it is even possible to complete that task.

WHAT IS MEANT BY 'MALINGERING'?

Within the *Diagnostic and Statistical Manual of Mental Disorders (DSM)*,[15] malingering is classified as a condition that may be a focus of clinical attention. According to the DSM, malingering is the intentional production of false or grossly exaggerated physical or psychological symptoms, motivated by external incentives, such as avoiding military duty, avoiding work, obtaining financial compensation, evading prosecution or obtaining drugs. The DSM specifies that malingering should be strongly suspected if there is any combination of a medicolegal context, marked discrepancy between the person's claimed disability and the objective findings, lack of cooperation with assessment and treatment, and the presence of antisocial personality disorder. The *International Classification of Diseases (ICD)*[16] categorises malingering in the Z codes—factors influencing health status and contact with health services (Z00–Z99)—and defines malingering (conscious simulation) simply as 'person feigning illness (with obvious motivation)'.

Neither of these definitions is very useful for diagnostic purposes, since they merely describe the behaviour of malingering without any practical guidance on decision-making in relation to the presence or absence of the characteristics proposed to be important. More useful conceptualisations recognise that malingering is a complex phenomenon with many 'shades of grey' in terms of the extent to which symptoms are actually produced *de novo* (i.e. symptoms arising in the absence of injury), exaggerated where they actually exist or reported in the absence of any genuine symptoms. The DSM and ICD definitions also fail to recognise the role of combined external incentives and internal psychological processes, and the extent to which compensation systems may act to encourage prolonged symptom reporting and disability.

Resnick[17] identified several types of malingering. He stated that *pure malingering* is the feigning of disease when it does not exist at all. *Partial malingering* is the conscious exaggeration of existing symptoms or the fraudulent allegation that prior genuine symptoms are still present. *False imputation* refers to the claimant ascribing actual symptoms to a cause consciously recognised by the patient as having no relationship to the symptoms. These distinctions have strong face validity in terms of the clinical presentation of patients following MVCs and, logically and intuitively, partial malingering or symptom magnification are likely to be the most prevalent forms of malingering using Resnick's framework. Main[18] argues that clinicians have a role in identifying symptom exaggeration (partial malingering) but that decisions about deception (pure malingering) should be the responsibility of the judicial system.

Rogers[19, 20] has proposed an explanatory model of malingering. He suggested that malingering may occur for one of three reasons, because malingering persons are:

1. mentally disordered
2. bad/criminal or
3. attempting to meet their objectives in adversarial circumstances (i.e. adapting to their circumstances).

The mentally disordered or pathogenic model proposes that malingering occurs because of a mental disorder. There is little evidence to support such a model except in selected psychiatric conditions, such as factitious disorder. The criminological model, on which the DSM criteria are arguably based, is rejected by Rogers as it assumes that malingering is perpetrated by a 'bad person, in bad circumstances, who is behaving badly' (p 8).[20] Given that many 'good' people regularly malinger (e.g. to take a day off work or to avoid a social event), the argument that malingerers are inherently bad people does not stand up to scrutiny in everyday life.

The adaptational model proposes that malingering is an adaptive response to adversarial circumstances in which the individual has a substantial personal investment. This argument is philosophically interesting as it implies that malingering is, in a sense, a product of our litigious society in many cases. Anecdotally, it fits with the author's own experience in medicolegal contexts—patients frequently describe being sent for assessments to antagonistic, disbelieving and sceptical health professionals where the patient feels pressured to 'prove' that their complaints are genuine and, in so doing, may well engage in abnormal illness behaviours with exaggerated disability. This presentation merely serves to reinforce the view of the sceptical assessor that the patient is malingering.

A fascinating study examined the number of claims for whiplash injury in a Canadian province after changing from a system of tort to a no-fault insurance system.[21] The authors found that the number of whiplash claims fell by almost 30% and the claims were resolved, on average, some 200 days earlier. Longer time to completion was associated with higher initial pain intensity and depression in the claimant but also with non-patient factors, such as engaging the services of a lawyer or seeing health practitioners who were more likely to offer active interventions, perhaps 'validating' the illness perception. They concluded that the type of insurance system profoundly affects the frequency and duration of whiplash claims. However, it is argued that most people filing insurance claims are not malingerers—rather, their behaviour reflects a complex interaction between biological factors, psychological reactions and appraisals, social forces, legal influences and financial incentives.[22]

APPROACHES TO DETECTION OF MALINGERING

Lanyon[23] has outlined a number of models for describing and understanding malingering and other forms of deception, from which methodologies for detecting malingering can be derived. According to Lanyon, traditional approaches to the detection of malingering have been based on a 'global-signs-of-lying' model, which assumes that certain universal, physiologically mediated signs correlate with attempts to deceive. Examples of detection strategies based on this model include the polygraph test and voice stress analysis. Lanyon described the basic characteristics of this model as follows:

1. the signs are independent of any particular context or content, so that the same signs are potentially observable no matter what kind of lies are being told
2. the signs themselves are universal in that everybody shows them
3. the signs are evidenced in psychophysiological measurement
4. people have limited ability to inhibit these signs even if they know about them.

Clearly, the model assumes that lying will produce psychophysiological arousal, which can be measured. An implicit assumption, therefore, is that lying is an emotion-producing activity. Another implicit assumption is that the physiological arousal observed on measurement is directly attributable to the lying. However, there is extensive evidence that physiological measures such as polygraphy are unreliable, and that results are open to multiple interpretations.[24, 25]

Two other models identified by Lanyon are *accuracy of knowledge* (including lack of uncommon knowledge, erroneous stereotypes and over-endorsement) and *personal influence*. *Accuracy of knowledge* refers to the assumption that successful deception requires the deceiver to have accurate knowledge of the target condition. This knowledge has two aspects: factual content and personal behaviour. Persons who are successful at deceiving know the facts about the target condition and also behave like a person who has the target characteristics. This leads directly to an assessment approach for detecting deception, that is, the assessment of a person's level of relevant knowledge of the target condition that the person is attempting to simulate. This is, therefore, a cognitive (knowledge-based) model of deception rather than an affective or autonomic model of deception. Successful detection is based on the identification of those characteristics about which the person's knowledge is most likely to be inaccurate.

Lanyon further delineated the accuracy of knowledge model into three subareas, as outlined below.

1. *Lack of uncommon knowledge* refers to characteristics of the target condition that involve uncommon knowledge that few people would tend to know. It refers, therefore, to items with high empirical validity but low face validity. Thus, people trying to feign a complex disorder may be 'caught' by this method because they do not have enough knowledge about the complexities of how the disorder presents.
2. *Erroneous stereotypes* refer to the idea that people hold common but erroneous beliefs about various disorders. Such items have high face validity but low empirical validity. Detecting deception using this method requires that the person is not highly knowledgable about the target condition. A person who adopts a 'split personality' when attempting to feign schizophrenia may be detected by this method, as the person is reflecting an erroneous stereotype about the clinical picture of schizophrenia.
3. *Over-endorsement* refers to symptoms that have both high face validity and high empirical validity but the deceptive responder lacks information about the normal prevalence of such characteristics. Thus, a symptom questionnaire may contain items that have high face validity for a particular disorder and have high empirical validity for some individuals in the target group, but simulators may endorse all of the symptoms when a member of the target group would endorse only a proportion of them. A person attempting to deceive may not know the normative number of items to endorse and may endorse too many. For example, a person who endorses hallucinatory symptoms in every sensory modality when attempting to feign schizophrenia may be detected by this method, since visual hallucinations occur much less frequently than is commonly believed and hallucinations in the olfactory and gustatory senses are very rare.

These approaches (and others) have been the subject of a good deal of research on malingering over the past 20 years.

However, a significant weakness of malingering research has been the challenge of determining an appropriate 'gold standard' measure against which to evaluate the utility of diagnostic tests. In diagnostic testing, the gold standard would be another established test that accurately identifies a group with, and without, the condition under study (known-groups design). The problem in malingering research is that confirmed malingerers are exceedingly rare. This drawback has been addressed through the use of simulation designs, where a group responds to a test 'as if' they had the condition under study. However, there are several problems with this design; for example, the extent to which a simulation adequately reflects the reality of a clinical situation and the extent to which a simulation design can reflect the magnitude of the incentive in the malingering group.

DIFFERENTIAL DIAGNOSIS OF PSYCHOLOGICAL DISORDERS WHERE SYMPTOM PRODUCTION OR MAGNIFICATION IS A FEATURE

Some of the DSM disorders that may resemble malingering because of the unexplained symptom patterns have been identified.[26] These are briefly outlined below.

Somatoform disorders are a group of disorders characterised by symptoms suggesting physical disorders but without demonstrable organic findings to explain the symptoms. There is positive evidence, or a strong presumption, that the symptoms are linked to psychological factors or conflicts.

These include *conversion disorder*, which is characterised by a symptom(s) suggestive of a neurological disorder that affects sensation or voluntary motor function, but is not fully explained by any known general medical condition. The symptom is not consciously or intentionally produced, and is severe enough to impair functioning or to require medical attention.

Hypochondriasis is characterised by persistent health-related worry and magnification of symptoms, despite appropriate medical reassurance and lack of findings on physical or laboratory examination.

Somatisation disorder is characterised by multiple physical complaints not fully explained by any known general medical condition.

Pain disorder is characterised by the presence of pain at one or more parts of the body and is of sufficient severity to warrant medical attention. However, the pain is not intentionally produced and psychological factors are judged to have an important role in the onset, severity, exacerbation or maintenance of the pain (DSM-IV).[15] This condition is of particular interest in the assessment of pain malingering (and of chronic pain more generally). The central distinction of *pain disorder* as a psychiatric illness is the psychogenic process—pain may present in the absence of any form of injury, may be unresponsive to usual medical management, and there are strong clinical indicators of underlying psychological conflict.

Factitious disorders are also relevant in the differential diagnosis. Factitious disorders are a group of disorders characterised by intentional production or feigning of physical or psychological symptoms or signs. The motivation here is related to a need to assume the sick role (e.g. to solicit attention or sympathy) rather than to seek obvious secondary gains, such as economic rewards.

The essential distinction between each of these disorders and malingering is intentionality and motivation—malingering involves the intentional production or exaggeration of symptoms. In contrast, somatoform disorders reflect an underlying psychological disorder and the symptom magnification is a reflection of that disordered thinking. Factitious disorder does involve intentional symptom production, but the motivation reflects an intrapsychic need rather than a financial motivation. In a review of the relationship between somatisation and secondary gain in chronic pain,[27] it was concluded that there was little scientific evidence to support a causal relationship between these variables.

EMPIRICAL STUDIES OF MALINGERING AND SYMPTOM MAGNIFICATION IN PAIN

Despite the enormous clinical interest in the assessment and treatment of chronic pain, and the burgeoning applied research in the area of malingering, there has been relatively little overlap between the two fields. This is quite remarkable when one considers that a high proportion of people with chronic pain are eligible for compensation or disability payments, but it perhaps reflects the inherent difficulty in identifying deception in a condition that is highly subjective and highly variable in experience and presentation. A review of all approaches to detection of deception is beyond the scope of this chapter (but see useful overviews[28, 29]). The studies to be reviewed here fall into three domains:

1. unusual response patterns on pain questionnaires or on scales designed to detect deceptive responses (pain malingering scales)
2. unusual responses on psychometric and neuropsychological tests
3. physical/medical anomalies or inconsistencies.

Most of the studies have used either simulation designs—typically, a group of healthy people are asked to perform 'as if' they have chronic pain—or a known-groups design—the group memberships are known and, thus, any differences can be ascribed to the group membership. This usually involves comparison of a non-litigating pain group to a litigating or presumed malingering pain group.

Unusual response patterns on pain questionnaires and pain malingering scales

Research on the use of psychological symptom questionnaires has focused mainly on identifying either unusual symptom patterns or general over-endorsement of symptoms among simulators or presumed malingerers. Leavitt[30] developed a list of pain descriptors in order to study whether pain simulators would choose different words to describe their (simulated) pain. He found that a moderately high level of correct classification of simulators could be achieved. He subsequently developed this paradigm further by asking patients with actual pain to exaggerate their pain and complete the pain descriptor scale. He concluded that it was more difficult to detect symptom exaggeration in those who already suffered pain, achieving only 64% correct classification rate for pain patients who exaggerated their pain, in comparison to 82% correct classification for people without pain.[31] Leavitt obtained data from a large sample of patients with chronic pain using the pain descriptor scale.[32] He then asked orthopaedic physicians to rate the patients independently for their level of organic pathology and likelihood of malingering. He found that those who were identified by the pain descriptor scale as being simulators (10.4% of the sample) were more likely to be rated by physicians as having less organic pathology and greater symptom exaggeration. However, not all patients identified as simulators were free of organic pathology, indicating that at least some malingerers have some pain but exaggerate its intensity rather than invent symptoms outright.

Three studies have investigated the Illness Behaviour Questionnaire.[33] Clayer et al.[34] compared healthy controls, pain patients and pain simulators, and identified 21 items (the Conscious Exaggeration, or CE, scale) that differentiated the simulator group. The same group subsequently studied 10 suspected malingerers who were independently assessed by psychiatrists. There was a reasonable correlation between psychiatrists' judgments of malingering and classification according to the CE scale, with sensitivity at 69% and specificity at 100%. The authors concluded that results from the CE scale cannot provide a reliable basis for medicolegal decisions.[35]

In another study, the CE scale was administered to a large sample of pain patients engaged in litigation or receiving compensation but found no difference between litigators and a pain sample not involved in litigation or receiving compensation.[36] Fishbain and colleagues[37] similarly found that the CE scale did not differentiate pain patients with and without several secondary gain variables. There is, therefore, little evidence for the use of the CE scale for the detection of pain malingering.

Although it is widely used in clinical practice, only a few studies have examined the utility of the Multidimensional Pain Inventory (MPI).[38] An early study compared pain simulators with a pain clinical sample and found that the simulators scored in a significantly more pathological direction.[39] In another study, the MPI was evaluated along with other pain measures in a study of simulated pain. Simulators were instructed to portray themselves as either coping well or coping poorly. Robinson et al.[40] concluded that the simulators could portray themselves in a convincing manner as coping either well or poorly. Although not examining symptom simulation per se, Bruehl and colleagues[41] developed a scale (Variable Responding, or VR) to identify random responding on the MPI, which has the potential for use in malingering research. Thus far, however, there is insufficient evidence to evaluate the utility of the MPI as an aid to identifying malingered pain.

Two studies have looked at the McGill Pain Questionnaire (MPQ)[42] in pain malingering. In one study, simulators could describe the affective distress associated with pain but overstated their pain in comparison to a clinical sample.[43] In another study which looked at the MPQ, Truscott concluded that a number of infrequently endorsed items (the pain infrequency [INF] scale) in a general pain population was moderately successful at differentiating pain patients with compensation in comparison to those without compensation.[44] The author concluded that the INF scale is promising as a measure of exaggerated pain, although he was making an unproven assumption that the group seeking compensation was more likely to contain exaggerators/malingerers. The MPQ warrants further research in terms of its use in malingering assessment.

One study examined the utility of the Symptom Checklist 90-Revised (SCL-90-R)[45] in detecting pain malingering specifically in whiplash. Wallis and Bogduk[46] compared a group of whiplash patients with chronic pain to a group that was asked to simulate chronic pain arising from a whiplash injury. They found that the genuine clinical group showed characteristic elevations on the Somatisation, Obsessive–Compulsive and Depression scales. In comparison, the simulating group displayed a generalised elevation across the range of clinical scales on the SCL-90-R. The simulating group could be differentiated from the clinical group on the basis of their elevated scores, although the authors did not provide information about the scale's only validity indicator, the Positive Symptom Total (PST) scores, or about the diagnostic cut-off scores for identifying simulation on the clinical scales.

A subsequent study also examined symptom checklist (SCL) responses in a group of pain simulators compared with a group of mixed chronic pain patients.[47] The simulators exceeded the pain group on all of the clinical scales of the SCL-90-R, tending to greatly overestimate the degree of psychological distress in pain patients. Simulators had consistently extreme elevations and were more likely to obtain a T-score over 70 on each of the clinical scales. About 80% of the respective groups could be identified with a PST total T-score of 74. These findings remain to be replicated by others.

Two studies have examined the Pain Patient Profile (P3),[48] a measure of psychological distress associated with chronic pain which has scales for depression, anxiety, somatic complaints and a validity scale (based on infrequent endorsement of Validity scale items in the normative sample). McGuire and Shores[49] found that a group of pain simulators did not differ on the P3 validity scale compared with the pain group, but scored significantly higher than the pain group on the P3 clinical scales (depression, anxiety, somatisation). The simulators were more likely to obtain an 'abnormal' score (T-score >55) on all of the clinical scales, with positive and negative predictive powers of about 70% and 80%, respectively, for individual subscale scores, and 100% positive predictive power when all three clinical scale scores exceeded 60 (but with slightly reduced negative predictive power).[49]

The same authors subsequently compared a chronic pain group answering honestly, a chronic pain group that was asked to exaggerate their complaints (partial malingering using Resnick's model) and a control group (non-pain patients attending a psychologist) that was also asked to simulate pain.[50] Both groups of simulating participants were more likely to obtain an abnormal T-score on the clinical scales. The Validity scale was able to differentiate the exaggerating pain group from the honest pain group. The authors concluded that a Validity score above 11 and T-scores over 70 on the clinical scales should alert the clinician to the possibility of symptom magnification.

Studies with the Minnesota Multiphasic Personality Inventory (MMPI-2)[51] have identified a typical response profile for chronic pain patients. However, attempts to use the MMPI validity scales to identify pain malingering have yielded inconsistent results. For example, Butcher and colleagues[52] examined the prevalence of elevated Fake Bad Scale (FBS) scores in a wide range of clinical populations but found inconceivably high rates of malingering, such that they recommend against the use of the FBS and contend that the scale actually reflects general maladjustment among people with genuine psychological and psychiatric problems. In contrast, another study found that probable pain malingerers and non-malingerers could be reliably differentiated using MMPI validity scales and elevations on the Hysteria and Hypochondriasis clinical scales, although the sample sizes were relatively small.[53] In reviewing the MMPI validity scales, Arbisi and Butcher[54] concluded that the MMPI is useful for comparing an individual patient's pain profile with that of large groups of patients with chronic pain and to screen for impression management using one of the better-validated MMPI validity scales, which suggests that an elevated score on the validity scales is indicative of deliberate misrepresentation.

The results of these studies indicate that several pain symptom questionnaires (e.g. the SCL-90, the MPI, the MPQ and the P3) and questionnaire-based validity tests (e.g. the MMPI validity scales) may have utility in identifying unusual response patterns among claimants of chronic pain. However, further research is required with each of these measures.

Malingered cognitive impairment in pain patients

As indicated earlier, cognitive complaints are often reported in whiplash patients and cognitive impairment may also be reported among general patients with chronic pain. Questions may arise about the nature and validity of such cognitive deficits. In an early study,[55] a measure of malingered memory impairment suggested a high level of underperformance in pain patients, even those who were *not* in litigation. The authors concluded that the cognitive complaints in non-malingering whiplash patients are more likely related to chronic pain, fatigue and depression, rather than organic brain damage. In a known-groups study,[56] 29 patients with probable malingered neurocognitive impairment based on failure of cognitive screening tests for malingering (using the guidelines of Slick et al.[57]) were also administered measures of pain and disability. A measure of pain perception, the Modified Somatic Perception Questionnaire, correctly classified over 90% of the probable malingerers, but this remains to be replicated.

In an effort to identify cognitive tests that may be used to identify malingering in pain patients, a number of studies have sought to show that performance on several cognitive tests is unaffected by pain. The rationale for this approach is that if performance is not usually affected, then poor performance may be taken as an indicator of deliberate poor performance on the test. A study on a forced-choice test of malingered memory impairment (Test of Memory Malingering, or TOMM[58]) showed that performance was unaffected by laboratory-induced pain.[59] However, short-term experimental pain and chronic pain are clearly different phenomena, not least because of the impact of chronic pain on mood, fatigue and everyday attentional demands. Thus, this finding needs to be demonstrated in patients with chronic pain. Nevertheless, symptom validity testing using forced choice memory testing (where below-chance performance based on binomial theory indicates deliberately poor performance) is a robust approach that has been demonstrated to differentiate genuine cognitive complaints from simulated cognitive complaints and presumed malingerers. It, therefore, has potential as a measure of suspect performance among pain claimants.

Several studies have focused on the Wechsler scales. Studies of the WAIS/WMS Digit Span using the Reliable Digit Span score (highest digits forward score plus highest digits backward score) show that digit span performance is not affected by laboratory-induced pain[60] and that a low score (< 7) differentiated patients with chronic pain, pain malingerers and people with brain injury.[61, 62] A study of the WAIS-III Processing Speed Index (PSI) showed that laboratory-induced pain and chronic pain had a minimal effect on test performance and that unusually low scores suggest deliberate suboptimal performance.[63] More recently, a comprehensive examination of the Working Memory Index (WMI) of WAIS-III showed that, although some pain patients evidenced attentional problems on the WMI, significant impairment (<70 WMI score) is suggestive of intentional underperformance.[64]

In the area of neuropsychological evaluation, there is a growing awareness of the benefit of multiple indicators of dissimulation. A study that evaluated the ability of three measures of symptom validity to identify malingering in brain injury and in chronic pain concluded that joint classification accuracy was superior to that of any of the tests used alone.[65] This is consistent with the guidelines of Slick et al.[57] and of the recent guidelines on evaluation of effort, response bias and malingering.[66] A recent practice guideline on effort testing in the assessment of cognitive functioning provides a very useful overview of the most widely used indices of suspicious response patterns.[67]

There is strong evidence that symptom validity testing can differentiate deliberate suboptimal performance. Also, test profiles using specific equations on common tests, such as the Wechsler scales, has potential utility for identifying dissimulated cognitive impairment in people with chronic pain.

Physical/medical anomalies or inconsistencies

Studies using methods other than questionnaires include a number of evaluations of Waddell's non-organic signs:[68] a number of physical findings that purport to be indicative of malingering, such as apparent exaggerations, inconsistencies and physiologically improbable performance.[69]

In a systematic review of the relationship between Waddell's signs and malingering or secondary gain, Fishbain at al.[70] concluded that there was no evidence of an association between the signs and a finding of malingering. In another review,[71] it was concluded that Waddell's signs are, in fact, an organic phenomenon and that the signs cannot be used to discriminate organic and non-organic problems. An earlier review by the same authors[72] suggested that forced choice testing for sensory loss, clinical examination and grip strength tests was unreliable in identifying the malingering subject. However, isokinetic testing was considered to have potential for discriminating maximal and submaximal effort. For a detailed update of muscle strength, range of motion and velocity of motion tests, see Robinson and Danneker.[73]

A DECISION-MAKING TEMPLATE FOR POSSIBLE AND PROBABLE MALINGERING

Cunnien[74] has proposed a clinical decision model for establishing a finding of malingering. He stated that *all* of the following (A, B, C, D) must be present to confirm malingering:

A. psychological or physical symptoms are clearly under voluntary control as manifested by *one or more* indicators:
   1. patient acknowledgment of voluntary control or deceit
   2. gross symptom production that is inconsistent with physiological or anatomical mechanisms
   3. direct observation of illness production
   4. discovery of paraphernalia or substances explaining the production of physical symptoms
   5. confirmatory laboratory testing (e.g. absence of electroencephalographic [EEG] abnormalities during an observed 'seizure')

B. clinical certainty that illness production occurs in response to:
   1. pursuit of financial gain, shelter or drugs, or
   2. avoidance of work, military duty, prosecution or legal consequences

C. another disorder, if present, cannot explain current symptoms

D. evidence of desire to assume the sick role, if present, cannot explain the totality of current symptoms.

An examination of Cunnien's criteria clearly highlights the problems inherent in identifying malingering. With regard to criterion A1, patients will rarely openly acknowledge deceitful behaviour, especially if they stand to lose from such an admission. Criterion A2 lends itself to psychological assessment, and indeed is the basis for the current paradigm for identifying symptoms that are likely to be malingered (the 'fake bad' methodology), although it is also true that many people with genuine complaints (e.g. pain, memory impairment, mental illness) have no discernible organic disease. Criteria A3 and A4 are unlikely to be met in the context of most medicolegal evaluations that occur in the practitioner's office. However, close surveillance in a supervised environment may enable one to satisfy these criteria. Criterion A5 is virtually impossible where psychological symptoms are concerned, as most psychological symptoms do not have physical or biological correlates which can be measured. Furthermore, it has been shown that physiological reactions can be faked[75] or distorted. Criteria B1 and B2 can be based only on an assumption that the presence of the external motivators are causing the symptoms. Without the client's admission that he or she is faking, one can probably never have 'clinical certainty'. Criterion C may be achievable under some circumstances, although there are many situations where patients have multiple medical investigations for unusual symptoms, without ever discovering the cause of the symptoms, and in the absence of any external motivation to malinger symptoms. Criterion D is again dependent on the patient's admission of his/her motivation.

Cunnien has suggested that the clinical decision model for malingering requires the specific finding of voluntariness in combination with clinical certainty, and that clinical certainty about intentionality implies patient acknowledgment of external motivations, corroboration by external sources, or strong evidence that symptoms began in conscious response to external events.

Bianchini and colleagues[76] point to the fact that in injuries in which pain is central, the person may also experience emotional, behavioural and cognitive symptoms, which may form part of the basis for the claim. Thus, the claim may focus on the combined impact (disability) arising from these variables. Consequently, Bianchini et al.[76] argue that the question should not only be about the veracity of the pain complaint or the extent of the pain problem, but the overall degree of disability attributed to the pain. Drawing on Slick et al.'s guidelines for malingered cognitive impairment,[57] they proposed the definition of Malingered Pain-Related Disability (MPRD) as 'the intentional exaggeration or fabrication of cognitive, emotional, behavioural or physical dysfunction attributed to pain for the purposes of obtaining financial gain, to avoid work, or to obtain drugs'. Their point is valid—few cases of pain-related disability focus only on the extent of the pain and its consequences—the impact of emotional reactions, relationship disturbance, loss of opportunity and future estimates of combined disability (to name but a few) typically feature in medicolegal claims. Thus, a definition of malingered pain which incorporates the broad areas influenced by pain seems logical, and it suggests that the diagnostic criteria for pain malingering must also be broad. As has been suggested by several commentators, decisions should be based on multiple sources of information and higher numbers of positive indicators are likely to have better predictive validity than single indicators.

As a conclusion that a person is malingering is at the upper end of clinical responsibility due to the risk of damage to personal reputation and the potential to deprive a person of compensation where it is genuinely deserved, the threshold for decision-making must be set higher than the decision that a person is answering honestly. While significantly more empirical work is required, it is suggested that diagnostic decisions regarding pain malingering might be based on the following criteria:

1. corroborated evidence of an accident or injury *and*
2. a claim that pain is present *and*
3. the presence of an incentive *and*
4. unusually elevated scores on *at least* one validated pain questionnaire using published cut-off scores yielding at least 80% correct classification *and*
5. unusually elevated scores on *at least* one well-established validity scale using published cut-off scores yielding at least 80% correct classification *and*
6. where there is no question of a genuine organic brain impairment, unusually elevated scores on *at least* one well-established psychometric validity test using published cut-off scores yielding at least 80% correct classification.

The greater the number of malingering indicators, the more confidence clinicians can have in their diagnosis. A conclusion that malingering is present should never be made on the basis of only one unusual test score or clinical indicator. Furthermore, the clinical impression that overstating of health problems is a matter of degree (i.e. a continuous or dimensional variable) rather than a dichotomous variable (malingering versus not malingering) has been shown empirically in a recent study.[77] The refinement of existing detection strategies and the development of more sophisticated methodologies, including interdisciplinary assessment, are likely to lead to more reliable conclusions.

References

1. Côté P, Cassidy DJ, Carroll L, et al. A systematic review of the prognosis of acute whiplash and a new conceptual framework to synthesize the literature. *Spine* 2001;26:E445–8.
2. Sterner Y & Gerdle B. Acute and chronic whiplash disorders – a review. *J Rehabil Med* 2004;36(5): 193–209.

3. Elliott JM, Noteboom JT, Flynn TF, Sterling M. Characterization of acute and chronic whiplash associated disorders. *J Orthop Sports Phys Ther* 2009;39(5):312–23.
4. Mayou R, Bryant B, Ehlers A. Prediction of psychological outcomes one year after a motor vehicle accident. *Am J Psychiatry* 2001;158:1231–8.
5. Kessels RPC, Aleman A, Verhagen WIM, van Luijtelaar ELJM. Cognitive functioning after whiplash injury: a meta-analysis. *J Int Neuropsychol Soc* 2000;6:271–8.
6. Fishbain DA, Cutler RB, Rosomoff HL, Rosomoff RS. Chronic pain disability, exaggeration/malingering, and submaximal effort research. *Clin J Pain* 1999;14: 244–74.
7. Rigler J. Ueber die Verletzungen auf Eisenbahnen Insbesondere der Verletzungen des Rueckenmarks. Berlin: Reimer Publishing, 1879.
8. Miller H. Accident neurosis. *Br Med J* 1961;1:19–25.
9. Bellamy R. Compensation neurosis: financial reward for illness as nocebo. *Clin Orthop Relat Res* 1997;336:94–106.
10. Fraser RD. Compensation and recovery from injury. *Med J Aust* 1996;165:71–2.
11. Weintraub MI. Chronic pain in litigation: what is the relationship? *Neurol Clin* 1995;13:341–9.
12. Hackett TP. Pain and prejudice: why do we doubt that the patient is in pain? *Anesth Prog* 1971; May-June:54–9.
13. Merskey H, Bogduk N, eds. Classification of pain. 2nd edn. Seattle: International Association for the Study of Pain, 1994.
14. Cronje RJ & Williamson OD. Is pain ever 'normal'? *Clin J Pain* 2006;22:692–9.
15. American Psychiatric Association. Diagnostic and statistical manual of mental disorders. 4th edn. Washington, DC: American Psychiatric Press, 2000.
16. World Health Organization. International classification of diseases. 10th edn. Geneva: World Health Organization, 2007.
17. Resnick PJ. Guidelines for the evaluation of malingering in posttraumatic stress disorder. In: Simon RI, ed. Posttraumatic stress disorder in litigation: guidelines for forensic assessment. Washington, DC: American Psychiatric Press, 1995.
18. Main CJ. The nature of chronic pain: a clinical and legal challenge. In: Halligan PW, Bass C, Oakley DA, eds. Malingering and illness deception. Oxford: Oxford University Press, 2003, pp 171–81.
19. Rogers R. Development of a new classificatory model of malingering. *Bull Am Acad Psychiatr Law* 1990;18:323–33.
20. Rogers R. Introduction. In: Rogers R, ed. Clinical assessment of malingering and deception. 2nd edn. New York: Guilford Press, 1997, pp 1–22.
21. Cassidy JD, Carroll LJ, Côté P, et al. Effect of eliminating compensation for pain and suffering on the outcome of insurance claims for whiplash injury. *N Engl J Med* 2000;342:1179–86.
22. Deyo R. Pain and public policy. *N Engl J Med* 2000;342:1211–13.
23. Lanyon RI. Detecting deception: current models and directions. *Clin Psychol: Sci Pract* 1997;4:3 77–87.
24. Iacono WG & Patrick CJ. Polygraphy and integrity testing. In: Rogers R, ed. Clinical assessment of malingering and deception. 2nd edn. New York: Guilford Press, 1997, pp 252–81.
25. British Psychological Society. A review of the current scientific status and fields of application of polygraphic deception detection. Leicester: BPS, 2004.
26. LoPiccolo CJ, Goodkin K, Baldewicz TT. Current issues in the diagnosis and management of malingering. *Ann Med* 1999;31:166–74.
27. Fishbain DA. Somatization, secondary gain, and chronic pain: is there a relationship? *Curr Pain Headache Rep* 1998;2:101–8.
28. Arnoff GM, Mandel S, Genovese E, et al. Evaluating malingering in contested injury or illness. *Pain Pract* 2007;7:178–204.
29. McDermott BE & Feldman MD. Malingering in the medical setting. *Psychiatr Clin North Am* 2007;30: 645–62.
30. Leavitt F. Pain and deception: use of verbal pain measurement as a diagnostic aid in differentiating between clinical and simulated low back pain. *J Psychosom Res* 1985;29:495–505.
31. Leavitt F. Detection of simulation among persons instructed to exaggerate symptoms of low back pain. *J Occup Med* 1987;29:229–33.
32. Leavitt F. Predicting disability time using formal low back pain measurement: the low back pain simulation scale. *J Psychosom Res* 1991;35:599–607.
33. Pilowsky I & Spence N. Manual for the illness behaviour questionnaire. 3rd edn. Adelaide: University of Adelaide, 1994.
34. Clayer JR, Bookless C, Ross MW. Neurosis and conscious symptom exaggeration: its differentiation by the Illness Behaviour Questionnaire. *J Psychosom Res* 1984;29:495–505.
35. Clayer JR, Bookless-Pratz C, Ross MW. The evaluation of illness behaviour and exaggeration of disability. *Br J Psychol* 1986;148:296–9.

36. Mendelson G. Measurement of conscious symptom exaggeration by questionnaire: a clinical study. *J Psychosom Res* 1987;31:703–11.
37. Fishbain DA, Cutler RB, Rosomoff HL, Steele-Rosomoff R. Does the Conscious Exaggeration Scale detect deception within patients with chronic pain alleged to have secondary gain? *Pain Med* 2002;3: 39–46.
38. Kerns RD, Turk DC, Rudy TE. The West Haven-Yale Multidimensional Pain Inventory (WHYMPI). *Pain* 1985;23:345–56.
39. Bruehl S, Lofland KR, Husfeldt B. Detection of response bias on the Multidimensional Pain Inventory. Paper presented at the American Pain Society 15th Annual Scientific Meeting, Washington, DC, 1996.
40. Robinson ME, Myers CD, Sadler IJ, et al. Bias effects in three common self-report pain assessment measures. *Clin J Pain* 1997;13:74–81.
41. Bruehl S, Lofland KR, Sherman JJ, Carlson CR. The Variable Responding Scale for detection of random responding on the Multidimensional Pain Inventory. *Psychol Assess* 1998;10:3–9.
42. Melzack R. The McGill Pain Questionnaire: major properties and scoring methods. *Pain* 1975;1:277–99.
43. Chastain DC & Cassisi JE. Cervical pain and distress in acute and simulated soft tissue neck injury. Paper presented at the American Pain Society 14th Annual Scientific Meeting, Los Angeles, California, 1995.
44. Truscott D. Assessing exaggeration of chronic pain reports with the McGill Pain Questionnaire: the pain infrequency (INF) scale. Paper presented at the 8th World Congress on Pain, Vancouver, Canada, 1996.
45. Derogatis LR. SCL-90-R: administration, scoring and procedures manual II for the revised version. Towson, MD: Clinical Psychometric Research, 1992.
46. Wallis BJ & Bogduk N. Faking a profile: can naïve subjects simulate whiplash responses? *Pain* 1996;66:223–7.
47. McGuire BE & Shores EA. Simulated pain on the Symptom Checklist 90-R. *J Clin Psychol* 2001;57:1589–96.
48. Tollison DC & Langley JC. Pain Patient Profile manual. Minneapolis: National Computer Services, 1995.
49. McGuire BE & Shores EA. Pain Patient Profile and the assessment of malingered pain. *J Clin Psychol* 2001;57:401–9.
50. McGuire BE, Harvey A, Shores EA. Simulated malingering in pain patients: a study with the Pain Patient Profile. *Br J Clin Psychol* 2001;40:71–9.
51. Butcher JN, Dahlstrom WG, Graham JR, et al. MMPI 2: manual for administration and scoring. Minneapolis: University of Minnesota Press, 1989.
52. Butcher JN, Arbisi PA, Atlis M, McNulty JL. The construct validity of the Lees-Haley Fake Bad Scale: does this scale measure somatic malingering and feigned emotional distress? *Arch Clin Neuropsychol* 2003;18:475–85.
53. Bianchini KJ, Etherton JL, Greve KW, et al. Classification accuracy of MMPI-2 validity scales in the detection of pain-related malingering. *J Forensic Neuropsychol* 2004;4:65–81.
54. Arbisi PA & Butcher JN. Psychometric perspectives on detection of malingering of pain: use of the Minnesota Multiphasic Personality Inventory-2. *Clin J Pain* 2004;20:383–91.
55. Schmand B, Lindeboom J, Schagen S, et al. Cognitive complaints in patients after whiplash: the impact of malingering. *J Neurol Neurosurg Psychiatr* 1998;15:435–49.
56. Larrabee GJ. Exaggerated pain report in litigants with malingered neurocognitive dysfunction. *Clin Neuropsychol* 2003;17:395–401.
57. Slick DJ, Sherman EMS, Iverson GL. Diagnostic criteria for malingering cognitive dysfunction: proposed standards for clinical practice and research. *Clin Neuropsychol* 1999;13:545–61.
58. Tombaugh T. Test of Memory Malingering manual. New York: MultiHealth Systems, 1996.
59. Etherton JL, Bianchini KJ, Greve KW, Ciota MA. Test of Memory Malingering performance is unaffected by laboratory-induced pain: implications for clinical use. *Arch Clin Neuropsychol* 2005;20:375–84.
60. Etherton J, Bianchini K, Ciota M, Greve K. Reliable Digit Span is unaffected by laboratory-induced pain. *Assessment* 2005;12:101–6.
61. Etherton J, Bianchini K, Greve K, Heinly M. Sensitivity and specificity of Reliable Digit Span in malingered pain-related disability. *Assessment* 2005;12:130–6.
62. Greve K, Bianchini K, Etherton JL, et al. The Reliable Digit Span Test in chronic pain: classification accuracy in detecting malingered pain-related disability. *Clin Neuropsychol* 2009;24:137–52.
63. Etherton J, Bianchini K, Heinly M, Greve K. Pain, malingering and performance on the WAIS-III Processing Speed Index. *J Clin Exper Neuropsychol* 2006;28:1218–37.
64. Etherton J, Bianchini K, Ciota M, et al. Pain, malingering and the WAIS-III Working Memory Index. *Spine J* 2009;6:61–71.
65. Greve K, Ord J, Curtis K, et al. Detecting malingering in traumatic brain injury and chronic pain: a comparison of three forced-choice symptom validity tests. *Clin Neuropsychol* 2008;22(5):896–918.

66. Heilbronner RL, Sweet JJ, Morgan JE, et al. American Academy of Clinical Neuropsychology Consensus Conference Statement on the neuropsychological assessment of effort, response bias and malingering. *Clin Neuropsychol* 2009;23:1093–129.
67. British Psychological Society. Assessment of effort in clinical testing of cognitive functioning for adults. Leicester: BPS, 2009.
68. Waddell G, McCulloch K, Kummel E, Venner RM. Nonorganic physical signs in low-back pain. *Spine* 1980;5:117–25.
69. Scalzitti DA. Screening for psychological factors in patients with low back problems: Waddell's nonorganic signs. *Phys Ther* 1997;77:306–12.
70. Fishbain DA, Cutler R, Rosomoff HL, Rosomoff RS. Is there a relationship between nonorganic physical findings (Waddell Signs) and secondary gain/malingering? *Clin J Pain* 2004;20:399–408.
71. Fishbain DA, Cole B, Cutler RB, et al. Structured evidence-based review of the meaning of nonorganic physical signs: Waddell signs. *Pain Med* 2003;4:141–81.
72. Fishbain DA, Cutler R, Rosomoff HL, Rosomoff RS. Chronic pain disability, exaggeration/malingering, and submaximal effort research. *Clin J Pain* 1999;14:244–74.
73. Robinson ME & Danneker EA. Critical issues in the use of muscle testing for the determination of sincerity of effort. *Clin J Pain* 2004;20:392–8.
74. Cunnien AJ. Psychiatric and medical syndromes associated with deception. In: Rogers R, ed. Clinical assessment of malingering and deception. 2nd edn. New York: Guilford Press, 1997, pp 23–46.
75. Orr SP, Pitman RK, Lasko NB, Herz LR. Psychophysiological assessment of post-traumatic stress disorder imagery in World War II and Korean combat veterans. *J Abnorm Psychol* 1993;102:620–4.
76. Bianchini KJ, Greve KW, Glynn G. On the diagnosis of malingered pain-related disability: lessons from cognitive malingering research. *Spine J* 2005;5:404–17.
77. Walters GD, Berry DTR, Lanyon RI, Murphy MP. Are exaggerated health complaints continuous or categorical? A taxometric analysis of the Health Problem Overstatement Scale. *Psychol Assess* 2009;21:219–26.

CHAPTER 17
Case descriptions

Michele Sterling, Trudy Rebbeck, Justin Kenardy

The preceding chapters of this book have provided an in-depth discussion of the whiplash condition, ranging from the epidemiology, mechanisms of injury, physical and psychological characteristics through to compensation and the legal factors with which many injured people will be involved. The aim of this chapter is to bring this knowledge together in three distinct case presentations that outline the heterogeneity of the whiplash condition.

In order to illustrate the varied clinical presentation of patients with whiplash and the assessment required, two case studies of acute whiplash are presented in order to emphasise the importance of this stage of the injury. At this early stage, effective assessment and management may help to prevent the development of chronicity in those at risk. The third case presentation is that of a patient with chronic whiplash. In order to illustrate the 'overall' management of whiplash, in-depth discussion of specific management is not provided; instead, interested readers are provided with appropriate references for more detailed discussion of specific techniques.

CASE DESCRIPTION 1: ACUTE WHIPLASH

Patient interview and history

Jane is a 32-year-old woman who is married with one two-year-old child. She works full-time as a personal assistant to a chief executive officer of an advertising company.

History: Jane was on her way home from work 10 days ago when her car was struck from behind while stopped at a red traffic light. Jane felt slight pain in her neck at the time of the accident and, after organising the car to be towed away, she went home. That night she could feel her neck getting stiff and when she awoke the next morning, she could barely turn her neck. Jane took the following two days off work (sick leave) as she found sitting at the computer aggravated her neck pain. Even though her pain then improved and she returned to work, Jane reported that by the end of the day, her neck pain was worse. Jane is usually very active and goes to gym classes three times a week, as well as playing hockey on the weekends, but has not been able to do so since the car accident. However, she has been able to ride a stationary bike at home for about 15 minutes at a time. Jane presents to the physiotherapist 10 days after the accident as she feels that her neck should be better by now and she is worried since a friend of hers experienced a similar injury and was unable to play any sport for 12 months. She also asked whether or not she should lodge a compensation claim for her injury.

Jane has not had any radiological investigations. She has taken paracetamol as necessary with some reported relief. Jane's sleep is not disturbed by pain.

Current symptoms and function

Pain: Left-sided neck pain (visual analogue scale [VAS]: 5/10), left-sided frontal headache (VAS: 4/10). There was no reported dizziness, paraesthesia or anaesthesia.

Her functional status, as measured by the Patient-Specific Functional Scale (PSFS),[1] is outlined below. For this instrument, 0/10 means unable to perform the activity and 10/10 means able to perform the activity at pre-injury levels:

- Picking up child: 4/10
- Working at office desk (> 30 minutes): 6/10
- Reading (> 30 minutes): 6/10

Neck Disability Index (NDI):[2] 28/100, indicating mild-to-moderate levels of pain and disability.[3]

On listening to Jane's responses in the patient interview, the clinician decided that there were no indications of post-traumatic stress symptoms, depression or pain-related distress, such as fear of movement—Jane is attempting to exercise within her pain limits and she has returned to work. On this basis, no additional questionnaires were administered. There was also little to suggest the presence of central hyperexcitability in Jane's clinical presentation.

Physical examination

Jane's posture was unremarkable. Her range of left cervical rotation was limited to 50 degrees and the movement reproduced her neck pain. All other directions of movement were full and pain-free. The physiotherapist noted several indications of impaired muscle control of the neck and upper quadrant,[4] including: poor control of return from cervical extension, altered muscle recruitment patterns with craniocervical flexion in supine (craniocervical flexion test) and impaired control of the scapula with arm movement. On manual examination of the cervical spine, local hyperalgesia over the left C2–C3 segment was noted. Clinical neurological examination (sensation, muscle power, reflexes) was normal and there was full and pain-free elbow extension with the brachial plexus provocation test. This test has been proposed as a useful clinical test of centrally augmented motor responses evident by bilaterally limited elbow extension with the test.[5]

Indications of prognosis

Jane's reported pain levels and NDI scores are moderate and the presence of moderate levels of pain and disability is a prognostic indicator for poor functional recovery.[6, 7] However, Jane's levels of psychological distress are low; there is no evidence of central hyperexcitability and neck range of movement is not markedly restricted. Therefore, it would be expected that Jane should recover well.

Management plan

At this stage, the physiotherapist should be able to undertake the management of this patient. There is little to indicate that referral to other healthcare providers is indicated.

Educational management should include providing: assurance about prognosis and that full recovery is expected; awareness of mechanisms underlying the condition; an explanation to Jane of the proposed management plan (see below) and its expected effects.

Physical management should be a multimodal approach. This would primarily involve improvement of cervical movement, retraining of motor control, progressing rapidly to functional and weight-bearing activities. This approach to management has been shown to be beneficial for patients without signs of central hyperexcitability.[8] Gentle manual therapy at the C2–C3 level could also be included for its hypoalgesic effect on the cervical spine.[9] As pain and disability decreases, a graduated cardiovascular fitness program could be introduced, with the aim of restoring full sporting activities.

In this case, this is little to indicate a prolonged recovery. Therefore, it would be expected that improvements would be seen quickly (as determined by clinically relevant changes on pain and functional outcomes) and that physiotherapy treatment would not be of a long-term nature. In response to Jane's question about claim lodgement, she could be advised not to lodge a claim and reassured that treatment sessions will be minimal. Claim lodgement in a patient following Jane's favourable recovery trajectory has been shown to be associated with a significant worsening of the clinical pathway.[10]

CASE DESCRIPTION 2: ACUTE WHIPLASH

Patricia is a 38-year-old woman who is married with two children aged 15 and 10 years. She works part-time (three days a week) as an administration assistant.

Patient interview and history

History: Six weeks ago, Patricia was involved in a motor vehicle crash, in which her car was hit on the rear passenger driver's side by a car that ran a red light. She felt immediate sharp pain in her neck. The car was extensively damaged and she was taken to hospital, where X-rays revealed no fracture or dislocation, and she was sent home with analgesics. Patricia went to her general practitioner the next day as her pain had spread into her right arm and was reaching an intolerable level. She was prescribed diclofenac and paracetamol and codeine (forte) and advised to take a week off work. After this time, Patricia then attempted to return to work but this exacerbated her pain; she could not concentrate and was experiencing some lightheadedness. She has since not returned to work. She is not sleeping well due to neck pain and reports that she cannot get to sleep due to thoughts about the accident. Prior to the accident, Patricia led a busy life with part-time work and caring for her children. She usually finds time to walk approximately 5 kilometres, three times a week, but has been unable to do this since the accident. Patricia has returned to her general practitioner for further advice. She feels that the pain is getting worse, is worried that something is seriously wrong with her neck and that she will never be able to return to her former busy lifestyle.

Current symptoms and function

Pain: Constant neck (VAS: 8/10) and right arm (VAS: 6/10) pain. Intermittent paraesthesia (VAS: 3/10) in the right hand.

Her functional status as measured by the PSFS[1] is outlined below.

- Sitting longer than 10 minutes: 2/10
- Turning head to look over right shoulder: 1/10
- Washing-up: 1/10

NDI:[2] 52/100, indicating moderate-to-severe levels of pain and disability.[3]

The general practitioner notes clues in Patricia's interview that are suggestive of post-traumatic stress (not sleeping due to thoughts about the accident) and pain-related psychological responses, for example, catastrophisation (there is something seriously wrong). For these reasons, the general practitioner opts to administer the Impact of Events Scale-Revised (IES-R)[11] and the Pain Catastrophising Scale (PCS) tests.[12] Patricia's scores were moderate for the intrusion and hyperarousal subscales of the IES-R and her score on the PCS was 32, which is consistent with pain catastrophising.[13] The general practitioner also noted features that are suggestive of the presence of central hyperexcitability of nociceptive processing, such as pain at night, and that Patricia's pain is easily provoked. In view of these reports, the S-LANSS was also administered and Patricia scored 24 on this instrument. A score over 12 is an indication of a neuropathic component to the pain.[14]

Physical examination

Patricia sat protectively cradling her right arm. Her cervical range of movement was markedly limited in all directions and all movements increased her pain. Clinical neurological examination (muscle power and reflexes) was normal but allodynia was noted with sensation testing of the right arm. The general practitioner was unable to palpate Patricia's cervical spine due to the presence of allodynia. A thermoroller preset at 20°C was reported as painful.

Indicators of prognosis

There are several adverse prognostic indicators associated with this clinical presentation. In addition to moderate-to-high levels of pain and disability,[6, 7] there is evidence of central hyperexcitability (S-LANSS score >12[14] and cold allodynia), marked neck movement restriction and moderate levels of post-traumatic stress, as well as catastrophisation. These factors have all been shown to have prognostic capacity.[13, 15]

Patricia is at risk of developing chronic pain and disability as a result of her injury. It is important that any treatment plan takes this into account.

Management plan

This is a critical time for Patricia's condition. The complex nature of her condition indicates that an interdisciplinary approach to her management will be required. It is now six weeks post injury and the patient is reporting moderate levels of post-traumatic stress symptoms. A psychological referral should be instigated such that further evaluation of the patent's psychological status is undertaken. Guidelines recommend that short-term, trauma-focused cognitive behavioural therapy delivered by a clinical psychologist should be commenced.[16] The general practitioner also plays a role in the patient's psychological management and it is important that clear information is provided to the patient without further adding to her distress or catastrophising the condition, and to include the patient in any treatment decisions to be made. The general practitioner will also need to consider Patricia's level of pain and aim to decrease this via the re-evaluation of her medication. While there are few investigations of pharmacotherapy for whiplash, adjuvant agents that are aimed at modulating nociceptive processing may need to be considered (see Chapter 5).

Patricia also demonstrates moderate-to-high levels of disability and marked loss of function. She has marked restriction of neck movement and likely will manifest impairments in muscle control and postural control, such as balance loss, which has been shown to be associated with reports of dizziness.[17] While at this stage, emphasis should be placed on the psychological and nociceptive processing aspects of the condition, it is important that treatment is also directed at improving movement and function. This may take the form of advice and encouragement to commence gentle exercises of the neck, as well as general activity as tolerated by pain, taking care not to overly provoke symptoms and potentially exacerbate central hyperexcitability.[18] The general practitioner may decide to refer Patricia to a practitioner experienced in the management of musculoskeletal pain or opt to provide basic advice in the first instance, with later referral when psychological symptoms and central hyperexcitability have decreased to some extent.

Due to the complexity of this whiplash presentation, it is clear that a more concerted approach to management is required. It is likely that the length of treatment time and the number of treatments will be greater than those required for case study 1. In both cases, progress should be monitored with validated outcome measures and treatment adapted in view of the individual patient's progress.

It can be seen that such an integrated approach to the management of this patient requires collaborative communication between various healthcare providers involved in her management.

SUMMARY OF CASES 1 AND 2

These two distinct clinical descriptions contrast the spectrum of clinical presentations that may be seen in individuals in the period shortly after whiplash injury. Case 1 demonstrates a much more straightforward case, with clear signs of a positive prognosis. In this case, the patient should be able to be successfully managed with minimal short-term care from a single practitioner experienced in the assessment and management of musculoskeletal pain.

In contrast, case 2 is much more complex, with the additional presence of psychological distress and central hyperexcitability. Several signs indicate that this patient is at risk of developing a chronic pain condition. These signs (moderate-to-high pain and disability, post-traumatic stress, pain-related distress and features indicative of central hyperexcitability) are potentially modifiable and initial treatment efforts should be directed towards this goal. Clearly, this patient will require an interdisciplinary approach to management, with close collaboration occurring between practitioners and, of course, the patient and her family.

CASE DESCRIPTION 3: CHRONIC WHIPLASH

Patient interview and history

George is a 42-year-old single man who worked full-time as a teacher. George has been sent by the insurance commission of his local jurisdiction for assessment by a specialist practitioner who reviews whiplash cases showing poor recovery.

George was involved in a motor vehicle crash 12 months ago. His car was stationary at traffic lights when a vehicle hit the rear of his car. He was able to drive the car and drove home. The next day he attended his general practitioner, who referred George to physiotherapy. George recalled that, initially following the accident, he was aware of the following symptoms: headache, neck pain, low back pain and shoulder pain.

Treatment and progress to date

George was initially referred to physiotherapy and attended on a couple of occasions. His pain level remained at fairly constant levels over the next few months. A few months later he suddenly 'twisted' his neck and was unable to move. After that incident, all of his symptoms worsened. He attended the general practitioner, who prescribed medications, including opioids. An X-ray was also taken, which confirmed no bony injury. George was then once again referred to physiotherapy and attended at least once per week. However, if his symptoms were worse, he would attend at least two to three times per week, and has continued ever since.

George recalled that physiotherapy treatment has consisted of the following: manual therapy, traction, heat and interferential treatment, and massage. When asked about the effect of treatment, George stated that it reduces pain to a low level for the remainder of the day following treatment but then the pain returns to its previous level. Overall, when directly asked how he would rate recovery on a scale of 0% (not at all recovered) to 100% (completely recovered), George stated that, overall, he feels 20% recovered on a good day, but otherwise 10% recovered when he is having a bad day. In addition to the physiotherapy treatment, George has also consulted an orthopaedic surgeon, who took scans, which showed 'bulging discs'.

George was working full-time as a teacher prior to the accident. He returned to full-time work three weeks after the accident. However, when his symptoms worsened, he reduced work by one day, and then continued to reduce work until two months ago, when he stopped completely. At present, George is receiving physiotherapy and continues to take opioid medication.

When asked about his beliefs regarding the cause of the pain and what he needed to recover, George stated he understood that he is suffering from a 'chronic pain syndrome'. He stated that he was scared of the pain and copes with it by lying down, watching movies and with massage and heat (possibly indicating a reliance on passive-coping strategies). George would like to return to sport and work, but is not sure how to achieve this.

Current symptoms and function

George describes his current ongoing symptoms as follows:

- Left-to-right sided neck pain, constant and at a level of 7–8/10, with intermittent 'spasms' increasing the pain to 10/10
- Daily constant headaches, intensity 6–9/10
- Bilateral tingling in the arms occurring once per week
- Low back pain (4/10)
- Unsteadiness at times when walking

His functional status, as measured by the PSFS,[1] is outlined below.

- Work: 0/10
- Playing baseball: 0/10
- Walking: 0/10 (10 minutes)
- Social (going out with friends): 0/10
- Sitting at the computer: 1/10 (30 minutes)

Functional Rating Index: 38/40, indicating severe self-reported disability due to back and neck pain.

Due to George's long-term condition and his obvious distress, poor function and lack of participation in his usual life activities, the clinician opted to include additional psychological measures.

George completed the following questionnaires:

- Pain Self-Efficacy Questionnaire:[19] 20/60, indicating low self-efficacy or confidence in performing activities while in pain.
- The Coping Strategies Questionnaire (castastrophising subscale):[20] 31/36 (86%), indicating poor coping strategies and high levels of pain catastrophisation.
- Patient Health Questionnaire-9 (PHQ-9):[21] score of 12, indicating a moderate level of depression, no suicidal ideation.
- IES-R:[11] high levels of post-traumatic stress symptoms on the avoidance and hyperarousal scales.
- S-LANSS:[14] 22, indicating a likely neuropathic component to the pain.

Physical examination

George sat with his left shoulder elevated. Cervical range of movement was markedly restricted in all directions and George reported that any movement exacerbated his neck pain. Neurological examination of the upper limbs revealed normal responses to deep tendon reflex testing. The Babinski and clonus tests were unremarkable. George reported decreased light touch sensation (hypoaesthesia) in the upper limbs, which was non-dermatomal in distribution. He reported pain to light touch (allodynia) over the posterior cervical spine. Attempts to evaluate muscle strength in the upper and lower limbs were unsuccessful due to pain. George reported pain with the application of thermorollers at 20°C. A pressure algometer was used to measure mechanical pain thresholds and these were decreased in the upper and lower limbs. Poor motor control of both the cervical flexors and extensors, as well as the shoulder girdle muscles, was noted.[4]

Interpretation of examination

George continues to report ongoing high levels of pain and disability and his overall quality of life is poor. He is not working, has limited social interaction and does not participate in previous activities he enjoyed prior to his accident. George has moderate levels of post-traumatic stress and depressive symptoms, as well as significant behavioural and psychological responses to pain—pain catastrophisation and poor self-efficacy. There is evidence of central hyperexcitability of nociceptive processing via the presence of allodynia, generalised mechanical hyperalgesia, hypoaesthesia and S-LANSS scores of greater than 12.

Management plan

George's condition appears to be deteriorating. The main concerns for management should be his severe psychological distress, particularly the depressive symptoms and post-traumatic stress. The presence of these factors requires further evaluation and management by a clinical psychologist. Prescription of antidepressant medication should also be considered. Due to the potential risk of these factors to his current and future well-being, they should be the priority of management. Pain-related beliefs and responses to pain would also be addressed, but as a secondary priority at this stage. In tandem with psychological support, a review of George's medication by a pain specialist is required as he continues taking opioids with little apparent benefit. It is also possible that this may be increasing his hyperalgesia.[22]

Once depression and post-traumatic stress are starting to improve and it is judged that George is ready, physical rehabilitation strategies should be introduced. Since past physiotherapy techniques have been more of a passive nature, focus should be placed on more graded active interventions following the principles of cognitive behavioural therapy, with goals being activity-focused rather than pain-focused. The therapist should draw on and reinforce skills and strategies learned through the cognitive behaviour therapy, such as relaxation, and behavioural activation. There is some evidence of efficacy for such an approach for patients with chronic whiplash associated disorders.[23] However, the clinician should carefully monitor the patient for any signs of provoked central nociceptive processing, such as increased hyperalgesia or pain, and ensure that this is taken into account and prevented by careful progression of the exercise program. Education about pain physiology may be useful to assist George in self-monitoring his physical progress; this form of education has been shown to be effective for people with chronic low back pain.[24]

In summary, George's complex clinical presentation indicates that an interdisciplinary approach to the management of his whiplash condition will be required. Due to the chronicity of George's condition, a pain management centre may be the most appropriate model of care, where the clinicians are experienced in the management of chronic pain. However, George's presentation suggests that this may need to be a 'staged' approach, where the psychological and pain aspects of his condition are managed first, then followed by physical rehabilitation. This may assist to prevent overwhelming George with assessment and management by multiple healthcare providers and allow time for him to absorb the information provided.

CONCLUSION

This chapter provides detailed accounts of the clinical presentations of three various possible whiplash presentations. It outlined possible management approaches based on the presentation of the patients, in terms of their pain, disability, function, physical and psychological impairments. The presentations were purposely used to demonstrate the heterogeneity of the whiplash condition, where some people will have a relatively straightforward presentation (case 1) compared to others, which creates a challenge for those involved in their management (cases 2 and 3). It was not the intention of this chapter to outline specific treatment approaches but rather to draw attention to when different services may be required. It is hoped that this chapter will help the reader to achieve the main objective of this book—to improve the diagnosis, assessment and subsequent management of individuals post whiplash injury.

References

1. Westaway M, Stratford P, Binkley J. The patient-specific functional scale: validation of its use in persons with neck dysfunction. *J Orthop Sports Phys Ther* 1998;27(5):331–8.
2. Vernon H. The neck disability index: patient assessment and outcome monitoring in whiplash. *J Musculoskelet Pain* 1996;4(4):95–104.
3. MacDermid J, Walton D, Avery S, et al. Measurement properties of the Neck Disability Index: a systematic review. *J Orthop Sports Phys Ther* 2009;39(5):400–17.
4. Jull G, Sterling M, Falla D, et al. Whiplash, headache and neck pain: research based directions for physical therapies. Edinburgh: Elsevier, 2008.
5. Sterling M. Testing for sensory hypersensivity or central hyperexcitability associated with cervical spine pain. *J Manipulative Physiol Ther* 2008;31:534–9.
6. Kamper S, Rebbeck T, Maher C, et al. Course and prognostic factors of whiplash: a systematic review and meta-analysis. *Pain* 2008;138(3):617–29.
7. Walton D, Pretty J, MacDermid J, Teasell R. Risk factors for persistent problems following whiplash injury: results of a systematic review and meta-analysis. *J Orthop Sports Phys Ther* 2009;39(5):334–50.
8. Jull G, Sterling M, Kenardy J, Beller E. Does the presence of sensory hypersensitivity influence outcomes of physical rehabilitation for chronic whiplash? A preliminary RCT. *Pain* 2007;129(2):28–34.
9. Sterling M, Jull G, Wright A. Cervical mobilisation: concurrent effects on pain, sympathetic nervous system activity and motor activity. *Man Ther* 2001;6(2):72–81.
10. Sterling M, Hendrikz J, Kenardy J. Developmental trajectories of pain/disability and PTSD symptoms following whiplash injury. *Pain* 2010;150(1):22–8.
11. Weiss D & Marmar C. The impact of events scale – revised. In: Wilson J & Keane T, eds. Assessing psychological trauma and PTSD. New York: Guilford Press, 1997:98–135.
12. Sullivan M, Bishop S, Pivik J. The pain catastrophizing scale: development and validation. *Psychol Assess* 1995;7:524–32.
13. Sullivan M, Stanish W, Sullivan M, Tripp D. Differential predictors of pain and disability in patients with whiplash injury. *Pain Res Manag* 2002;7(2): 68–74.
14. Bennett M, Smith B, Torrance N, Potter J. The S-LANSS score for identifiying pain of predominantly neuropathic origin: validation for use in clinical and postal research. *J Pain* 2005;6(3):149–58.
15. Sterling M, Jull G, Vicenzino B, et al. Physical and psychological factors predict outcome following whiplash injury. *Pain* 2005;114:141–8.
16. Forbes D, Creamer M, Phelps A, et al. Australian guidelines for the treatment of adults with acute stress disorder and posttraumatic stress disorder. *Aust N Z J Psychiatry* 2007;41:637–48.
17. Treleaven J, Jull G, Low Choy N. Standing balance in persistent whiplash: a comparison between subjects with and without dizziness. *J Rehabil Med* 2005;37:224–9.
18. Sterling M & Kenardy J. Physical and psychological aspects of whiplash: important considerations for primary care assessment. *Man Ther* 2008;13(2):93–102.
19. Nicholas M. The pain self-efficacy questionnaire: taking pain into account. *Eur J Pain* 2007;11:153–63.
20. Rosenstiel A & Keefe F. The use of coping strategies in chronic low back pain patients: relationship to patient characteristics and current adjustment. *Pain* 1983;17:33–44.

21. Duffy F, Chung H, Trivedi M, et al. Systematic use of patient-rated depression severity monitoring: is it helpful and feasible in clinical psychiatry? *Psychiatr Serv* 2008;59(10):1148–54.
22. Angst M & Clark D. Opioid-induced hyperalgesia: a qualitative systematic review. *Anesthesiology* 2006;104:570–87.
23. Stewart M, Maher C, Refshauge K, et al. Randomised controlled trial of exercise for chronic whiplash associated disorders. *Pain* 2007;128(1–2):59–68.
24. Moseley G, Nicholas M, Hodges P. A randomised controlled trial of intensive neurophysiology education in chronic low back pain. *Clin J Pain* 2004;20(5):324–30.

CHAPTER 18
Future directions

Michele Sterling and Justin Kenardy

At the time of the Quebec Task Force review, there would not have been enough research data available on which to base a book such as this. The past 15 years, in particular, have seen a rapid growth in research and, consequently, knowledge of whiplash associated disorders (WAD). We now know that whiplash can be a remarkably complex condition in some individuals, with disturbances in nociceptive processing, motor and postural control, as well as psychological distress clearly evident. However, this improved understanding of the condition is yet to be translated to improved health outcomes for injured people or to a significant reduction in costs. While the expanded interest in whiplash among researchers, clinicians and others is gratifying, it is clear that we still have much ground to cover. The ultimate goal is to devise a rational approach to developing satisfactory treatments, particularly for those at high risk of developing chronic pain and disability.

Despite there still being significant gaps in our knowledge, the progress documented in this book is significant and encouraging. Thus, it is fitting to conclude this book with some examples of the many fields of work requiring future attention.

INTERVENTION TRIALS

There seem to be several obvious areas where trials of intervention are urgently required. The first of these would be the clear lack of trials investigating pharmacotherapy for patients with whiplash at both the acute and chronic stages. There is now convincing evidence of augmented central nociceptive processing that is present from soon after injury,[1] persists in and predicts those individuals with poor functional recovery,[2] and is associated with non-responsiveness to standard physical rehabilitation approaches.[3] Other conditions showing similar phenomena (e.g. fibromyalgia) have undergone extensive investigation as to the effects of various pharmacotherapies to the extent that some medications are now approved by the US Food and Drug Administration for use in this condition.[4] There are also a far greater number of trials investigating pharmacotherapy for low back pain[5] than whiplash. Furthermore, initially higher levels of pain and/or disability are the most consistent predictors of poor health outcomes following whiplash injury.[6–8] Guidelines for acute pain management advocate the importance of early pain relief following injury,[9] yet whiplash guidelines do not make this a priority of treatment as there are no high-quality trials available on which to base recommendations.[10, 11]

In addition to pain, post-traumatic stress is also common in people with whiplash.[12] There is emerging evidence that administration of an opiate[13] and beta blockers[14] administered very soon after a traumatic injury can prevent the development of post-traumatic stress disorder (PTSD), and these may also be novel approaches in the management of patients with acute whiplash and symptoms of post-traumatic stress. Thus, trials of pharmacotherapy for whiplash should be a research priority.

There is now available a large volume of research on the psychological sequelae of whiplash injury, as can be seen from the discussions of Chapters 8 and 13. In contrast, there are few treatment trials of psychological interventions or combined psychological and physical management approaches for WAD. Again, this is in contrast to the data available in other musculoskeletal conditions, such as low back pain. Some whiplash studies have combined a cognitive behavioural type of approach delivered by a physiotherapist in conjunction with an exercise program,[15, 16] making it difficult to tease out the relative efficacy of both components. Few studies have investigated the effects of a psychological-based intervention delivered by a clinical psychologist. In view of recent findings of the presence of PTSD symptoms and depression in some patients with whiplash (Chapters 8 and 13), it would seem important that future studies investigate the effectiveness of treatments targeted at PTSD and depression. As outlined in Chapter 13, effective treatments, such as trauma-focused cognitive behaviour therapy, exist for the management of PTSD, and preliminary data indicate that PTSD treatment may potentially have an effect not only on PTSD symptoms but also on pain and disability.[17] This would also seem to be an area ripe for research, where there is much supporting evidence on which to base a case for such trials.

Most clinical guidelines recommend the provision of education and advice as part of the management of WAD.[10, 11, 18] Individual studies have investigated various educational approaches, such as the provision of information pamphlets[19] or educational videos,[20] but when taken together in a systematic review, the results are disappointing in that there was moderate evidence of no difference on pain and disability for various forms of advice focusing on return to activity.[21] Thus, it would seem that we are no closer in understanding the most effective education to provide to whiplash-injured people and the most effective way to deliver that advice. Since the provision of education and advice forms the mainstay of most management approaches, albeit physical or psychological, then it would seem a priority that further investigation of this area is required.

Most exercise approaches to both acute and chronic whiplash have delivered only modest effects.[3, 16, 22] Some studies have investigated approaches that, while efficacious for non-traumatic neck pain, have provided disappointing results when translation to the whiplash condition is attempted.[3] In the study by Jull et al.,[3] it was shown that those participants with higher levels of pain and disability and sensory hypersensitivity indicative of augmented central nociceptive processing responded poorly to an intensive 10-week program of specific exercise. It may be that more creative approaches to physical rehabilitation are required for whiplash, particularly for those with a more complex clinical presentation.

The whiplash subgroup with sensory hypersensitivity also shows sympathetic nervous system and motor disturbances[1, 23] that are similar to features of complex regional pain syndrome (CRPS) type 1.[24] Altered central representation of perceptual, motor and autonomic systems has been implicated as possible mechanisms underlying the pain of CRPS.[25] Treatment approaches that broadly aim to restore altered cortical representation, such as graded motor imagery and mirror visual feedback, have been shown to decrease pain and disability associated with CRPS,[26] and sensory discrimination training can also decrease the pain and disability of CRPS.[27] The similarities of the manifestations of CRPS and complex whiplash suggest that investigation of such approaches is warranted.

DO SOME PATIENTS HAVE A PRE-EXISTING RISK OF DEVELOPING CHRONIC PAIN AFTER WHIPLASH INJURY?

The co-occurrence of disturbed nociceptive processing, stress responses—both physiological and psychological, marked motor changes and moderate-to-high levels of pain and disability in some patients with whiplash may not be coincidental. It has been argued that these responses are interrelated and develop in response to a common stressor—the motor vehicle crash (MVC).[28, 29] It may also be the case that some individuals have a pre-existing risk of developing chronic pain following a given injury or stressor. Animal studies have shown that an identical induced injury (chronic constriction injury of the sciatic nerve) evokes both pain and disability, including sleep disruption and disrupted social behaviours, in only a subgroup (approximately 30%) of rats.[30] The authors suggest that disabilities evoked by the injury reflect a specific and select neurobiological response to injury that may be related to genetic differences in neural and glial adaptations in the periaqueductal grey regions of the brain.[30] Preliminary evidence in whiplash-injured humans suggests that genetic variations in the function of catechol-o-methyltransferase (COMT, an enzyme involved in the degradation of catecholamines) may influence vulnerability to acute and chronic WAD symptoms after an MVC (Chapter 9).[31] Additionally, population-based studies have demonstrated that pre-collision factors of perceived health and health-seeking behaviour are predictive of the development of widespread bodily pain (not specifically whiplash) following an MVC.[32]

Taken together, these studies indicate that some people, for possibly genetic reasons, are more predisposed to tip into a hyperexcitable systemic-type state following an injury. These hypotheses require further evaluation, although it is not clear what should be done for individuals who may fit this scenario. It may be that they require earlier and targeted interventions towards settling the hyper-responsiveness, via decreasing either the stress responses or levels of pain, as outlined earlier.

IMPROVING PROGNOSTIC MODELS

While predictive studies have certainly improved our understanding of injured people at risk of poor recovery, there is still some way to go before we have clear modifiable risk factors that can be targeted with early interventions. There are now several systematic reviews available on the prognosis following whiplash injury and all of them comment on the general variable quality of prognostic studies.[6–8, 33]

Various factors have been noted, including: inconsistencies between studies in time from injury until baseline data collection, time to follow-up and use of various and, sometimes, unvalidated outcome measures.[8] The most consistent predictive factors are initially higher pain and disability levels, which were identified by every systematic review.[6–8, 33] However, these factors alone, while having high sensitivity, have been shown to have relatively low specificity to predict those individuals who will develop persistent symptoms.[2] Other factors, such as sensory measures and psychological distress, when added to the pain levels, have improved the specificity of a predictive model,[2] but these factors require further validation before they are universally accepted. This is also the case for other identified prognostic factors, which require validation in independent cohorts before they become commonplace in clinical practice.[34] Additionally, Kamper et al.[7] concluded that the inadequate reporting of prognostic associations represents a major barrier to meaningful interpretation of the literature. These authors argue that statistical significance was often reported without detailing the magnitude or clinical relevance of any association.[7]

In order to provide more precise and interpretable data on prognostic indicators for recovery, it is important that future studies pay attention to methodological quality criteria, use validated measures to determine all outcomes and report the magnitude of all prognostic associations, significant or otherwise. Additionally, the use of more sophisticated analysis techniques, such as trajectory group-based modelling, would be advantageous in shedding light on clinical pathways of recovery and non-recovery following whiplash injury.[35]

IDENTIFICATION OF A PERIPHERAL LESION

Despite some promise shown in some magnetic resonance imaging studies where craniocervical ligament damage may be present,[36] we have not come much closer to being able to locate a peripherally injured structure in the necks of whiplash-injured people. There are two sides of the argument as to whether or not to continue the quest to identify such lesions.

It is known that there is generally poor correlation between features present on radiology and patient-reported symptoms for a variety of conditions, including arthritis,[37] low back pain[38] and whiplash.[39, 40] Thus, even if a lesion could be identified, treatment approaches would be directed towards the physical impairments and psychological factors identified on individual patient assessment. In other words, the treatment approach would be no different whether a peripheral lesion can be identified or not.

However, the identification of some injuries may change a usual approach to treatment. For example, a small fracture within a zygapophyseal joint that is not viewable via radiology (at present)[41] may be better managed with early rest followed by a gradual return to activity and not full early return to activity. Similarly, the identification of damaged neural structures, such as blood within the dorsal root ganglia,[41] has implications for the prescription of early medication for neuropathic pain. The identification of injured structures may also validate the patient's condition, and this could alleviate some of the associated distress. Therefore, a better understanding of each potentially injured tissue may help improve the diagnosis and treatment of whiplash injuries, and research efforts in this area should continue. With the continued development of higher resolution imaging techniques, this may be a fruitful area in the near future.

CONCLUSION

The above-mentioned suggestions for future research and management directions for whiplash are not meant to be exhaustive and there is no doubt that other areas also require further investigation. The knowledge and understanding of the enigmatic whiplash condition has come a long way in recent times but we still have a way to go in order to improve outcomes for injured people. Improved outcomes for these patients will require close cooperation between researchers, clinicians and policy makers. It is hoped that the body of work in this book lays the foundation to really move forward in the management of whiplash and not to be held back by preconceptions of this condition.

References

1. Sterling M, Jull G, Vicenzino B, Kenardy J. Sensory hypersensitivity occurs soon after whiplash injury and is associated with poor recovery. *Pain* 2003;104: 509–17.
2. Sterling M, Jull G, Vicenzino B, et al. Physical and psychological factors predict outcome following whiplash injury. *Pain* 2005;114:141–8.
3. Jull G, Sterling M, Kenardy J, Beller E. Does the presence of sensory hypersensitivity influence outcomes of physical rehabilitation for chronic whiplash? A preliminary RCT. *Pain* 2007;129(2): 28–34.

4. Rao S. Current progress in the pharmacological therapy of fibromyalgia. *Expert Opin Investig Drugs* 2009;18(10):1479–93.
5. Chou R & Huffman L. Medications for acute and chronic low back pain: a review of the evidence for an American Pain Society/American College of Physicians clinical practice guideline. *Ann Intern Med* 2007;147(7):505–14.
6. Carroll L, Holm L, Hogg-Johnson S, et al. Course and prognostic factors for neck pain in whiplash-associated disorders (WAD). Results of the Bone and Joint Decade 2000–2010 Task Force on Neck Pain and Its Associated Disorders. *Spine* 2008;33(42):583–92.
7. Kamper S, Rebbeck T, Maher C, et al. Course and prognostic factors of whiplash: a systematic review and meta-analysis. *Pain* 2008;138(3):617–29.
8. Walton D, Pretty J, MacDermid J, Teasell R. Risk factors for persistent problems following whiplash injury: results of a systematic review and meta-analysis. *J Orthop Sports Phys Ther* 2009;39(5):334–50.
9. Macintyre P, Scott D, Schug S, et al. Acute pain management: scientific evidence. Melbourne: ANZVA & FPM, 2010.
10. Motor Accident Authority (NSW). Guidelines for the management of whiplash associated disorders. Sydney: NSW, 2007.
11. South Australian Centre for Trauma and Injury Recovery. A clinical pathway for best practice management of acute and chronic whiplash-associated disorders. Adelaide: TRACsa, 2008.
12. Sterling M, Hendrikz J, Kenardy J. Developmental trajectories of pain/disability and PTSD symptoms following whiplash injury. *Pain* 2010;150(1):22–8.
13. Holbrook T, Galarneau M, Dye J, et al. Morphine use after combat injury in Iraq and post-traumatic stress disorder. *N Engl J Med* 2010;362(2):110–17.
14. Strawn J & Geracioti T. Noradrenergic dysfunction and the psychopharmacology of posttraumatic stress disorder. *Depress Anxiety* 2008;25(3):260–71.
15. Soderlund A & Lindberg P. Cognitive behavioural components in physiotherapy management of chronic whiplash associated disorders (WAD)—a randomised group study. *Physiother Theory Pract* 2001;17:229–38.
16. Stewart M, Maher C, Refshauge K, et al. Randomised controlled trial of exercise for chronic whiplash associated disorders. *Pain* 2007;128(1–2):59–68.
17. Jenewein J, Wittmann L, Moergeli H, et al. Mutual influence of PTSD symptoms and chronic pain among injured accident survivors: a longitudinal study. *J Trauma Stress* 2009;22(6):540–8.
18. Moore A, Jackson A, Jordan J, et al. Clinical guidelines for the physiotherapy management of whiplash associated disorder. London: The Chartered Society of Physiotherapy, 2005.
19. Kongsted A, Qerama E, Kasch H, et al. Education of patients after whiplash injury: is oral advice any better than a pamphlet? *Spine* 2008;33(22): E843–8.
20. Oliveira A, Gevirtz R, Hubbard R. A psycho-educational video used in the emergency department provides effective treatment for whiplash injuries. *Spine* 2006;31(15):1652–7.
21. Haines T, Gross A, Burnie S, et al. Patient education for neck pain with or without radiculopathy. *Cochrane Database Syst Rev* 2008;(4):CD005106.
22. Rosenfeld M, Seferiadis A, Gunnarsson R. Active involvement and intervention in patients exposed to whiplash trauma in automobile crashes reduces costs. *Spine* 2006;31(16):1799–804.
23. Sterling M, Jull G, Vicenzino B, et al. Development of motor system dysfunction following whiplash injury. *Pain* 2003;103:65–73.
24. Rijn M, Marinus J, Putter H, van Hilten J. Onset and progression of dystonia in complex regional pain syndrome. *Pain* 2007;130:287–93.
25. Moseley G. Graded motor imagery for pathologic pain: a randomized controlled trial. *Neurology* 2006;67: 2129–34.
26. Daly E & Bialocerkowski A. Does evidence support physiotherapy management of adult complex regional pain syndrome type one? A systematic review. *Eur J Pain* 2009;13(4):339–53.
27. Moseley G & Wiech K. The effect of tactile discrimination training is enhanced when patients watch the reflected image of their unaffected limb during training. *Pain* 2009;144(3):314–19.
28. Ferrari R, Russell A, Carroll L, Cassidy D. A re-examination of the whiplash associated disorders (WAD) as a systemic illness. *Ann Rheum Dis* 2005;64(9):1337–42.
29. McLean S, Clauw D, Abelson J, Liberzon I. The development of persistent pain and psychological morbidity after motor vehicle collision: intergrating the potential role of stress response systems into a biopsychosocial model. *Psychosom Med* 2005;67: 783–90.
30. Mor D, Bembrick A, Austin P, et al. Anatomically specific patterns of glial activation in the periaqueductal gray of the sub-population of rats showing pain and disability following chronic constriction injury of the sciatic nerve. *Neuroscience* 2008;166(4):1167–84.
31. McLean S, Diatchenko L, Reed C. Catechol-O-methyltransferase (COMT) met/met genotype influences cortisol response and pain symptoms after minor motor vehicle collision (MVC). American Pain Society Meeting, Tampa Bay, Florida, 2008.

32. Wynne-Jones G, Jones G, Wiles N, et al. Predicting new onset of widespread pain following a motor vehicle collision. *J Rheumatol* 2006;33:968–74.
33. Scholten-Peeters G, Verhagen A, Bekkering G, et al. Prognostic factors of whiplash associated disorders: a systematic review of prospective cohort studies. *Pain* 2003;104(1–2):303–22.
34. Altman D, Vergouwe Y, Royston P, Moons K. Prognosis and prognostic research: validating a prognostic model. *Br Med J* 2009;338:b605.
35. Jones B & Nagin D. Advances in group-based trajectory modeling and an SAS procedure. *Sociological Methods Res* 2007;35(4):542–71.
36. Krakenes J & Kaale B. Magnetic resonance imaging assessment of craniovertebral ligaments and membranes after whiplash trauma. *Spine* 2006;31(24):2820–6.
37. Keefe F & Somers T. Psychological approaches to understanding and treating arthritis pain. *Nat Rev Rheumatol* 2010;6:210–16.
38. Sheehan N. Magnetic resonance imaging for low back pain: indications and limitations. *Ann Rheum Dis* 2010;69(1):7–11.
39. Elliott J, Sterling M, Noteboom T, et al. The clinical presentation of chronic whiplash and the relationship to findings of MRI fatty infiltrates in the cervical extensor musculature: a preliminary investigation. *Eur Spine J* 2009;18(9):1371–8.
40. Ichihara D, Okado E, Chiba K, et al. Longitudinal magnetic resonance imaging study on whiplash injury patients: minimum 10-year follow-up. *J Orthop Sci* 2009;14(5):602–10.
41. Taylor J & Taylor M. Cervical spinal injuries: an autopsy study of 109 blunt injuries. *J Musculoskelet Pain* 1996;4(4):61–79.

Index

Page numbers followed by 'f' denote figures; those followed by 't' denote tables